The Primary Care Toolkit

Larry C. James · William T. O'Donohue
Editors

The Primary Care Toolkit

Practical Resources for the Integrated
Behavioral Care Provider

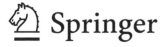 Springer

Editors
Larry C. James
Mililani, HI
USA
larry.james@us.army.mil

William T. O'Donohue
Department of Psychology
University of Nevada
Reno, NV
USA
wto@unr.edu

ISBN: 978-0-387-78970-5   e-ISBN: 978-0-387-78971-2
DOI 10.1007/978-0-387-78971-2

Library of Congress Control Number: 2008933582

Printed on acid-free paper

springer.com

Contents

Contributors

Kevin Alschuler, M.S.
Department of Psychology, Eastern Michigan University, Ypsilanti MI 48197, Kalschul@emich.edu

Laura L. Bauer, Ph.D.

Michelle Byrd, Ph.D.
Department of Psychology, Eastern Michigan University, Ypsilanti, MI 48197, USA, mbyrd@emich.edu

Blake Chaffee, Ph.D.
Vice President, Integrated Healthcare Services, TriWest Healthcare Alliance, Phoenix, AZ, USA, bchaffee@triwest.com

Michael A. Cucciare, Ph.D.
VA Palo Alto Healthcare System and Stanford University School of Medicine, CA 94025, USA, cucciare@hotmail.com

Amanda Drews, Ph.D.
Semel Institute and Resnick Neuropsychiatric Hospital, Los Angeles, CA, USA

Melanie P. Duckworth, Ph.D.
Department of Psychology, University of Nevada, Reno, Reno, NV 89557, USA, melanied@unr.edu

Erika Gerber, B.A.
Department of Psychology, University of Nevada, Reno, Reno, NV 89557, USA, mail@erikagerber.com

Lisa Hagen Glynn, B.S.
Department of Psychology, University of New Mexico, Albuquerque, NM 87131, USA, lglynn@unm.edu

Holly Hazlett-Stevens, Ph.D.
University of Nevada, Reno, NV, USA, hhazlett@unr.edu

Robert E. Jackson, Ph.D.
Director, Primary Care Behavioral Health Clinics, Tripler Army Medical Center, HI, USA, doc.jackson@yahoo.com

Larry C. James, Ph.D.
Department of Psychology, Tripler Army Medical Center, Mililani, HI 96789, USA, jamesbdaddy@aol.com

Erica M. Jarrett, Ph.D.
Chief, Primary Care Psychology Service, Department of Internal Medicine, Walter Reed Army Medical Center, Washington, DC, USA, erica.jarrett@amedd.army.mil

Dianne Lavin, Psy.D., RN, FNP-C
Schofield Barracks Family Practice Clinic, Schofield Barracks, HI, USA, ddlavin001@hawaii.rr.com

Ranilo Laygo
Assistant Professor, Center on Disability Studies, Honolulu, HI 96822, USA, ranilo@hawaii.edu

Eric R. Levensky, Ph.D.
Clinical Psychologist, Department of Behavioral Medicine Program, New Mexico VA Health Care System, Albuquerque, NM 87108, USA, levensky@unm.edu

Tony Lezzi, Ph.D.
Department of Behavioral Medicine Service, London Health Sciences Centre, Ontario, N6A 4G5, London, tony.iezzi@lhsc.on.ca

Jason Lillis, Ph.D.
Stanford University School of Medicine, Stanford, CA 94025, USA
jasonlillis22@gmail.com

Simone K. Madan, Ph.D.
Division of General Internal Medicine, University of California, San Francisco, CA, USA

Brie A. Moore, Ph.D.
CareIntegra, Inc./University of Nevada Reno, Reno, NV 89519, USA, brieamoore@yahoo.com

William T. O'Donohue, Ph.D.
Department of Psychology, University of Nevada, Reno, Reno, NV 89519, USA, wto@unr.edu

Megan Oser, M.A.
University of Nevada, Reno, NV, USA, meganoser@gmail.com

Christine N. Runyan, Ph.D.
Mid-State Health Center, Plymouth, NH, trunyan@midstatehealth.org

Jason Satterfield, Ph.D.
Director, Behavioral Medicine, Associate Professor of Clinical Medicine, University of California, 400 Parnassus Ave, A405, San Francisco, CA 94143-0320, jsatter@medicine.ucsf.edu

Richard P. Schobitz, Ph.D.
Deputy Director, Behavior Medicine Division, Office of the Chief Medical Officer, TRICARE Management Activity, Schobitz@hotmail.com

M. Todd Sewell, M.A.
Department of Psychology, University of Nevada, Reno, Reno, NV 89557, USA, wto@unr.edu

Lauren Woodward Tolle
Department of Psychology/296, University of Nevada, Reno, Reno, NV 89557-0296, USA, ltolle@unr.nevada.edu

Aditi Vijay, M.A.
Department of Psychology, University of Nevada, Reno, Reno, NV 89557, USA, aditi.vijay@gmail.com

Introduction

James and Folen (2005) and O'Donohue, N. Cummings, Cucciare, Runyan and J. Cummings (2005) have pioneered and reconceptualized how clinical psychologists, medical practitioners, hospital chief executive officers, and many health care administrators for large health care systems think about the delivery of behavioral health services. Their seminal works have provided a solid research and conceptual foundation to answer the question *why would you place a psychologist in a primary care clinic?* In particular, Cummings's and O'Donohue's research has documented the efficacy, cost savings, improvements in the patients' quality of life, and provider satisfaction. Clearly, their research and conceptual models have set the gold-standard for any behavioral health professional seeking to implement services in the primary care setting.

However, the field needs a hands-on or "toolkit" for the everyday behavioral health practitioner in the primary care setting. The present volume entitled *The Primary Care Toolkit* is specifically targeted at the applied practitioner intending to deliver services in the primary care setting. Our book is plush with helpful handouts and reference materials for the practitioner. The book will serve as a how to guide for psychologists, physicians, graduate students, and health care administrators alike. The first of its kind, our handbook offers chapters on the mainstay diseases in the primary care clinic such as chronic pain, depression, anxiety, coronary heart disease, diabetes, ADHD, smoking cessation, asthma, dementia, and the somatizer. Rather than simply describing the medical illness as is done in most primary care texts, our authors provide the reader with helpful information on assessment and treatment of the condition within the primary care clinic and offers handouts and references as well. For the CEOs, department heads and health care administrators, we offer guidance on how to determine the need and what administrators need to understand and expect, and provide detailed information on a training program. Often, one of the most difficult things for behavioral health practitioners to accomplish is to determine appropriate financial models for cost-effectiveness, quality improvement/management, treatment compliance, and the appropriate use of Current Procedural Terminology (CPT) codes, in particular, for the primary setting. Our book will provide the reader with "how to" chapters on these important areas of the primary care practice. We have included materials for medical colleagues as well as a chapter on training the PCP in integrated care and core competencies relating to medical personnel. Often, behavioral health care professionals may tend to not focus on marketing and communication devices. Thus, we have included practical chapters on patient education materials and the in-house newsletter, which will take the reader through how to make their services known, accessible, and relevant to the market and clinical needs of the primary care arena.

A major message of this book is that integrated care is not the co-location of a traditional mental health professional in a medical setting. This is a very common misconception that leads to problematic practice. Traditional mental health certainly has its proper role; i.e. as a specialty service. The relationship between a primary care psychologist and a traditional specialty care psychologist is much the same as the relationship between a family practice physician and a cardiologist. Neither replaces the other, and each has an important set of functions and core competencies. And when properly functioning, they work synergistically.

Integrated care has gained increasing interest over the past few decades. When health care service delivery models are examined, integrated care is often one of the central ways that health care delivery is recommended to be reformed (witness the President's New Freedom Commission Report, or the Task Force Report for the Department of Defense). Yet, graduate programs are not producing anything close to the number of graduates needed to perform competently in integrated care. In fact, in clinical psychology there are less than five programs producing graduates. Because of the lack of competently trained professionals and because of the wide range of definitions of "integrated care," the parachuting of the traditionally trained mental health professional is probably the most frequent way integrated care is being implemented. This is most unfortunate. This sort of poorly designed integrated care is largely unevaluated: hence its outcomes are unknown. However, there is reason to be pessimistic. Integrated care can acquire a bad name by the unfulfilled expectations brought about by this bastardizing of quality integrated care.

This book also shows the skill sets needed for competent integrated care. Population management, consultation liaison skills, stepped care, efficient assessment and screening, evidence-based brief and targeted practice, triage, chronic-disease management, medical literacy, team-building skills, knowledge of quality improvement, psycho-educational groups, treatment adherence and life-style changes are some of the core competencies of integrated care that are not commonly known by traditional mental health professionals. We do not believe this book is a replacement for sound training in these skills, but it will hopefully help the student of integrated care take some steps in the right direction.

Part I
Tools for Getting Started

How to Determine the Need: A Readiness Assessment System

Megan Oser and William T. O'Donohue

The Possibility of Integrated Health Care

Health care organizations are facing increasing pressure to improve their quality of care while reducing costs. Integrating behavioral health care within primary care settings has provided better and more efficient patient care using fewer resources at less cost. Accordingly, the three goals of integrated care include (a) producing healthier patients; (b) producing healthier patients with more efficient use of resources; and (c) removing barriers to access by offering more convenient and less stigmatizing services (O'Donohue, Cummings, & Ferguson, 2003). However, integrating behavioral health care within primary care clinics first requires a careful analysis.

To implement an integrated behavioral health care system within a primary care institution is a process that may be difficult without first identifying possible gaps within the existing health care organization that might obstruct the implementation of the new system of integrated care. Because integrated care systems are currently evolving, primary care organizations must strategically plan how to position themselves for the future of integrated care. Before implementing changes in functioning, structure, and/or future objectives, a health care organization should assess its readiness to adopt and create these major changes (Nelson, Raskind-Hood, Galvln, Essien, & Levine, 1999).

Conceptually, readiness to adopt integrated care may be characterized as the level of fit between a behavioral health care system and the primary care institution. A higher level of readiness leads to a lower level of risk and a more successful integrated care implementation process and outcome. A lack of information about readiness for change increases uncertainty for decision-makers and decreases their ability to make effective decisions that will mitigate risks associated with the adoption of integrated care (Snyder-Halpern, 2001). Conversely, health care organizations with attributes that contribute to a readiness and ability to adapt to changing environments

M. Oser (✉)
University of Nevada, Reno, NV, USA
e-mail: meganoser@gmail.com

L.C. James, W.T. O'Donohue (eds.), *The Primary Care Toolkit*,
DOI 10.1007/978-0-387-78971-2_1, © Springer Science+Business Media, LLC 2009

and that can incorporate new technologies, such as behavioral health care, are more likely to be successful in engaging patients and keeping them healthy (Lehman, Greener, & Simpson, 2002).

A readiness assessment identifies the potential challenges that might arise when implementing new procedures, structures, and/or processes within the current organizational context. Furthermore, through the identification of the "gaps" within the existing organization, the readiness assessment affords the opportunity to remedy these gaps either before or as part of the implementation plan (Poats & Salvaneschi, 2003). In this chapter, a readiness assessment instrument is presented that identifies the strengths and weaknesses of a health care organization, toward the goal of saving the health care organization costly time and effort when adopting an integrated care model.

The First Vital Steps

The assessment of the readiness of health care organizations to adopt new processes and technologies is a vital first step that prevents unpleasant and costly problems after implementation. An organization should have a basic understanding of its environment and its ability to make changes. Strategic planners need to understand the environment and state assumptions about the various changes that could occur, assess the ability to make the necessary changes to thrive within an integrated care model, reinforce the organization's vision, and support the organization's long-term financial capabilities. For understanding the environment, a health care organization should identify its distinctive competencies and areas of weakness, conduct interviews with internal and external stakeholders, and identify environmental opportunities and threats. Ultimately, such assessments provide information on key industry and market drivers that affect the likely success of the proposed integrated care initiative (Belt & Bashore, 2000). The following general questions will help to provide a broad perspective of the issues that the health care organization may face during a prospective transformational process:

- Are the organization's executives committed to the initiative?
- Is the organization prepared to budget a sufficient amount of funding to implement successfully and to maintain the new system?
- Are the physicians and other clinicians willing to devote sufficient time and effort so that the ultimate solution will serve their needs?
- Are the clinicians ready for a collaborative working environment?
- Are the service levels necessary to support the use of integrated care in health care environments clearly defined (Poats & Salvaneschi 2003)?

Lessons Learned

Clearly, the integration of behavioral health care into a primary care setting can be a daunting process. The case of Oregon's transition to a managed care model for Medicaid-funded substance abuse treatment provides an example of the need to assess for readiness to successfully implement a system of behavioral health care (D'Ambrosio, Mondeaux, Gabriel, & Laws, 2003). Although initially this transition might have appeared more simplified because only one component of behavioral health care was integrated into a primary care setting, this process was difficult and many problems arose before, during, and after the transition. The state of Oregon neither adequately assessed the Oregon Healthcare System's readiness to integrate behavioral health care, nor did it use this information to strategically and systematically plan to remedy the gaps that existed in the health care organization before implementing the substance abuse program. The major lessons learned from this transition in the state of Oregon include (a) the early facilitation of communication and relationship-building among the key stakeholders would likely have initiated the identification, discussion, and resolution of an array of issues that later created problems; (b) the establishment of uniform reporting and paperwork requirements would have substantially reduced the confusion and burden that befell the providers, and (c) systematic enforcement of contractual requirements and procedural guidelines may have led to more consistent operating procedures (e.g., increased referrals to behavioral health services by primary care physicians). The authors report, "Despite preparation at the state and provider levels, the transition to a managed care service model created more chaos and problems in a three-year period than had occurred in Oregon's substance abuse treatment system in decades" (D'Ambrosio, Mondeaux, Gabriel, & Laws, 2003).

Integrated Care Readiness Assessment

The readiness assessment instrument presented on the next several pages is designed to identify potential barriers to an organization's readiness for integrated care. Organizations can use this instrument in an effort to avoid problems encountered by the Oregon Healthcare System, for example, which will potentially save health care organizations costly time and effort.

The Organization Readiness for Integrating Behavioral Health into Primary Care instrument (Dyer, Eskelsen, Martin, & Ullrich, 2003) is a guide that provides an overview of elements suggestive of organizational success in integrating primary care and behavioral health. This instrument serves as the foundation for the proposed readiness assessment instrument outlined in the next several pages and was adapted to reflect the readiness constructs reviewed in this chapter as well as the full integrated care model.

Characteristics of Readiness to Implement an Integrated Health Care System

(1) The first readiness characteristic to be considered is organizational readiness. Organizational readiness includes the following:

- A high level of executive commitment to the integrated care initiative from key decision-makers;

- An understanding of the financial investment and time commitment that integrated care requires;
- Consensus throughout the organization that the integrated care initiative is aligned with organizational goals;
- Physicians' and clinicians' support for the initiative and their understanding of its value; and
- Clinicians' skill at working in a collaborative medical team.

(2) The second group of factors to consider when assessing an organization's readiness to change are Staff characteristics: Crucial to the dimension of staff characteristics is physician adoption of the integrated care initiative. Patterns of physician adoption include the following:

- The physicians affiliated with the organization believe that it is relatively easy to care for patients at the facility and that integrated care will improve this experience;
- The relationship between the physicians and the organization's administration and other clinicians is open and collaborative;
- Physicians actively participate in initiatives that promote leading clinical practices; and
- Some physicians are willing to take leadership roles while implementing an integrated care system by taking responsibility for focusing on key objectives and helping to promote the system within the physician community.

  Another key feature of staff characteristics may be conceptualized as knowledge readiness. Knowledge readiness, as defined by Snyder-Halpern (2001), reflects both general and specific kinds of knowledge required by health care decision-makers.

- General knowledge includes previous health care organization innovation patterns and decision-making processes.
- Specific knowledge encompasses such aspects as integrated clinical practice standards, the impact of current clinical practice standards on current practice processes and patient outcomes, and integrated care innovation characteristics—particularly in terms of team function, contracts, and licensing. Staff skill readiness identifies aspects such as clinician training needs and approaches to the customization of integrated care innovation from a clinician-centered perspective. Staff skill readiness typically includes
- Clinicians' background and skill level,
- Previous experiences with integrated care,
- Perceptions of the ability of integrated care to support intended clinical practices and its benefits,
- Degree of satisfaction with existing patient care,
- Degree of desired and perceived involvement in the integrated care innovation process,
- Level of commitment to the health care organization, and
- Idiographic responses to change.

(3) The third factor to be considered is resource readiness, which is the health care organization's ability to logistically support the implementation of integrated care. This assessment requires that health care decision-makers be knowledgeable about the type and availability of organizational resources required for initial customization and execution processes of integrated care as well as its ongoing maintenance. Resource readiness encompasses a wide range of assets such as money, space, availability of training, supervisors, and consultation services (Snyder-Halpern, 2001).

Benefits of Adopting Integrated Care

The next logical step following the formal readiness assessment is the assessment of the opportunities that successful implementations of a new technology, in this case integrated care, can deliver. Identifying improvement opportunities helps health care organizations to understand both the qualitative and quantitative benefits that can be achieved with integrated care.

Implementation and adoption of integrated care can afford improvement in the quality and safety of patient care, medical cost offset, and improvement in market share. By improving the delivery of patient care and reducing the workload of physicians, the performance and job satisfaction of care providers will improve, and thus improvement in market share may be realized. These overall improvements will strengthen the competitive position of the health care institution within its community (Poats & Salvaneschi, 2003).

Gap Analysis

The above questionnaire can be used to identify gaps and to develop strategies to address these. The more honestly and completely this questionnaire is filled out, the more likely future integrated care efforts will be successful. Gaps should not be viewed as "failures" or as fatal, but rather as inevitable (deal with perfectionism or denial here) and in the spirit of quality improvement as the target to be achieved. While it is true that sufficient gaps or key gaps (no management support) may result in delays, other gaps can just be successfully remedied. A first step should be an honest analysis of the severity, the number, and the likelihood/timeline that gaps can be ameliorated.

Some of these gaps may be addressed without technical assistance; others may not. It can be cost-effective to consult with experts in the field on how to remedy some of the gaps whose solutions are not immediately evident or that resist initial attempts at resolution. There are some useful primers on setting up an integrated care clinic: O'Donohue, et al. (2005) have written *Integrated Care: A Guide for Effective Intervention.* Also Patricia Robinson's and Jeff Reiter's (2006) *Behavioral Consultation and Primary Care: A Guide to Integrating Services* is an excellent resource. There are also three integrated care websites that provide useful

Readiness assessment for integrating behavioral health care

I. Health Care Organizational Factors:	Not Planning	Being Studied or prepared	Seeking approval or consensus	In place	In place with plans for improvement
1. Descriptions of job expectations	☐ 0	☐ 1	☐ 2	☐ 3	☐ 4
2. Defining service pathways (i.e., service needs in population to support use of integrated care)	☐ 0	☐ 1	☐ 2	☐ 3	☐ 4
3. Organizing population programs	☐ 0	☐ 1	☐ 2	☐ 3	☐ 4
4. Physician focus groups	☐ 0	☐ 1	☐ 2	☐ 3	☐ 4
5. Aligning integrated care with primary care organizational goals	☐ 0	☐ 1	☐ 2	☐ 3	☐ 4
6. Policies & Procedures Manual for Primary Care Integration	☐ 0	☐ 1	☐ 2	☐ 3	☐ 4
II. Motivation of Staff to Integrate Behavioral Health Care:	Very Weak	Weak	Neither Weak nor Strong	Strong	Very Strong
1. Involvement of key staff in change process	☐ 0	☐ 1	☐ 2	☐ 3	☐ 4
2. Involvement of skeptics of integration in the design and implementation process	☐ 0	☐ 1	☐ 2	☐ 3	☐ 4
3. Physicians' belief that integrated care will improve patient care	☐ 0	☐ 1	☐ 2	☐ 3	☐ 4
4. Willingness and ability of key staff to influence colleagues	☐ 0	☐ 1	☐ 2	☐ 3	☐ 4
III. Clinical Services and Training:	Not Planning	Being Studied or prepared	Seeking approval or consensus	In place	In place with plans for improvement
1. Protocol for training current staff and/or hiring new staff	☐ 0	☐ 1	☐ 2	☐ 3	☐ 4
2. Consultation patterns between behavioral health care provider (BCP) and primary care provider (PCP)	☐ 0	☐ 1	☐ 2	☐ 3	☐ 4
3. Brief and evidence-based interventions	☐ 0	☐ 1	☐ 2	☐ 3	☐ 4
4. Training and credentialing Staff in offering primary care	☐ 0	☐ 1	☐ 2	☐ 3	☐ 4
5. Preparatory workshops and training to increase understanding of the integrated care initiative	☐ 0	☐ 1	☐ 2	☐ 3	☐ 4
6. Skill-based training for BCPs and PCPs	☐ 0	☐ 1	☐ 2	☐ 3	☐ 4
7. Determine reporting and supervisory relationships	☐ 0	☐ 1	☐ 2	☐ 3	☐ 4
IV. Financial:	Not Planning	Being Studied or prepared	Seeking approval or consensus	In place	In place with plans for improvement
1. Identifying payment mechanisms for behavioral health providers	☐ 0	☐ 1	☐ 2	☐ 3	☐ 4
2. Identifying methods of risk-sharing with partners	☐ 0	☐ 1	☐ 2	☐ 3	☐ 4

IV. Financial (Cont.):	Not Planning	Being Studied or prepared	Seeking approval or consensus	In place	In place with plans for improvement
3. Developing agreements for distribution of cost savings	☐ 0	☐ 1	☐ 2	☐ 3	☐ 4
4. Incentives for staff to perform according to organizational standards	☐ 0	☐ 1	☐ 2	☐ 3	☐ 4

V. Operational:	Not Planning	Being Studied or prepared	Seeking approval or consensus	In place	In place with plans for improvement
1. Inclusion as provider in health plans	☐ 0	☐ 1	☐ 2	☐ 3	☐ 4
2. Patient access to BCP and referral procedures established	☐ 0	☐ 1	☐ 2	☐ 3	☐ 4
3. MIS to track flow of patients(i.e., who is referring and types of treatment provided)	☐ 0	☐ 1	☐ 2	☐ 3	☐ 4

Quality Improvement Systems:

	Not Planning	Being Studied or prepared	Seeking approval or consensus	In place	In place with plans for improvement
4. Measures for patient satisfaction	☐ 0	☐ 1	☐ 2	☐ 3	☐ 4
5. Feedback forms for evaluation of BCPs to maintain a standard of care	☐ 0	☐ 1	☐ 2	☐ 3	☐ 4
6. Quarterly evaluation of PCP satisfaction	☐ 0	☐ 1	☐ 2	☐ 3	☐ 4
7. Tracking medical utilization change targeting high utilizers	☐ 0	☐ 1	☐ 2	☐ 3	☐ 4
8. Employing structured case discussions weekly	☐ 0	☐ 1	☐ 2	☐ 3	☐ 4
9. Monthly review of interventions for impact	☐ 0	☐ 1	☐ 2	☐ 3	☐ 4
10. Sampling of outcomes (clinical, financial) over regular time periods	☐ 0	☐ 1	☐ 2	☐ 3	☐ 4
11. Empirically supported measures used to track patient outcomes	☐ 0	☐ 1	☐ 2	☐ 3	☐ 4
12. Dissemination of patient outcomes to Integrated Care teams regularly	☐ 0	☐ 1	☐ 2	☐ 3	☐ 4

Resources:

	Not Planning	Being Studied or prepared	Seeking approval or consensus	In place	In place with plans for improvement
13. Space/co-location for BCPs	☐ 0	☐ 1	☐ 2	☐ 3	☐ 4
14. Making available of training, supervisors, and consultation services	☐ 0	☐ 1	☐ 2	☐ 3	☐ 4

VI. Administrative:	Not Planning	Being Studied or prepared	Seeking approval or consensus	In place	In place with plans for improvement
1. Billing and coding system	☐ 0	☐ 1	☐ 2	☐ 3	☐ 4
2. Scheduling templates	☐ 0	☐ 1	☐ 2	☐ 3	☐ 4
3. Charting and documentation requirements	☐ 0	☐ 1	☐ 2	☐ 3	☐ 4
4. Documentation quality improvement system (i.e., regularly reviewing all documentation for meeting standards)	☐ 0	☐ 1	☐ 2	☐ 3	☐ 4

resources. Triwest.com's behavioral health portal provides information on clinical guidelines for the behavioral health provider and the physician as well as patient self-management resources. Careintegra.com provides information about medical cost offset, behavioral pathways to medical utilization, and other books and resources that can be useful. Another useful site is http://www.behavioral-health-integration.com. This site offers moderated discussions regarding integrated care as well as other useful resources for filling any gaps identified. Finally, there are a number of well-known experienced integrated care consultants in the field who can assist with this (e.g., Kirk Strosahl's and Patti Robison's mountviewconsulting.com; Nick Cummings and William O'Donohue's careintegra.com, Sandy Blount's collaborativecare.com). These experts can provide a variety of levels of consulting that can vastly improve learning curves by teaching about their "lessons learned."

Conclusions

It is important to recognize that integrated care is not just parachuting traditional mental health into a medical care clinic. Such an assumption is a typical mistake and will result in a number of problems (unfulfilled expectations, scheduling jams, no medical cost offset, etc). Integrated care requires specially trained (and temperamentally inclined) behavioral health clinicians, physicians trained to work with these individuals, administrators to support this system, key resources, and a financial model to sustain these efforts. Quality is based on the notion of designing (and continually redesigning) systems that increasingly produce better outcomes. Quality is rarely achieved by minimizing initial design efforts. We hope that with this readiness assessment method and with resources to fill any gaps identified, an organization's integrated care efforts will be successful.

References

Belt, J., & Bashore, E. (2000). Managed care strategic planning: The reality of uncertainty. *Healthcare Financial Management, 54*(5), 38–42.

D'Ambrosio, R., Mondeaux, F., Gabriel, R. M., & Laws, K. E. (2003). Oregon's transition to a managed care model for Medicaid-funded substance abuse treatment: Steamrolling the glass menagerie. *Health Social Work, 28*(2), 126–36.

Dyer, R., Eskelsen, N., Martin, E., & Ullrich, C. (2003). *Organization Readiness for Integrating Behavioral Health into Primary Care.* Criterion Health, Inc. Available at: http://www.criterionhealth.net/default.aspx

Lehman, W., Greener, J., & Simpson, D. (2002). Assessing organizational readiness for change. *Journal of Substance Abuse Treatment, 22*, 197–209.

Nelson, J., Raskind-Hood, C., Galvin, V., Essien, J., & Levine, L. (1999). Positioning for partnerships: Assessing public health agency readiness. *American Journal of Preventative Medicine, 16*, 103–117.

O'Donohue, W., Cummings, N., & Ferguson, K. (2003). Clinical integration: The promise and the path. In Cummings, N., O'Donohue, W., & Ferguson, K. (Eds.), *Behavioral Health as Primary Care: Beyond Efficacy to Effectiveness* (pp. 15–30). Reno, NV: Context Press.

Poats, J., & Salvaneschi, M. (2003). *Health Care Technology: Innovating clinical care through technology.* [On-line]. Available: www.hctproject.com/documents.asp?d_ID=1827

Snyder-Halpern, R. (2001). Indicators of organizational readiness for clinical information technology/systems innovation: A Delphi study. *International Journal of Medical Informatics, 63*(3), 179–204.

What Administrators Should Know About the Primary Care Setting

Larry C. James

What does the health care manager need to know about the primary care integration model and the primary care (PC) setting? However, the *a priori* question and knowledge for the health care managers should be the fact that the mental health care system in the United States is costly, ineffective, out of date, does not employ modern technology, and, above all else, is broken (James & Folen, 2004; Richardson & Corrigan, 2002; Cummings, Cummings, & Johnson, 1997; Strosahl, 1994). These authors clearly cite how the traditional mental health system has failed its patients and the referral providers. In fact, most Americans receive their mental health care from their primary care physician rather than a psychologist or psychiatrist (Narrow, Reiger, Rae, Manderscheid, & Locke, 1993). In fact, 67% of all psychotropic medications are prescribed by primary care providers, 90% of the top ten common medical complaints in primary care have no organic or medical basis, and 70% of all primary care visits have psychosocial concerns. Richardson authored the 'Institute of Medicine report' (Richardson & Corrigan, 2002) which concluded the mental health system is ineffective, has a broken referral system, is plagued by a stigma problem, and does not meet the needs of the mental health patient. These data beg the question, why not provide behavioral health care in the primary care setting?

Administrators who are less than pleased with their current mental health system, model, and resources, given the data, should transform their old mental health system to the new primary care integration model. Several authors (James & Folen, 2004; O'Donohue, Byrd, Cummings, & Henderson, 2005); Cummings, Cummings, & Johnson, 1997; Frank, McDaniel, Bray, & Heldring, 2004; Strosahl, 2005), although each somewhat unique from one another, all have pioneered a novel approach to integrate clinical psychology services into the primary care setting. These authors have developed primary care behavioral health models centered around the pivotal components of healthcare: patient access, quality treatment, cost effectiveness, and collaboration with referral providers.

L.C. James (✉)
Department of Psychology, Tripler Army Medical Center, Mililani, HI 96789, USA
e-mail: jamesbdaddy@aol.com

L.C. James, W.T. O'Donohue (eds.), *The Primary Care Toolkit*,
DOI 10.1007/978-0-387-78971-2_2, © Springer Science+Business Media, LLC 2009

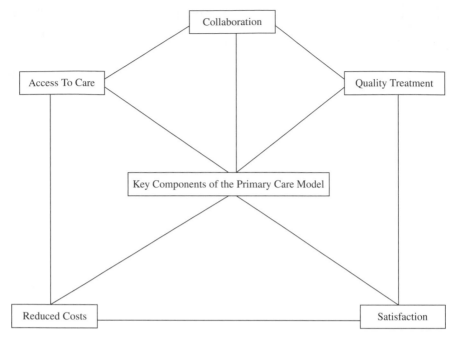

Fig. 1 Key components of the primary care model

Administrators should know that there are four motivating factors to deliver behavioral health services in the primary care setting. Figure 1 illustrates the key components of the model, and each is described separately below.

Patient Access and Costs

James (2005) provided anecdotal examples of the many access-to-care problems in the traditional mental health care system. In this study, James surveyed 50 patients who were new referrals to his clinic. James's anecdotal study found that, on average, it took approximately 14 months for a mental health patient to actually be seen by the psychologist or psychiatrist in the traditional model. In other words, from the moment the primary care physician sent a patient to the mental health clinic, in most of the cases, he/she did not receive any treatment for 14 months.

While surveying the patients he was amazed at the many practical reasons for the delay in treatment and the many hurdles in access to behavioral health care. He found that in many cases, the patients rather than the provider (or his/her staff) held the responsibility to deliver the consult to the mental health clinic. Then, usually it would take 6 to 8 weeks, if not even longer, for an appointment with a psychiatrist. James found that by that time, most patients would acquire help from resources within his or her community; for example, patients would seek services from their pastor, a community organization, friends, or spouse.In many cases, however, patients would suffer quietly without treatment.

Patients reported to James that there were many other practical problems that simply impeded their access to mental health treatment. Patients felt embarrassed to present themselves at the mental health clinic. The clinics were usually located in a separate building or remote from the primary care clinic. Hence, patients felt that they could not go to the mental health clinic "unnoticed." They reported a "stigma," which was identified by the Institute of Medicine (2001) as a major barrier to care.

Patients reported that there was always limited parking or it was difficult to contact the mental health clinic by phone to schedule an appointment. Thus, many of the patients just simply gave up in their quest for formal mental health care and sought help from resources in the community. James reasoned that providing behavioral health care directly in the primary clinics would immediately increase access to care and avoid the practical barriers described above.

Reducing Costs

Hospital administrators should be cognizant of the fact that the traditional model is not only broken with regard to access, but that it is more costly (Coffey et al., 2000). Balesterieri, Williams and Wilkinson (1988) demonstrated that locating behavioral health care in the primary care setting improved outcomes and reduced costs. Pignone et al. (2002) found that this model illustrated an improved recognition of depression as well as an overall improvement of health outcomes. Laygo et al. (2003) found a 21% reduction in medical utilization the year after behavioral health contact in an integrated care setting. In a randomly controlled trial involving over 120,000 patients, Cummings, O'Donohue, and Ferguson (2002) found a 40% reduction in 18 months following a high utilizer outreach program. Cummings, O'Donohue, and Ferguson (2002) provide a review of medical cost offset associated with integrated care. Lorig et al. (1999) in a randomized trial found that perhaps a chronic disease self-management program can improve health status while reducing hospitalization. Programs as such can easily be provided in primary care settings whereby the PC psychologist plays an active part in the disease management.

Quality Treatment, Satisfaction and Collaboration

What happens when behavioral care is located directly in the primary care clinic? Are providers and patients more satisfied? Is this model more cost effective? Von Korff et al. (1998) conducted a large scale study examining the effects of a collaborative and integrative model of care and found the collaborative model to be significantly more cost effective. Laygo et al. (2003) found both high physician (4.9/5) and patient satisfaction (4.6/5) with integrated care. James (2006) in a large federal system in Hawaii found that the PC lowered the patient "no show" rate, improved access and patient and provider satisfaction. James found that when he provided specific PC training for the psychologists and placed staff in PC clinics, the results were impressive. The referring physicians welcome feedback on their patients the same day, and on some occasions were able to consult with the psychologist while the psychologist evaluated the patient.

James and his staff were frustrated with the old model of mental health care. He described it as disjointed, ineffective, costly and also noted that the mental health staff showed little interest in providing a fast, innovative, cost-effective, and user-friendly service.

What Should the Administrator Keep from the Old Model?

One is not asserting that the old mental health model be completely discarded. Rather, it is believed that there is some value in the old model. The PC model is designed for the patient who is early in the disease process and is amenable to receiving services in the PC setting. Perhaps some family physicians would rather suggest that the seriously impaired schizophrenic, borderline personality disorder patient, and/or the unstable bipolar manic receive services in the psychiatry clinic on the other side of the hospital. One can reasonably argue that patients as such may be too disruptive and unstable to be treated in the PC setting.

Therefore, patients with serious mental health conditions may be better served in the traditional mental health clinic. Why? There are several practical reasons that by and large center around safety. For the seriously mentally ill and unstable mental health patient, having to restrain a patient is not unusual, and intense verbal confrontations with staff can be common. The PC setting is not equipped for this nor are the staff in such settings trained for such encounters.

Now, having said this, the author is very familiar with community hospitals that serve primarily an indigent, urban population that provides services to the seriously mentally ill directly within the primary care clinic. In these community hospitals, the psychiatrists are utilized as consultants, and the primary care provider prescribes all medications. Perhaps, it may simply depend on the comfort level of the PC staff.

All mental health care for children and family therapy would typically be provided in a child and adolescent clinic or a family clinic. Some authors, such as Frank, McDaniel, Bray, and Heldring (2004) provide models to deliver all behavioral health care directly in the primary care clinics. In particular, Dr Susan McDaniel describes many cases of conducting family therapy in the PC setting. McDaniel discusses providing treatment with families that would traditionally be seen in psychology clinics, psychiatry department, or the social work department. These authors have adopted a model that meets the needs of a varied type of patients. It was once thought that patients with serious mental health conditions could only be treated in the traditional mental health clinic.

Given this evidence, ideally one can argue to expand the existing PC model and integrate in child and family psychologists who would welcome the opportunity to work in the PC setting. Etherage (2005) describes a PC behavioral health model he had implemented into a large federal health care system in Maryland where exists a large pediatric population. He provided the PC model training to pediatric psychologists at his hospital and found the transition to be a success. He concluded that when behavioral health services were delivered directly in the pediatric clinics, referral time improved, patient and provider satisfaction increased, and outcome improved.

Summary

Administrators will need to weigh the pros and cons of each model, the PC model or the traditional mental health model, to identify which one best suits their needs. However, the PC model is effective, yields more provider and patient satisfaction, reduces costs, and offers a safe and efficacious clinical outcome.

References

Balesterieri, M., Williams, P., & Wilkinson, G. (1988). Specialist mental health treatment in general practice: A meta-analysis. *Psychological Medicine, 18*, 711–717.
Coffey, R., Mark, T., King, E., Harwood, H., McKusick, D., Genuardi, J., et al. (2000). *National estimates of expenditures for mental health and substance abuse treatment, 1997* (SAMHSHA Publication No. SMA-00-3499). Rockville, MD: Substance Abuse and Mental Health Services Administration.
Cummings, N. A., Cummings, J. L., & Johnson, J. N. (1997). *Behavioral Health in Primary Care*. Madison, Connecticut: Psychosocial Press.
Cummings, N. A., O'Donohue, W., & Ferguson, K.(Eds.) (2002). *The impact of medical cost offset on practice and research: Making it work for you*. Reno, NV: Context Press
Etherage, J. R. (2005). Pediatric behavioral health consultation: A new model for primary care. In L. C. James, & R. A. Folen (Eds.), *The Primary Care Consultant: A new frontier for psychologists in hospitals and clinics* (pp. 173–190). Washington, DC: American Psychological Association Press.
Frank, F. G., McDaniel, S. H., Bray, J. H., & Heldring, M. (2004). *Primary Care Psychology*. Washington, DC: American Psychological Association Press.
James, L. C., & Folen, R. A. (2005). *The Primary Care Consultant: The next frontier for psychologists in hospitals and clinics*. Washington, DC: American Psychological Association Press.
James, L. C. (2005). Integrating Clinical Psychology into the Primary Care Setting. A paper presented at The Hawaii Psychological Association Convention. Honolulu, Hawaii.
James, L. C. (2006). Integrating clinical psychology into primary care. *Journal of Clinical Psychology, 60*, 1207–1211.
Laygo, R., O'Donohue, W., Hall, S., Kaplan, A., Wood, R., Cummings, J., et al. (2003). Preliminary results from the Hawaii integrated healthcare project II. In. N. Cummings, O'Donohue, W., & Ferguson, K. (Eds.), *Behavioral health as primary care: Beyond Efficacy to effectiveness*. Reno: Context Press.
Lorig, K. R., Sobel, D. S., Stewart, A. L., Brown, B. W., Bandura, A., & Ritter, P. (1999). Evidence suggesting that a chronic disease self-management program can improve health status while reducing hospitalization. A randomized trial. *Medical Care, 37*, 5–14.
Narrow, W., Reiger, D., Rae, D., Manderscheid, R., & Locke, B. (1993). Use of services by persons with mental health and addictive disorders: Findings from the National Institutes of Mental Health epidemiologic catchment area program. *Archives of General Psychiatry, 50*, 95–107.
O'Donohue, W. T., Byrd, M. R., Cummings, N. A., & Henderson, D. A. (2005). *Behavioral Integrative Care: Treatments that Work in the Primary Care Setting*. New York: Brunner-Routledge.

Pignone, M. P., Gaynes, B. N., Rushton, J. L., Burchell, C. M., Orleans, C. T., Marlow, C. D., et al. (2002). Screening for depression in adults: A summary of the evidence for the U.S. preventive services task force. *Annals of Internal Medicine, 136*, 765–776.

Richardson, W. C., & Corrigan, J. M. (2002). Shaping the Future. The IOM Newsletter. Vol. 1(4). Winter edition.

Strosahl, K. D. (1994). Entering the new frontier of managed health care: Gold mines and land mines. *Cognitive and Behavioral Practice, 1*, 5–23.

Strosahl, K. D. (2005). Training behavioral health and primary care providers for integrated care: A core competence approach. In W. T. O'Donohue, M. R. Byrd, N. A. Cummings, & D. A. Henderson (Eds.), *Behavioral Integrative Care: Treatments that work in the primary care setting* (pp. 15–52). New York: Brunner-Routledge.

Von Korff, M., Katon, W., Bush, T., Lin, E., Simon, G. E., Saunders, K., et al. (1998). Treatment costs, cost offset and cost-effectiveness of collaborative management of depression. *Psychosomatic Medicine, 60*, 143–149.

Financial Models for Integrated Behavioral Health Care

Blake Chaffee

Integrated behavioral health care or "integrated care" is a distinct service delivery model aimed at early identification and appropriate intervention with that portion of medical/surgical patients presenting with behavioral health issues. The clinical rationale for integrated care and the potential for medical cost offset savings have been clearly substantiated in available research (Cummings, 2007; O'Donohue, Ferguson & Cummings, 2002), but the financial models supporting it as part of health care operations rather than as a demonstration program have been less fully explored. This chapter discusses the financial considerations for health care organizations in implementing integrated care and models to support it.

Integrated care is a service delivery model different from the specialty behavioral health care with different clinical and administrative requirements. Integrated care is not simply hiring and placing behavioral health professionals in primary care settings. Integrated care is a systematic program. Providers in integrated care settings need additional training and support in areas such as medical literacy, chronic-disease management, consultation/liaison services, pharmacology, stepped-care interventions, relapse prevention, group treatments, self-management interventions, and quality improvement, among other skills (O'Donohue, Cummings & Ferguson, 2003). Training is essential to the success of this delivery system, as few behavioral health providers have the skill set to perform competently in integrated care settings. Psychologists have frequently been recruited for integrated care because their graduate training and skill set most closely approximate the training requirements mentioned above, but research shows that the type of provider (psychologist, social worker, psychiatrist) is not a significant factor in achieving the medical cost-offset effect.

Not only is the clinical skill set of the provider different, the administrative support requirements for integrated care also differ. There are two major models of integrated care: the consultative model (James & Folen, 2005) and the Biodyne model (Laygo et al., 2003). Essentially, the psychologist practices delivering triage,

B. Chaffee (✉)
Vice President, Integrated Healthcare Services, TriWest Healthcare Alliance, Phoenix, AZ
e-mail: bchaffee@triwest.com

L.C. James, W.T. O'Donohue (eds.), *The Primary Care Toolkit*,
DOI 10.1007/978-0-387-78971-2_3, © Springer Science+Business Media, LLC 2009

brief assessment, and targeted interventions. The psychologist's time is often scheduled in 15- and 30-minute increments to ensure availability. Referrals and scheduling are completely different from those in specialty behavioral health. For example, in the Biodyne model, the integrated care psychologist frequently receives referrals in real time via the "hallway handoff," where a primary care physician walks a patient down the hall to see the psychologist or brings the psychologist into the exam room, introduces him/her to the patient and then steps out to see the next patient.

Maintaining the availability of the psychologist to accommodate additional referrals from the primary care physicians with whom they work is essential to the success of integrated care. Functioning in a traditional specialty behavioral health care delivery model while co-located in a primary care clinic would quickly result in the behavioral health professional's psychotherapy schedule filling to capacity. The behavioral health professional would then not be available to see additional new referrals or to consult with the primary care physician.

The Biodyne model of integrated care resolves these problems by employing research-based psychotherapy protocols focused on resolving specific presenting problems in brief treatment episodes, rather than on extensive therapy for more general goals (Laygo et al., 2003). In addition, structured psycho-educational groups for managing chronic medical conditions, stress management, and anger management are utilized to increase the patient's self-management skills. More severe mental disorders would be referred for behavioral health specialty care in the specialty behavioral health clinic or the network.

Melek (1999) discussed integrating behavioral health care into commercial managed care and recognized the need for "new models of reimbursement and risk-sharing. . .for successful integrated systems of care to better align the incentives between the behavioral and medical healthcare providers" (p. 9). Melek argued that the reimbursement and risk-sharing arrangements for both behavioral health care and medical health care providers in integrated care should be aligned to motivate them to deliver cost-effective, efficient services. Further, the financial model should:

- encourage early diagnosis and appropriate treatment of behavioral disorders in the primary care setting;
- provide for educational and prevention programs related to behavioral and medical wellness; and
- be fair to all participants.

Melek then presented models for reimbursement and risk-sharing in three specific settings:

- Integrating full-time behavioral health care into a heavily capitated PCP group that participates in risk pools in a mature managed care marketplace.
- Integrating part-time behavioral health care into a mixed capitation and fee-for-service PCP group without existing risk-sharing arrangements in a less mature managed care marketplace.
- Integrating full-time behavioral health care into a multi-specialty group with a global capitation in a moderately mature managed care market.

In the first model, the behavioral health providers (BCP) would be salaried and would also participate in risk-pool sharing and risk and productivity adjustments in the same manner as their primary care provider (PCP) colleagues. Funding for psycho-educational and preventive programs implemented by the BCPs would be funded via the capitated revenues received by the integrated provider group or could be negotiated with payers and managed care plans on the basis of savings in future medical care costs. This model aligns the financial and operational risks and incentives most closely. If, for example, having the BCPs in the primary care clinic actually leveraged the PCPs' time by allowing them to readily refer cases with behavioral health issues via "hallway hand-offs," then the PCPs would be available to see more patients. Potentially, a significant physician-leveraging effect might allow the PCPs to enlarge the number of patients enrolled to them, increasing the capitated revenues the integrated provider group might receive. Additionally, the BCPs functioning in an integrated care model might allow the group to achieve savings through medical cost offsets paid through their risk pools. Melek (2001) provides an actuarial analysis of the potential effect on the integrated provider group's revenues over the first two years, estimating a 12% increase in revenue in the first year and an 8.3% increase between the first and second years. These funds could be used to cover the start-up costs of implementing the integrated care model and provide additional profits to all members of the integrated care group.

In the Melek's (2001) second model, the PCP group receives a straight capitation payment per member per month for its managed care business, does not participate in any additional risk-sharing arrangements with its payers, and has a significant volume of fee-for-service (FFS) business. The providers, including the BCPs would be salaried, but would participate in member risk adjustments and productivity adjustments within the group. The BCPs negotiate a risk-sharing arrangement with the PCPs based on their ability to leverage the PCPs' time: The BCPs would share in any additional capitated revenue from enlargements in the PCPs' patient panels. The BCPs might also share in any medical FFS revenue resulting from referrals they provide to the PCPs from their FFS clients. Melek's actuarial analysis for this model estimates a 4% increase in the integrated care group's total revenue in the first year and a 3.9% increase in the second year.

Melek's (2001) third model posits BCPs joining a multi-specialty group practice that is capitated for all professional services and pharmacy costs. The group also participates in an external risk pool for facility costs. The PCPs and BCPs are salaried, and the BCPs participate in all risk-sharing arrangements. Melek does not provide an actuarial analysis for this model.

Melek's (1999; 2001) two discussions focus on capitated models of health care delivery. Capitated models dominate the managed care HMO (health maintenance organization) industry and staff model HMOs and have also been applied to federal programs, including Medicare and Medicaid. Preferred provider organizations (PPO) are much more likely to utilize some version of fee-for-service reimbursement, primarily because their membership has the option of utilizing any provider in the PPO network without referral from their PCP, making capitation unworkable. Government's direct care programs such as the medical systems of the military service branches and the veterans administration (VR) are also not currently funded in a capitated mode. Where are the financial incentives for the development of integrated care in those systems? Melek (1999; 2001) did address how integrated care can work with FFS reimbursement, and the larger point is this: The same integrated care principles that apply within a capitated payment model, e.g. physician leveraging and medical cost offset, still apply in other payment models. The crucial point to note, however, is that the effects of these integrated care principles may be more difficult to demonstrate and may not have the same effect on provider behavior when not as directly connected to provider reimbursement, for both the PCP and BCP. In other words, the principles of integrated care may be most clearly evident in the capitated model at the provider group level where payer and provider risk and incentives may be best aligned. This does *not* mean that integrated care cannot be implemented in larger-scale systems such as the military, the VA, or network PPOs, but that such implementations should carefully attend to the alignment of provider and payer risks and incentives.

Melek's (1999; 2001) analyses of capitated and mixed payment models contain the essential elements that make integrated care most effective, i.e. payer risk and incentives, provider risk and incentives, physician leveraging, and medical cost offset. To these, this author would add "access to care" which is really a secondary effect of physician leveraging. In Melek's (1999; 2001) descriptions, when the BCPs leverage their PCPs' time by allowing them to readily refer cases with behavioral health involvement, thereby freeing them to see other patients, the other, new patients the PCP is able to see really represent additional access to care in the PCP's clinic. In Melek's (1999; 2001) examples, the physician leveraging effect motivates the integrated group as a whole, the individual PCP, and the individual BCP because the additional capacity or access created translated directly into increased revenue or personal reimbursement. This increased capacity or increased access to care produced by physician leveraging will not have the same effect in other noncapitated health care systems *unless* the payer and provider risk and incentives are as fully aligned.

In a network PPO with primarily FFS provider reimbursement, the payer attempts to limit financial risk by discounting provider reimbursements, monitoring utilization, and case managing high-risk or high-utilizing cases. From the payer's point of view, integrated care would be appealing if its medical cost offset effects were demonstrable and tangible, but achieving those effects takes considerable investment of money and time. O'Donohue, Ferguson and Cummings (2002) discuss medical cost offset and the findings of over 30 years of studies, including meta-analyses. Although the literature provides ample evidence that medical cost offset/ savings have been significant in a variety of settings, achieving those savings is not a foregone conclusion, and the commitment as to the financial and resource investment necessary to launch an integrated care program must be made *before* evidence can be obtained that savings will be realized.

Making this even more unlikely is the element of *time*. The time required to implement integrated care networkwide and then realize any medical cost offset/ savings would be at least three or more years, assuming that the PPO's claims-information systems would be able to track and evaluate accurately the pre- and post-integrated care costs. Despite the research findings, some health plans and medical managers may view the up-front investment as too large and the timeline to realizing medical cost offset savings as too long to justify taking the risk. So the risk to the PPO payer in investing the time and resources—personnel and financial—to implement and evaluate integrated care simply but effectively outweighs the potential benefits to health care system efficiency and finances. The potential payoff in increased quality of patient care and medical cost offset may be huge, but the operable word here in the minds of most health care managers will be "potential," while the time, effort, and costs on the front-end are very real.

For health plans operating network PPOs, *control* is also an issue in considering integrated care implementations. In staff model HMOs, the health plan employs the physicians and staff and determines how they operate. In a network PPO, the providers are independent practitioners who contract to provide services to a health plan's members. The typical network PPO provider will have a number of contracts with different health plans and typically will seek to limit the volume of patients from any single payer in order to maintain their independence and negotiating leverage. The health plan seeking to implement integrated care must therefore find other incentives to stimulate the development of integrated care in its network. As we have discussed previously, physician leveraging is the most powerful incentive for network providers to implement integrated care because it translates directly into increased provider/clinic revenue.

Scale is another potential obstacle to the implementation of integrated care. Most PPOs operate extensive networks, and implementing integrated care within a sufficient number of primary care practices to achieve any overall medical cost offset effect would be a huge—and probably expensive—logistical, educational, and management challenge. Add to this the *scope of the effort* required to implement integrated behavioral health care in a large PPO network. Most health plans do not have the technical expertise nor the personnel resources required to implement and sustain an integrated behavioral health program regionwide. There are several additional obstacles for any health plan considering such an initiative, including:

- The technical expertise and knowledge base for integrated care service delivery;
- The training of the behavioral care providers (BCP);
- Information system support to evaluate physician leveraging and medical cost offset.

We have alluded to the technical expertise and knowledge-base requirements earlier in describing integrated care as a distinct delivery system. Integrated care has been developed and implemented in a number of settings, and the "lessons learned" documented in a growing body of literature (O'Donohue, Ferguson & Cummings, 2002). Operational experience is invaluable, however, and most health plans do not yet have internal subject matter experts.

Research indicates that the type of behavioral health professional (psychologist, social worker or psychiatrist) delivering the integrated care interventions is not a significant factor in producing the medical cost offset effect (O'Donohue, Ferguson & Cummings, 2002). Psychologists are frequently employed in integrated care applications because their training and skill set most closely approximates the requirements of integrated care behavioral health professionals. Nevertheless, psychologists may not be sufficiently trained in the following areas to function effectively in an integrated care setting:

- Medical terminology
- Psychopharmacology
- Short-term, targeted interventions
- Brief session triage/assessment

Documenting physician leveraging and medical cost offset are not typical capabilities of health plan information systems, but are both requirements to demonstrate the efficacy of integrated care and justify the implementation and operational cost.

Despite the obstacles, there are incentives to the development and proliferation of integrated care approaches in network PPO and other FFS environments. In the years since Melek's (1999; 2001) discussions of integrated care in an FFS reimbursement model, an entirely new area of reimbursable services opened to integrated care providers with the introduction of health and behavior assessment codes (Current Procedural Terminology, 2007). Since January 1, 2002, codes for health and behavior assessment and intervention services apply to behavioral, social, and psychophysiological procedures for the prevention, treatment, or management of physical-health problems. Prior to the introduction of health and behavior assessment codes, such interventions rendered by psychologists or other behavioral health practitioners could not be reimbursed directly. The only options available to integrated care providers were to either diagnose the medical/surgical patient with mental disorder listed in the Diagnostic and Statistical Manual of Mental Disorders (DSM-IV) or use the DSM-IV diagnosis 316.00 Psychological Factors Affecting Physical Condition. Neither of these options applied to cases in which medical/surgical patients could benefit from behavioral techniques that could prevent, reduce, or help them manage the symptoms of their medical/surgical condition. Psychological Factors Affecting Physical Condition indicate that the patient exhibits psychological symptoms or behaviors that negatively affect the incidence, severity, or management of their physical condition. While this applies to a certain subset of the patients that providers in integrated care may see, it does not cover those patients who could benefit from psycho-educational approaches, skill training, or behavior modification aimed to increase their ability to self-manage their physical condition. The Health and Behavior Assessment Codes were specifically designed to allow behavioral health consultation in such cases, including:

- patient adherence to medical treatment;
- symptom management;
- health-promoting behaviors;
- health-related risk-taking behaviors; and
- adjustment to physical illness.

The American Psychological Association (APA) Practice Directorate described the codes as follows in its 2002 Internet announcement:

96150 – the initial assessment of the patient to determine the biological, psychological, and social factors affecting the patient's physical health and any treatment problems.

96151 – a re-assessment of the patient to evaluate the patient's condition and determine the need for further treatment. A re-assessment may be performed by a clinician other than the one who conducted the patient's initial assessment.

96152 – the intervention service provided to an individual to modify the psychological, behavioral, cognitive, and social factors affecting the patient's physical health and well-being. Examples include increasing the patient's awareness about his or her disease and using cognitive and behavioral approaches to initiate physician prescribed diet and exercise regimens.

96153 – the intervention service provided to a group. An example is a smoking cessation program that includes educational information, cognitive-behavioral treatment and social support. Group sessions typically last for 90 minutes and involve 8 to 10 patients.

96154 – the intervention service provided to a family with the patient present. For example, a psychologist could use relaxation techniques with both a diabetic child and his or her parents to reduce the child's fear of receiving injections and the parents' tension when administering the injections.

96155 – the intervention service provided to a family without the patient present. An example would be working with parents and siblings to shape the diabetic child's behavior, such as praising successful diabetes management behaviors and ignoring disruptive tactics.

Health and behavior assessment codes cannot be billed for psychotherapy services and cannot be billed on the same day as a psychiatric CPT code for the same patient. The provider must bill for the predominant service rendered. Health and behavior assessment codes are also billed in 15-minute units of service.

Health and behavior assessment codes clearly expand the service array that an integrated care provider may offer, thereby increasing the types of patients that can be served and the revenue that can be generated. Broadening the prospects for referrals from a PCP may increase the physician leveraging effect the BCP can provide. The introduction of health and behavioral assessment codes therefore offers provider groups with two service- and revenue-enhancing opportunities. Such incremental revenue may contribute to offsetting the implementation costs of integrated care and reducing perceived risk for managers contemplating integrated care start-ups.

The military health system has implemented integrated care in a variety of settings. The Army, Navy, and Air Force have all developed integrated care programs in some of their military treatment facilities, but all of the Services have had difficulty sustaining their integrated care delivery systems because of the duty assignment rotations and deployment requirements of their active duty providers. The Air Force program actually developed an internship-training program to address the different training requirements of integrated care and to provide a steady stream of trained BCPs for their integrated care clinics. In the military health system, the ultimate "payer" is the government. The financial risks and incentives obviously differ significantly in these settings from those in capitated commercial managed care programs. Nevertheless, US Air Force health system planners viewed the medical cost offset saving potential of integrated care as sufficiently compelling to launch its integrated behavioral health program (Primary Behavioral Health Care

Services Practice Manual, Version 2.0, March 2002). The Air Force viewed integrated care as a service-delivery model that would allow their co-located PCPs and BCPs to address the utilization and costs of patients with behavioral health issues in the primary care setting. Cost and utilization concerns were therefore the primary impetus for the development of integrated behavioral health care in the US Air Force medical system (Runyan, Fonseca & Hunter, 2003).

The fact that integrated care is a higher-volume practice than specialty behavioral health care has particular value within the military health system. Integrated care is an entirely different health service delivery system than the specialty behavioral health model in which most behavioral health providers are trained. When co-located, BCPs practice "behavioral health primary care" in a manner analogous to their PCP counterparts, their visit lengths decrease, and the number of encounters significantly decreases compared with specialty behavioral health. Integrated care is therefore by design a higher-volume practice model than specialty behavioral health care. The brief triage, assessment, and targeted interventions of integrated care are designed to address the behavioral health issues most commonly presented in primary care, e.g. anxiety, mild/moderate depression, and psychological factors related to physical conditions. Patients with more severe behavioral health conditions requiring more intensive services would be referred to the behavioral health specialty clinic by the integrated care provider. The higher volume of encounters generated by integrated care providers has particular value in the military health care system where productivity is measured in relative value units (RVU). The RVU system is typically utilized to measure provider, clinic, and department productivity, and budget decisions are frequently based on the results. Within these financial contingencies, the relatively high workload and the resulting RVU totals generated by integrated care providers become valuable commodities for the department claiming the workload. Workload allocation decisions within such a system can dramatically alter the development of integrated care. For example, if the psychology department of a medical center attempted to claim the workload of integrated care psychologists working in the primary care, family practice, adult medicine, pediatrics, internal medicine, or cardiology departments, there would be little incentive for those departments to collaborate in implementing or further developing integrated care. If, on the other hand, the psychology department negotiated workload-sharing arrangements with the various medical departments that reflected their respective contributions to the implementation and support of integrated care, the contingencies would be aligned to support the development of integrated care wherever the workload would support it. These contingencies are by no means unique to the military health system and are analogous to the financial contingencies in commercial managed care settings. The effects of these contingencies are important to be recognized and addressed in any integrated care application.

Military health system providers are all salaried, and they do not share in any incentive-compensation programs tied to the numbers of patients enrolled to them or to their productivity. As discussed above, military health system provider productivity is typically measured using the relative value unit (RVU) system rather than the financial indicators common in commercial health plans and private practice.

The benefits of high-volume workload accrue primarily to the department budgets rather than individual providers in the military health system. Nevertheless, RVU totals as measures of individual productivity can serve as powerful incentives to providers in military and other government direct care systems if they are considered in annual performance evaluations. A provider's RVU total may then become a meaningful incentive to achieve and maintain high workload volumes.

Access-to-care (physician leveraging) effects of integrated care have had primary appeal in the military health system. The author has been involved in the development of an integrated care pilot project at military health facilities in Hawaii (Chaffee & O'Donohue, 2007). The ability of the integrated care model to facilitate access to behavioral health consultation for service members with deployment-related behavioral health issues, including PTSD, was recognized and highly valued by military health system leaders. For active duty service members, referral to the mental health specialty clinic frequently remains fraught with issues of stigma and career concerns despite the military's significant efforts to address these concerns. Access to behavioral health consultation in the primary care clinic provided another channel for early identification and intervention with deployment-related behavioral health concerns.

As mentioned above, medical cost offset was a primary driver of the US Air Force integrated care program. This is not surprising when the military health system is viewed as analogous to a large-staff model HMO within which medical cost offset savings could be realized. What is especially noteworthy about the Air Force program is that medical cost offset was viewed as a real and sufficiently valuable effect that the Air Force proceeded with its implementation, despite all the problems and complexities associated with the scale of the US Air Force health system (Primary Behavioral Health Care Services Practice Manual, Version 2.0, March 2002). The Air Force viewed integrated care as an essential element of its "primary care optimization" initiative (Runyan, Fonseca & Hunter, 2003).

In summary, the focus on medical cost offset as the primary goal of integrated care in applications described in much of the previous literature is striking, although there are some notable exceptions such as Melek (1999; 2001). This focus may have had a limiting effect on the development and proliferation of integrated care more broadly in the health care delivery system, given the relative lack of importance of medical cost offset in financial models other than capitation. The US Air Force program is exceptional for its somewhat visionary recognition of the importance of medical cost offset in the military direct care system. This emphasis on medical cost offset may have overshadowed the potential of physician leveraging to drive integrated care development in capitated models, FFS arrangements, and government programs by providing revenue and/or productivity enhancement and increased access to care. Although it may be difficult to quantify operationally, the physician leveraging appears to have considerable value to medical managers (Chaffee & O'Donohue, 2007). This effect may be further enhanced by extending the array of reimbursable services integrated care providers can offer, and the health and behavioral assessment codes provide a basis for that. The physician leveraging effect has the advantage of being more quickly evident, and it can be evaluated over a shorter timeframe than medical cost offset. This advantage may allow the longer timeframe to achieve and evaluate medical cost offset effects to be seen as less of a deterrent to implementing integrated care. Broader recognition of how these elements may contribute to the financial viability of integrated care approaches in a variety of health care settings may make integrated care implementation more appealing, tilt the balance of cost–benefit decision-making in favor of integrated care, and promote its proliferation in the health care system.

Glossary

Integrated care: health care service delivery models that integrate behavioral health providers into primary care and/or specialty care settings and operations. BH providers are frequently co-located in medical clinics, and their scheduling and practice patterns may be altered from those of specialty behavioral health providers, e.g. seeing patients in brief (15–20 minutes) sessions vs. the traditional (45–50 minutes) psychotherapy visits.

Medical cost offset: Originated by Dr. Nick Cummings, medical cost offset denotes the savings in future medical costs following a behavioral health intervention minus the cost of that behavioral health intervention.

Specialty behavioral health care: Denotes the traditional care delivery model for behavioral health services as a separate medical specialty, typically accessed by referral from primary care physicians and its associated services including 60–90 minutes initial diagnostic evaluations, the traditional "50-minute hour" individual psychotherapy session, and group psychotherapy.

Capitation: The classic and probably still most common form of reimbursement in managed care. In a capitated arrangement a health plan or provider is pre-paid a per member per month fee to cover health care services to a particular population of beneficiaries, e.g. employees of a company, regardless of the actual number of services rendered. The capitation fee may cover all health care services or only specific services as when behavioral health services are contracted separately.

Fee-for-service: Probably the most common payment arrangement for health care providers. Under fee-for-service payment, a health care provider agrees to accept a particular fee for each particular service, usually expressed as some percentage of billed charges.

Risk adjustments: Changes in compensation amounts related to the actual or expected incidence of disease or health care utilization patterns in a population or population sub-group.

Productivity adjustments: Adjustments to provider compensation related to increases or decreases in his/her output measured in services rendered or patients seen.

Preferred provider organization (PPO): A group of primary care and specialty care providers contracted to deliver services to specific patient groups. PPO providers are typically community providers in independent practice who otherwise may or may not have any business or corporate connection to one another. Typically, primary care physicians in PPOs do not function as "gatekeepers" for specialty care referrals, and beneficiaries are free to consult physicians of their choice; however, the beneficiary's cost share will usually be less when utilizing network PPO physicians. PPO may also refer to the health plan arrangement under which such physicians deliver their services.

Physician leveraging: Any change in a physician's practice activities that allows the physician to be more productive or more patients.

Case management: A managed care intervention in which a case manager, typically a nurse or social worker, assists patients in organizing and securing the various health care services required to most effectively treat their medical and behavioral health conditions.

Relative Value Units (RVU): A representation of the resources needed to provide a medical service. In 1992, Medicare implemented the Resource-Based Relative Value Scale in an effort to establish a standard system for payment purposes by comparing the resources required for delivering various medical services. RVUs were assigned to the CPT codes for each service which standardized Medicare payments for that service nationwide. RVUs may also be utilized as a measure of provider productivity.

References

APA Practice Directorate announces new health and behavior CPT codes. (2002). Retrieved December 13, 2007, from http://www.apa.org/practice/cpt_2002.html

Chaffee, R. B., & O'Donohue, W. (2007) The TriWest Hawaii integrated care pilot project: Executive summary and final report.

Cummings, N. A. (2001) A new vision of healthcare for America. In N. A. Cummings, W. O'Donohue, S. C. Hayes, & V. Follette (Eds.), *Integrated behavioral healthcare: Positioning mental health practice with medical/surgical practice.* (pp. 19–37). New York: Academic Press.

Current procedural terminology (CPT) 2007. Chicago, IL: The American Medical Association, 2006.

James, L. C., & Folen, R. A. (2005) *The primary care consultant: The next frontier for psychologists in hospitals and clinics.* Washington, DC: The American Psychological Association.

Laygo, R., O'Donohue, W., Hall, S., Kaplan, A., Wood, R., Cummings, J., et al. (2003) Preliminary results from the Hawaii Integrated Healthcare Project II. In N. A. Cummings, W. T. O'Donohue, & K. E. Ferguson (Eds.), *Behavioral health as primary care: Beyond efficacy to effectiveness.* (pp. 111–144). Reno, NV: Context Press.

Melek, S. P. (1999) *Financial, risk and structural issues related to the integration of behavioral healthcare in primary care settings under managed care.* Denver, CO: Milliman & Robertson, Inc.

Melek, S. P. (2001) Financial risk and structural issues. In N. A. Cummings, W. O'Donohue, S. C. Hayes, & V. Follette (Eds.), *Integrated behavioral healthcare: Positioning mental health practice with medical/surgical practice.* (pp. 257–272). New York: Academic Press.

O'Donohue, W., Ferguson, K. E., & Cummings, N. A. (2002) Introduction: Reflections on the medical cost offset effect. In N.A. Cummings, W. T. O'Donohue & K.E. Ferguson (Eds.), *The impact of medical cost offset on practice and research: Making it work for you.* (pp. 11–25). Reno, NV: Context Press.

O'Donohue, W., Cummings, N. A., & Ferguson, K. E. (2003) Clinical integration: The promise and the path. In N. A. Cummings, & W. T. O'Donohue (Eds.), *Behavioral health as primary care: Beyond efficacy to effectiveness* (pp. 15–30). Reno, NV: Context Press.

Primary Behavioral Health Care Services Practice Manual, Version 2.0, March 2002. Produced for the Behavioral Health Optimization Project, US Air Force Medical Operations Agency, Population Health Support Division (AFMOA/SGZZ), Office for Prevention and Health Services Assessment (OPHSA), Brooks AFB, Texas 78235.

Runyan, C. N., Fonseca, V. P., & Hunter, C. (2003) Integrating consultative behavioral healthcare into the Air Force medical system. In N. A. Cummings, & W. T. O'Donohue (Eds.), *Behavioral health as primary care: Beyond efficacy to effectiveness* (pp. 145–163). Reno, NV: Context Press.

Essential Competencies of Medical Personnel in Integrated Care Settings

Christine N. Runyan

The inclusion of psychological services in medicine has existed within tertiary care and specialty care settings, such as inpatient consultation and oncology, for decades. The inclusion of behavioral health specialists within primary care settings is relatively recent, however. The growing need for well-trained and effective delivery of behavioral health services within primary care is due to several critical factors as discussed in prior chapters. This chapter will focus on the training and core competencies necessary for primary care medical providers, in order for an integrated service to become highly effective. A perspective on these competencies would be incomplete without first defining primary care and primary care providers.

According to the Institute of Medicine, *primary care* is "the provision of integrated, accessible health care services by clinicians who are accountable for addressing a large majority of personal health needs, developing a sustained partnership with patients, and practicing in the context of family and community." Webster's *New World Medical Dictionary* takes this a step further adding the concept of a medical home[1], defining primary care as a "medical home" for a patient, ideally providing continuity and integration of health care. The aims of primary care are to provide the patient with a broad spectrum of care, both preventive and curative, over a period of time and to coordinate all of the care the patient receives. The common thread among these well-adopted perspectives on primary care has to do with developing a provider–patient relationship over time. Distinct from specialists whose opinion may only be sought for isolated complaints or episodically over time, primary care providers seek to develop a long-standing relationship with their patients that necessarily requires attending to a wide variety of patients' needs along their developmental continuum. As such, several distinct medical disciplines serve as primary care providers, specifically: family practitioners; pediatricians; internists; obstetricians/gynecologists; and nurse practioners.

C.N. Runyan (✉)
Mid-State Health Center, Plymouth, NH
e-mail: trunyan@midstatehealth.org

[1] The concept of a medical home has primarily been adopted by pediatricians and pediatric associations, but has more recently been adopted as a goal for primary care as well.

L.C. James, W.T. O'Donohue (eds.), *The Primary Care Toolkit*,
DOI 10.1007/978-0-387-78971-2_4, © Springer Science+Business Media, LLC 2009

Family practitioners are physicians who have completed a family practice residency and are board certified, or board eligible, for this specialty. The scope of their practice is broad, including children and adults of all ages, and may include obstetrics as well. Pediatricians have completed a pediatric residency and are board certified/eligible, in this specialty. The scope of their practice includes the care of newborns, infants, children, and adolescents. Internists have completed a residency in internal medicine and are board certified or eligible, in this specialty. The scope of their practice includes the care of adults of all ages for many different medical problems. Obstetricians/gynecologists (OB/GYN), having completed a residency and being board certified/eligible, often serve as a primary care provider for women, particularly of childbearing age. Finally, depending on state laws, nurse practitioners (NP) and physician assistants (PA) can also serve as primary care providers and are more commonly doing so over the past decade. These practitioners complete advanced professional training as well as a certification process; they can write prescriptions, although the scope of this varies by state, and all are required to consult with physicians in their practice.

Similar to psychology graduate programs, internships, and post-doctoral fellowship programs that are accredited by the American Psychological Association, medical schools-run residency programs in each of the various disciplines also have an accreditation process. The Council on Medical Education (CME) formulates policy on medical education by recommending educational policies to the American Medical Association (AMA). A number of recent reports have raised concerns about process and product of the US medical education, especially the inadequacies in physicians' preparation for practice in a health care system that is newly focused on patient-centered care, the quality, and safety. Although US health care system has changed dramatically in the past century—including how care is organized, delivered, and financed—changes in physician education and training have been less far-reaching and innovative. In response to these concerns, the AMA launched the Initiative to Transform Medical Education (ITME) in 2005. ITME aims to promote excellence in patient care by implementing reforms in the medical education and training system across the continuum, from premedical preparation and medical school admission through physicians' continuing professional development. The transformation proposed by the ITME is best summarized in its June 2007 report to the AMA. While this report enumerates several goals, the expansion of knowledge or competencies within any specific content area—such as behavioral health—is not the focus of the report. However, one of the overarching goals is to enhance communication skills among physicians in training by modifying admissions criteria to give greater weight to emotional intelligence and by providing targeted educational and supervision experiences in complex communication styles that mimic provider–patient exchanges and include cultural awareness and competence. This goal, although not specific to behavioral health, certainly lends acknowledgement to the fact that in today's health care market, physicians are faced with complex communications with patients that extend beyond a reporting of isolated physical symptoms requiring a single prescription. Rather, this recommendation from this report suggests that the role of the physician is becoming exceedingly multifarious and while knowledge of anatomy and physiology may be learned, social skills and the ability to communicate effectively may not be as easily acquired.

After graduation from medical school, most physicians will complete a residency in an area of specialization, such as family practice or internal medicine. The Accreditation Council for Graduate Medical Education (ACGME) accredits residency programs, and the process of accreditation is designed to ensure a program's compliance with the program requirements of its specialty as well as a set of clearly delineated institutional requirements. Compliance is measured through periodic reviews and site visits. The ACGME is responsible for accrediting all programs leading to primary certification by the 24-member boards of the ABMS, as completion of an accredited program is required for primary board certification. That is, the ACGME evaluates the degree to which residency programs comply with program requirements for graduate medical education in family medicine, pediatrics, obstetrics and gynecology, and internal medicine. Despite all being disciplines of primary care, each of these specialties has a comprehensive list of program requirements, varying in aspects such as program length, scope of training, core competencies, core knowledge, and processes of evaluation (http://www.acgme.org/acWebsite/RRC_320/320_prIndex.asp). For example, the program requirements for family medicine, recently approved in July 2007, specify the duration of time a resident must receive training through a formal structured experience in the care of infants and children (4 months), maternity care (2 months), gynecology (1 month), and musculoskeletal and sports medicine (2 months). However, in the domain of mental health and human behavior, the program requirements only specify requisite knowledge and exposure, rather than time parameters. Specifically, the current requirements are as follows (ACGME Program Requirements for Graduate Medical Education in Family Medicine, Effective: July 1, 2007):

Residents must demonstrate knowledge of established and evolving biomedical, clinical, epidemiological and social-behavioral sciences, as well as the application of this knowledge to patient care. In the domain of Human Behavior and Mental Health, residents should acquire knowledge and skills in this area through a program in which behavioral science and psychiatry are integrated with all disciplines throughout the residents' total educational experience. (a) Training should be accomplished primarily in an outpatient setting through a combination of longitudinal experiences and didactic sessions. Intensive short-term experiences in facilities devoted to the care of chronically ill patients should be limited. (b) There must be faculty who are specifically designated for this curricular component who have the training and experience necessary to apply modern behavioral and psychiatric principles to the care of the undifferentiated patient. Family physicians, psychiatrists, and behavioral scientists should be involved in teaching this curricular component. (c) There must be instruction and development of skills in the diagnosis and management of psychiatric disorders in children and adults, emotional aspects of non-psychiatric disorders, psychopharmacology, alcoholism and other substance abuse, the physician/patient relationship, patient interviewing skills, and counseling skills. This should include videotaping of resident/patient encounters or direct faculty observation for assessment of each resident's competency in interpersonal skills. This will require sufficient faculty who participate on an on-going basis in the program, and in the FMC, in particular.

Although this requirement may appear quite extensive and comprehensive, if a program can demonstrate that their residents achieve sufficient exposure to the concepts of mental health and human behavior through other programmatic activities, no *specific* amount of didactic or experiential training is required. Fortunately, the presence of a behavioral scientist on the faculty of a family practice residency program is required. However, the type of behavioral scientist is not specified, such that a social worker, psychologist, or other behavioral scientist can fill this role, and furthermore, the degree of involvement by this person is unspecified and, thus, varies widely among residency programs. In reading through the complete list of program requirements for an accredited family practice residency, the multitude of competing demands is evident. Without the requirement for a specific and formal rotation in mental health and human behavior by the ACGME, substantial variability among providers; competencies, expertise, and comfort with mental health conditions makes perfect sense. Nonetheless, the requirements for family practice specialty are far more descriptive and comprehensive than any of the aforementioned disciplines of primary care. That is, none of the other residency programs – pediatrics, OB/GYN, or internal medicine – specifies any requirement for a behavioral scientist faculty member or for any minimum time required in a rotation geared toward mental health or human behavior. Given the minimal required education and training, it should not come as a surprise how frequently mental health conditions are not recognized and not treated in primary care settings. And yet, ask any practicing primary care provider what single category of complaints are most time-consuming or what single category of medications are most often prescribed, and the resounding answer will be psychological issues and psychotropic medications! So, when and where do primary care providers actually develop the expertise and experience for treating mood disorders, anxiety disorders, and childhood disorders such as ADHD? . . . On the job training.

Moreover, it is absolutely necessary for primary care providers to quickly develop this skill set due to a limited and laborious referral processes for specialty mental health services, the lack of feedback, and the dearth of psychiatric services available for consultation or treatment management nationwide. In some areas these barriers and the shortage of mental health providers is even more pronounced. For example, 35 states in the US fall below the average of 8.67 child and adolescent psychiatrists per 100,000 children and adolescents. Moreover, 190 metropolitan counties do not even have one child and adolescent psychiatrist (JAACAP Study, 2006). Though the focus of this chapter is not to recount the need for integrated services, the aforementioned concerns underscore the need for primary care providers to develop core competencies right alongside behavioral health specialists to ensure optimal and seamless integration.

Based on the experience in several different types of primary care settings (military, private practice, Federally Qualified Health Centers, and non-profit clinics), there are some generic, minimum competencies necessary for primary care providers to possess or acquire for the integrated services to succeed. It should be noted that every setting is unique, and this list is not meant to be exhaustive. The

Table 1 Core competencies for primary care providers in an integrated clinic

Knowledge Competencies	• Delivers care from a biopsychosocial perspective of illness and of wellness • Understands the model of behavioral health consultation, collaborative care, and the goals of integration • Knows how, who (types of patients) and when to refer to behavioral health
Clinical Competencies	• Delivers Evidence-Based Medicine for mental health condition; Relies on protocol driven care guidelines for pharmacotherapy • Able to expand scope of practice working with a behavioral health provider • Effective referrals - clearly communicates reason for referral to behavioral health and generates appropriate expectations for patients • Responsive to BHC's suggestions and feedback / Delays initiating medications until after initial BHC visit, if a protocol is established or when diagnostic uncertainly exists • Able to increase impact of behavioral health interventions by incorporating this into follow-up appointments • Effective Verbal and Written Communication
Program-Level Competencies	• Functions effectively as a team member • Conducts shared medical appointments as needed or requested • Receptive to shared medical groups in an area of interest, or in response to needs of the practice • Uses behavioral health screening to enhance recognition of BH needs and quality of care - Seamlessly integrates behavioral health services into routine medical care

requisite competencies are divided into three main domains: knowledge, clinical, and program-level competencies, and will be addressed in turn. A summary of these core competencies is provided in Table 1.

Knowledge Competencies

A vast majority of primary care providers have been trained in, or have come to believe in, the biopsychosocial model. Typically, however, the acute care model of medicine and the pressure to produce (i.e., treat more and more patients in shorter periods of time) does not allow most providers to promote the holistic model of health they may prefer, in their daily practice. Having behavioral health care providers on-site is often a welcome addition for most PCPs, allowing them to communicate the importance of the mind–body connection to their patients via the process of a simple in-house referral. However, if a provider does not readily accept the biopsychosocial model and practices medicine from a purely biological medical model, it is likely that few, if any, referrals will come from this provider.

The likelihood of adapting his or her practice to substantially include behavioral health is low; however, over time, these providers tend to use behavioral health in specific instances and if directly requested by their patients.

Beyond the biopsychosocial perspective, primary care providers working in integrated clinics should clearly understand the scope and nature of the behavioral health services offered. While it is best to avoid a situation in which the physician is confused about whom and what types of problems to refer, the main risk is that they sell the service to a patient based on inaccurate information, leading to expectations on behalf of the patient that cannot be met. In such instances, if a medical provider does not fully understand the role and scope of an integrated behavioral health service, encourage them to provide only the necessary information to their patients (i.e. name and appointment time).

It goes without saying that all primary care providers working with integrated behavioral health providers should clearly know how to refer in any given setting. That is, an easy mechanism for the PCP to refer patients to the internal behavioral health provider should exist and all PCPs should know how to use this process. Beyond this logistical knowledge, knowing who and when to refer to the behavioral health provider are equally critical, but a bit more complex. Typically, primary care providers are very good at identifying patients with mental health needs when the severity and intensity of these needs fall at the extreme end of the continuum— that is, patients with non-responsive depression, extreme anxiety, suicidal tendencies, and those with bipolar or psychotic disorders. However, most primary care providers will require training and assistance to identify the patients who do not present so clearly with behavioral health needs. For example, providers may not readily refer patients with fibromyalgia, vague pain complaints, chronic headaches, or physical pain, many of whom may be maintained on narcotic pain medication; patients with diabetes mellitus or borderline diabetes; patients with hypertension or other chronic medical conditions; patients using tobacco, excess alcohol, or other substances; patients with sleep problems; or children presenting with possible attention deficit hyperactivity disorder (ADHD). This list represents types of conditions for which the addition of a behavioral health provider is likely to enhance quality and effectives of the primary care provider's treatment plan. Prior to effective models of integrated and collaborative care, primary care providers have been acculturated to referring patients to mental health providers without getting routine feedback regarding their care or partnering to co-manage illness and improve outcomes. Thus, the mere presence of a mental health provider in a clinic probably will not immediately change a primary care provider's expectations. Time spent with and experience gained in a different model of care; rapid, routine feedback; and a care model that is not only responsive to collaboration, but requires it, will eventually change most primary care providers' assessment regarding which patients are good candidates for behavioral health care, and what to expect once they are referred to an on-site behavioral health provider. That is, a primary care provider's level of competency for being able to make good BH referrals increases over time and with experience.

Clinical Competencies

One of the core clinical competencies for primary care providers is to deliver evidence-based care for mental health conditions and to employ evidence-supported protocols for pharmacotherapy. Generally, this competency is directly and exponentially enhanced with the addition of a behavioral health consultant. For example, a referral for cognitive-behavioral therapy as a first-line treatment for panic disorder, rather than initiating a benzodiazapine, would constitute evidence-based care for mental health. Using protocols and outcome assessments to determine when a change in anti-depressant medication dosage or class is warranted is another example. Based on current data that suggests fairly poor implementation of evidence-supported clinical guidelines in primary care, the addition of a behavioral health consultant generally enhances this basic competency of primary care providers. Another extension of this competency is related to the various degrees of comfort and experience with prescribing psychotropic medications among PCPs. Some will prescribe medications across the spectrum of psychiatric diagnoses, including mood stabilizers and anti-psychotics. Others may agree to maintain a patient on these types of medications once prescribed and stabilized by a psychiatrist, but refuse to initiate patients on these medications. For those who fall on the conservative end of this continuum, most likely this is related to the lack of collaborative mental health specialists in their practice. Having a mental health provider with education and training in pharmacology who agrees to co-manage patients and share in the responsibility of routinely assessing for compliance, side-effects, and overall effectiveness of pharmacotherapy will be a new, and typically, welcome addition to most primary care providers. However, the legal and ethical burden remains on the PCPs, and it is their prescribing license that will be in jeopardy in the event of an adverse action. Thus, it may take some PCPs time and experience working with a behavioral health provider to broaden their own prescribing practices and their comfort in doing so with the addition of an integrated behavioral health provider.

Other core clinical competencies include the PCP's ability to make clear, effective referrals; be receptive to the BHC's feedback, and be capable of enhancing the impact of the behavioral interventions, be able to make a referral in a way that does not alienate the patient or cause skepticism for the behavioral health service is critical. The goal is to make the referral in a way that communicates the importance of total health care to the patient and the opportunity for them to meet with a behavioral health provider within the same clinic to address their needs. Particularly when there is an established relationship between the patient and the primary care provider, how the provider handles the referral to behavioral health sets the stage for the patient's receptivity, openness, and compliance with behavioral interventions. In fact, with effective referrals, patients are typically quite happy about seeing the BHC. Another of the core competencies for primary care providers includes being receptive to the BHC's feedback and implementing suggestions as appropriate. Similar to any other consultation request and subsequent feedback and recommendations a PCP may receive from a specialist, recognizing the BHC's unique expertise and having confidence in these recommendations is essential in an integrated clinic. One example may be for the PCP to postpone starting a medication until after the initial BHC consultation; another example includes taking a BHC's recommendation to increase a medication dosage or switch classes of anti-depressant medications if the desired improvements in PHQ-9 scores are not being demonstrated. Finally, being able to enhance the behavioral health provider's recommendations and interventions is a clinical competency that evolves over time. That is, when the medical provider has a follow-up appointment with a shared patient, he or she is expected to inquire about and reinforce the behavioral health interventions as well. This allows the patient to clearly experience a collaborative and team approach, knowing that both providers are aware of and on board with the patient's health care plan.

Program-Level Competencies

One of the most important competencies for any primary care provider working in an integrated clinic is the willingness and capacity to be a team member. That is, most physicians are used to being a solo practitioner or the team leader. While any prescriptions are clearly the ultimate responsibility of the physician, there may be times when the behavioral health provider serves more as the team leader. Another competency includes the ability to conduct a shared medical appointment. These can be used in situations where the patient and their primary care provider may be having difficulty communicating effectively about symptoms or a care plan. Another example may be when results from medical diagnostic tests have revealed a significant negative finding and are being presented to a patient. Although numerous examples of when and why such an appointment may be used, primary care providers may not be accustomed to having another provider present during their appointment or know how to capitalize on their expertise and presence. Ultimately, experience in these care delivery models may—and hopefully does—lead to shared medical groups. Finally, the routine use of screening measures to systematically assess depression, anxiety, alcohol misuse, and readiness to quit tobacco is another essential competency in a well-integrated primary care clinic. The provider's role in screening is to be familiar with the screening tools and to identify patients to be referred to the behavioral health consultant.

How Competencies Can Be Developed

A presentation delivered to a group of practicing primary care providers based on national statistics regarding the under-recognition and lack of evidence-based care typically delivered for psychological conditions in primary care settings is typically *not* the best way to gain acceptance as a team member in an integrated setting. That said, direct provider trainings and in-services can be an invaluable part of developing these competencies. No one likes to be told that they are not doing a good job. So, when training primary care providers to develop one or more of the core competencies previously discussed, capitalizing on how these skills will ultimately make their practice more efficient, easier, or more successful (outcomes) is a preferred approach. While using either national data or even local clinic data can be helpful, and provides evidence to PCPs that their trainer is well-informed on this topic, it is still wise to create an incentive for the providers to develop new skills and change their existing practice. Other ways to enhance primary care providers' core competencies include developing clinic-wide protocols for screening or treating specific conditions using clinical pathways and algorithms. This can reduce guess-work and allow primary care providers the ability to track patients into inte-grated services, thereby delivering evidence-based care as a function of a clinical protocol.

Beyond formal didactic training, protocol-driven medicine, and tactics such as a newsletter or weekly specials discussed elsewhere in this book, there are a few non-specific ways to help primary care providers develop competencies for an integrated care setting. First, if you produce good, quality work and are knowledgeable about pharmacology, differential diagnoses, and any areas that are highly applicable to the specific population within your clinic, your physician colleagues are more likely to listen to you and learn from you. Another way to increase their receptivity is to *be available*, always. Letting PCPs know that interruptions are acceptable and reacting appropriately to such interruptions will also increase PCPs' ability to work collaboratively with behavioral health providers. It will increase the likelihood that they will seek consultation on both an emergency and a regular basis, since they can be assured that the BHC will be responsive and available. Moreover, letting PCPs know whether their patients are doing well is an invaluable service—a BHC may be seeing the patient more regularly than the PCP, and the patients may not go back to their PCP for many months if they are improving. Thus, closing the loop and providing feedback on the success stories are welcomed by most PCPs, and highly encouraged. Finally, listening to the PCP's experiences, feedback, and suggestions after they have worked in the integrated clinic for a while is one of the best sources of data for making improvement in the service and identifying areas of low competency among the PCPs. That is, their feedback—both positive and negative—is likely to highlight some areas of unmet expectations and to evaluate whether this is due to flaws in the service delivery, inaccurate expectations on their part, or areas of low competency. Remember, PCPs are one of the BHC's most important customers—ensuring their satisfaction with the service will also ensure the livelihood and future success of the BHC's service itself.

In sum, most of the core competencies necessary for a primary care provider to practice within an integrated setting will not be taught through their medical-school education or residency training. In fact, it may be necessary for them to unlearn how they previously worked with mental health practitioners, once they are in an integrated setting. Fortunately, if done correctly, the learning curve is not very steep, as the vast majority of PCPs are not only welcoming of support regarding behavioral health needs, but some are downright desperate for such in-house expertise.

Integrated Care: Whom to Hire and How to Train

William T. O'Donohue

The key to integrated care, like most behavioral health care, is personnel. Without good clinicians, properly trained and properly supported, an integrated care delivery system will completely fail or, at best, fail to reach its potential. This raises the question of how to make decisions regarding whom to hire and how to train those that have been hired. This chapter will address these questions.

It is also important to realize at the outset that integrated care is not simply placing a conventionally trained specialty mental health professional in a medical setting. The medical setting requires skill sets that the conventionally trained mental health professional does not have. Examples of these skills include:

1. Medical literacy
2. Consultation liaison skills regarding medical problems as well as behavioral health problems
3. Screening
4. Population management
5. Chronic-disease management
6. Working in a medical team
7. Working within the fast-paced, action-oriented ecology of primary care
8. Behavioral medicine skills such as treatment adherence and chronic-disease management
9. Case management skills
10. Education for medical staff about integrated care
11. Stepped-care approaches to problems (self management, bibliotherapy, e-health, etc.)
12. Brief interventions
13. Group interventions

This specialized skill set thus requires specialized hiring and specialized training.

W.T. O'Donohue (✉)
Department of Psychology, University of Nevada, Reno, NV 89519, USA
e-mail: wto@unr.edu

L.C. James, W.T. O'Donohue (eds.), *The Primary Care Toolkit*,
DOI 10.1007/978-0-387-78971-2_5, © Springer Science+Business Media, LLC 2009

Whom to Hire?

This is an interesting question for the behavioral health-field in general. No studies have been done on the validity of hiring decisions in this field. One could hire and evaluate the quality of hiring decisions much more systematically. One could specify desired outcomes—from punctuality, to astute case formulation, to following evidence-based treatment protocols, to adapting to change, to being a good team player. Then, one could take possible predictors, prestige of the academic institution where they received their degree, number of years of experience, type of degree, stated specialty, quality of letters of recommendation, interview ratings, etc., and see how these factors are valuable at predicting these outcomes. But, this is rarely done. Instead evaluators rely on what might be generously called bootstrap methods, and then live with the results (perhaps their confirmation biases and other heuristics make them relatively happy with these).

What Type of Degree/Behavioral Health Professional?

A variety of professionals are doing integrated behavioral care. There are no studies showing any differential effect based on degree. This does not mean that there are no differential effects as the absence of evidence does not mean the absence of the effect. It just means that no data-based statements can be made. Here are my personal views based on informal observations (which again, could be wrong):

1. An excellent combination of degrees is seen in nurses with additional training in behavioral health. In one project I was fortunate to hire two nurse practitioners with Psy. Ds. They were excellent and took to the integrated primary care setting like ducks to water. They are medically literate; familiar with working on a medical, interdisciplinary team, familiar with the pace of primary care, familiar with a consultation liaison model; and usually comfortable with evidence-based protocols. However, they are rare. But if you can find one, and they are worth looking for, they can be excellent.
2. Doctorates vs. subdoctorates. I hypothesize that there are a few major advantages of hiring at the doctorate level. First, they can be called "doctor" during any hand off and this can be very significant to patients. Patients can feel less uncomfortable with sub-doctoral clinicians as "Dr" is the degree they expect to make key decisions and implement key treatments in their health care. Second, in fee-for-service models it can be necessary for someone to be at the doctorate level to receive reimbursement (although this varies across states and health plans). Finally, it is often the case that hiring at the doctoral level is not all that more expensive than hiring at the masters level.
3. Psychologists vs. other health professionals. I suggest that among all the diverse behavioral health care professionals it is only psychiatrists that do not make a

good fit. This will rarely be a practical issue, as they will not usually be interested in integrated care employment (especially given their current scarcity), but sometimes this issue does arise. Generally, what patients need in integrated care are skills that the typical psychiatrist does not have or is not interested in providing. The key skill that the psychiatrist has—prescribing psychoactive medication—can generally be achieved by the primary care physician and the non-medical integrated care professional, as training in psychopharmacology is key (see below). There are some exceptions to this—medical cocktails for bipolar—but this can be handled through a referral. The key skills needed in integrated care such as delivering chronic-pain management, treatment compliance interventions, lifestyle change interventions, group treatments for high prevalence problems like depression and chronic-disease management groups are not the key skills that a typical psychiatrist possesses, or is interested in acquiring. In addition, as they are in short supply, psychiatrists are expensive and thus make it harder to show medical savings. I have generally hired clinical psychologists for integrated care projects I have managed, and by and large I have been happy with this decision. I have found no differences in the performances of Psy.Ds vs. Ph.Ds. However, I am open to hiring other professionals such as social workers, particularly medical social workers.

4. Values and prior training reflected in the degree. I think it is critical to hire only individuals trained in and ready to practice in evidence-based psychotherapy and evidence-based assessment (Fisher & O'Donohue, 2006). There is no forum in which it is acceptable to practice what Nicholas Cummings calls one's "psychoreligion." In this context, where people's lives depend on good treatment, only those treatments that have been tested and have relatively known outcomes are to be practiced. Because the vast majority of evidence-based treatments are cognitive behavioral, I do assess the candidate's training and experience in practicing CBT techniques (O'Donohue, Fisher & Hayes, 2001). Fortunately, many (although not all) doctoral programs and practice settings also have this value and therefore this requirement; although it will winnow the number of candidates considerably, it will not make hiring too difficult. This data-based orientation is also critical because all integrated care should be practiced in a context of systematic quality improvement (see Chapter 9, this volume), and evidence-based practice increases the likelihood that the clinician will be open to quality improvement data.

5. There are a few programs in the nation that provide direct systematic training in integrated care. Among these are programs conducted by the University of Nevada, Reno, Forest Institute of Professional Psychology, Wright State, Argosy, Hawaii, and Eastern Michigan University. Graduates from programs like these are highly desirable. In addition, some pre-doctoral internships or post-doctoral training sites, particularly those in the VA system and in the military, provide integrated care experience. These again often produce excellent candidates. Finally, a close cousin to integrated care is behavioral medicine and health psychology. Individuals with these degrees can also be excellent candidates.

What Type of Prior Experience?

Of course it is ideal if someone could be hired who had provided high-quality integrated care services in the past, although finding someone like this is fairly rare. Some large health plans, such as the Kaiser Health plan of California, also provide integrated care.. Individuals with experience with the following settings are also desirable:

1. Individuals with quality prior experience in behavioral medicine and health psychology
2. Individuals who have worked in medical settings, particularly primary care.
3. Individuals who have worked with special populations that integrated care settings will serve (e.g. children in pediatrics or elderly in family medicine)
4. Individuals who have experience working in evidence-based delivery systems.
5. Individuals who have prior experience with business and, particularly, business aspects of health care.

What Are the Other Attitudes/Behaviors That Are Positive?

1. Ready to learn new things and can accept change. Integrated care is innovative and often requires changes, and is not a static system.
2. Have high energy and like fast-paced practice.
3. Can work with both medical and behavioral health cases.
4. Can manage cases well (e.g. make good referrals, follow up).
5. Can write and speak clearly and succinctly.
6. Are good at regulating emotions and distress.
7. Have some understanding of the cultures that clinic serves (e.g. the poor, the rural)
8. Have lived in the community for a while and know about resources relevant to problems encountered in the clinic.
9. Like the challenge of constant improvement and thus can take constructive suggestions for improvement.
10. Are smart—the Bill Gates principle—there is a lot of knowledge needed to practice well in integrated care.
11. Are free from pathology, especially Axis II. Informally screen for this.
12. Are not wedded to specialty care assessment and treatment models.

What Are the Other Attitudes That Are Negative Signs?

1. A belief that assessment must be a very involved process, e.g. all clients need an MMPI-2.
2. A disinterest in group psychotherapy
3. Problems with authority/concerns about status in a medical setting as in "I'm a doctor too so the M.D. should not be head of the team."

4. Concerns with the "medical model"
5. Problems in getting along with others.
6. Too much experience in large bureaucratic system where folks are used to "gaming the system" and not working hard
7. Problems seeing a lot of patients per day in short periods
8. Do not look reasonably healthy themselves. It is hard to sell healthy life styles when the provider looks like he/she does not follow one.
9. Problems with authority. The medical system is more authoritarian than the behavioral health system.
10. Not open to practicing in a stepped care model.
11. Not good at establishing a therapeutic relationship in about 10 minutes or less.
12. Strongly negative attitudes toward business, managed care, and the financial aspects of practice.

Research Agenda in Training

It would be useful to construct clinical and team scenarios that arise in integrated care and have a job candidate role-play his/her responses. One would also need a valid rating system to score these. Nicholas Cummings had such as system in his American Biodyne. He reasoned that one cannot tell how good a clinician actually is by his vita and an interview. One can put symptoms in these scenarios (e.g. depressive, borderline, etc.) and see if the clinician makes the right diagnosis. One can then ask for case-formulations and brief treatment plans to assess whether the candidate can translate assessment information into an evidence-based action plan that is properly nuanced. One can also then state that this is the first treatment session for a depressive individual and then let the job candidate take over the role-play. It would be interesting and important to develop a core set of these clinical scenarios (e.g. treatment compliance, chronic pain, life style change, etc.) and see exactly where the job candidate is. It would also be interesting to see how the candidate can handle the meta-issues that come up in therapy (behaviors that interfere with therapy, lack of motivation, ambivalence, very late or missing appointments, relapse) to see the candidate's skills in handling these kinds of important clinical problems.

Training in Integrated Care

Pre-graduate Training

We will discuss three major ways to gain training. The first method is mainly relevant for graduate students or, more precisely, applicants choosing a graduate program. As mentioned previously, there are some doctoral programs that have formal integrated care training. Nicholas Cummings and the author have developed a curriculum taught at the University of Nevada, Reno's doctoral program in Clinical Psychology. It consists of eight courses (six didactic courses and two practica) that students take in addition to their normal course work. It is designed to produce competent clinicians as well as leaders (e.g. administrators, entrepreneurs, researchers) in integrated care.

Integrated Care Curriculum at University of Nevada, Reno

1. Introduction to Health Care Delivery, Managed Care: A general survey of the health care crisis and responses to this such as managed care, epidemiology, medical economics, quality improvement, clinical outcomes, disease management, and consultation liaison services. This course is designed to give the students both the context that integrated care occurs in and a synoptic view of integrated care.
2. Economics of Health Care and Health Policy: This course is taught by a health care economist and introduces the student to the history of health care economics; the economic dimensions of the current health care crisis; an understanding of insurance, incentives, and perverse incentives in health care; advantages and disadvantages of schemes like universal health care; and other major economic tools and analysis of health care.
3. Business Basics: This course is usually taught by an MBA and is designed to allow the student to be business literate. Topics covered include the following:

   1. Marketing
   2. Business ethics
   3. Accounting
   4. Organizational behavior
   5. Quantitative analysis
   6. Finance
   7. Operations
   8. Entrepreneurship
   9. Strategic planning

4. Psychopharmacology: This course is the conventional psychopharmacology course taught in most programs.
5. Psychotherapy and Supervision in Organized Systems of Care: This course covers evidence-based assessments and interventions used in integrated care including motivational interviewing, chronic-pain management, treatment adherence, disease management, smoking cessation, diet and exercise, relapse prevention and stepped-care interventions for depression, anxiety and other commonly occurring mental disorders.
6. Medical Psychology: This course is designed to make the student medically literate. It is a brief course on common medical illnesses encountered in primary care (e.g. diabetes, COPD, asthma, coronary heart disease, Alzheimer's disease, cancers etc.), usually organized around organ systems. The course emphasizes

the pathophysiology, common medical treatments, and common psychological problems and treatments.

7. Behavioral Medicine: This is a traditional behavioral-medicine course focusing on the assessment and treatment of chronic pain, pre-surgery interventions, etc
8. Organized Systems of Care Practicum/Externship (2 semesters): One of these practica is clinical and the other is in business/administration.

Training at the Post-Graduate Level

The remainder of the chapter will assume that one has hired a conventionally trained mental-health professional. They know specialty care practice but they do not know integrated care. How do they learn these skills at the post-graduate level? There are a variety of options, each with its own set of advantages and disadvantages.

One method is to hire consultants who will come to your organization and impart training. Obviously this is not a very efficient method for a single practitioner but can be cost-efficient for multiple clinicians. Consultant costs are usually a few thousand dollars a day plus expenses. Two major consultants offering this training are CareIntegra (careintegra.com; the author is a principal in this company) and Mountainview Consulting (Patty Robinson and Kirk Strosahl, www.behavioral-health-integration.com). Training is often for a week or two initially. It is very important that this initial training be augmented with a tail that includes case consultation, and problem solving during implementation. Clinicians can drift back to conventional specialty care, and the trainer can help identify this early and solve problems. In addition, there are usually problems commonly encountered during implementation also (e.g. low initial referrals) where the trainer can provide invaluable help to resolve. Without this supportive timely problem-solving and monitoring, the integrated care system can fail or become needlessly controversial.

Described below is an example of a two-week training that occurred in a very successful integrated care project with the military. This project achieved high patient satisfaction, provider satisfaction, clinical outcomes, improvements in functioning, and evidence of increased physician efficiency (Chaffee, O'Donohue, & Laygo, 2007).

Two-Week Training Agenda and Required Readings

Day One	General introduction: Goals of the project, background, what is integrated care?, basic principles, population management, ecology of primary care, teamwork, and medical literacy
Day Two	Medical psychology: Becoming medically literate
Day Three	Practicing in a primary care team: Population management, epidemiology, chronic diseases, stepped care, consultation liaison services in primary care, depression, pain, anxiety, diabetes, lifestyle, treatment adherence, groups, managing referrals

Day Four	Practicing in a primary care team (continued)
Day Five	Psychopharmacology
Day Six	Biodyne model
Day Seven	Quality improvement and general discussion
Day Eight	Clinical role-plays (entire group): depression, PTSD, panic, marital problems, obesity, treatment compliance, ADHD, difficult patient, diabetes group
Day Nine	Clinical role-plays (continued) and practica
Day Ten	Clinical role-plays and practica (continued)

Required Readings

- *Brief Focused Psychotherapy* (Cummings & Sayama, Taylor and Francis)
- *Introduction to Integrated Care* (O'Donohue et al., Prometheus)
- *Evidence-Based Practice Guidelines* (Fisher & O'Donohue, Springer)
- *Primary Care Consultation* (James and Folen, APA Books)

This training was then augmented as needed by telephonic case consultation, biweekly group meetings, and bimonthly clinic visits looking at key parameters (schedules being filled, percentage of physicians making referrals, note review, satisfaction rating reviews). In addition, clinicians would indicate gaps in their training (e.g. protocols not covered) and were supported then by giving the protocols and materials.

A final way to gain integrated care skills are various post-doc training programs, some offering certificates. A list of these programs is available at: http://www.integratedprimarycare.com/training%20programs.htm

An example of an innovative certificate program is that has been recently developed and implemented by Alexander Blount at the Department of Family Medicine and Community Health at the University of Massachusetts Medical School. The cost currently is $1,600 per student, and they offer a few distance learning sites. The downside of these programs is that they do require multiple trips to a few distance learning sites (mainly east of the Mississippi) and the associated expenses in addition to the tuition. In addition it takes 6 months to complete the course, as each workshop is offered on one Friday per month. However, the topics they cover are relevant to integrated care. An example of two of the days of the six-day workshop:

Workshop 1: Primary Care Culture and Needs
Faculty: Ronald Adler, MD and Alexander Blount, EdD

Culture and Language of Primary Medical Care (2 hours)

- Primary care's role in health system
- Primary care vs. specialty medical care
- Content and sequence of the basic medical interview
- Recommended preventative care expected of primary care physicians
- Role-play: primary care interview with associated decision-making

Goal: Feel comfortable and oriented in a primary care setting.

Behavioral Health Needs in Primary Care (1 hour)
  - Mental health and substance-abuse rates
  - Behavioral health needs
  - Chronic illness mental and behavioral health needs
  - "Ambiguous" illnesses
  - Cultural impact on illness presentations
  - A typical morning in practice
  - Example of common "complex" cases

Goal: Conceptualizes how a behavioral health professional can help in a wide variety of primary care cases.

Consulting with MDs (3 hours)
  - Common physician perceptions of role of a BHP
  - Ways of impacting those perceptions
  - How physicians want to be approached
  - Determining what input from BHP is useful to the PCP
  - Terms for types of collaborative care
  - Co-located patterns of care
  - Integrated patterns of care
  - Practice dual interview
  - Practice talking in front of the patient for a hand off

Goals: Effectively uses the curb-side consultation model to communicate with a physician. Can speak sensitively and with clarity about a patient's situation with a physician in front of the patient.

Workshop 2: Evidence-based Therapies and Substance Abuse in Primary Care
Faculty: Jeffery Baxter, MD, Alexander Blount, EdD and Ben Miller, PsyD

Substance Abuse in Primary Care (3 hours)
  - Chronic illness vs. failure of will
  - Role of SA in common illnesses and health behaviors
  - The CAGE and other quick screens
  - Physician training in identifying and treating substance abuse
  - Chronic pain and the dilemmas of pain medication.
  - What a Behavioral Health Provider can add to the care in each case.
  - Evidence based approaches to substance abuse in primary care.

Goals: Can identify substance abuse problems of patients presenting medical complaints. Can work collaboratively to help patients with SA problems.

Evidence-based Therapies (3 hours)
  - Role of "evidence" in making treatments credible
  - Types of evidence available for approaches we use
  - CBT and the therapies of patient activation
  - Family and other multi-person approaches in primary care
  - The role of solution-focused interviewing in patient and provider change

- Role-plays to practice
- Working in brief visits and brief treatments

Goals: Able to briefly assess, engage, and intervene with adults with behavioral health needs in primary care, using methods supported by evidence. Able to briefly assess, engage, and intervene with children with behavior problems using methods supported by evidence.

Key Readings in Integrated Care

Although one cannot simply learn to be a good clinician simply by reading, reading is essential to becoming a good clinician. Very useful books in integrated care that should be part of any clinician's library include the following:

Cummings, N., Cummings, J. & Johnston, J. (1997). (Eds.) *Behavioral health in primary care: A guide for clinical integration.* New York: Psychosocial Press.
Cummings, N. A., O'Donohue, W., Hayes, S., & Follette, V. (Eds.) (2001).*Integrated health care: Positioning mental Health Practice with Medical/Surgical Practice.* San Diego, CA: Academic Press.
Cummings, N. A., O'Donohue, W., & Ferguson, K.(Eds)(2002). *The impact of medical cost offset on practice and research: Making it work for you.* Reno, NV: Context Press.
Cummings, N. O'Donohue, W., & Ferguson, K (Eds.). (2003). *Behavioral health as primary care: Beyond efficacy to effectiveness.* Reno, NV: Context Press.
Cummings, N., Duckworth, M., O'Donohue, W., & Ferguson, K. (Eds.). (2004). *Substance abuse in primary care.* Reno, NV: Context Press.
Cummings, N., O'Donohue, W. & Naylor, E. (2005). *Psychological approaches to chronic disease management.* Reno: Context Press.
Fisher, J.E. & O'Donohue, W. (Eds.). (2006). *Practitioners' guide to evidence-based psychotherapy.* New York: Kluwer Academic/Plenum Publishers.
Haas, L.J. *Primary care psychology.* Oxford: Oxford University Press.
James, L., & Folen, R. (2005).*The primary care consultant.* Washington, D.C.: APA Books.
O'Donohue, W., Fisher, J. E., & Hayes, S.C. (Eds.) (2003). *Cognitive Behavior Therapy: A step-by-step guide for clinicians.* NY: John Wiley.
O'Donohue, W., Byrd, M., & Cummings, N. A., & Henderson, D. (Eds.). (2004) *Treatments that work in primary care setting.* New York: Bruner-Mazel.
O'Donohue, W., Cummings, N., Cucciarre, M., Cummings, J., & Runyan, C.N. (2006). *Integrated behavioral healthcare: A guide for effective action.* New York: Prometheus.
O'Donohue, W. & Levensky, E. (Eds.). (2006). *Treatment adherence: A practitioner's guide.* Thousand Oaks, Sage Publications, Inc.
O'Donohue, W. Moore, B, & Scott, B (Eds.). (2007). *Handbook of pediatric and adolescent obesity treatment.* Routledge.
Robinson, P. & Reiter, J. (2006). *Behavioral consultation and primary care: A guide to integrating services.* New York: Springer.

Summary and Conclusions

Probably the most frequent mistake and the mistake most responsible for failures of integrated care delivery systems is to fail to realize that there is a training agenda. This chapter began with outlining the reasons for this training agenda: in a nutshell, integrated care is not simply placing a specialty care clinician in a medical setting. It then provided considerations for the hiring decision. Hiring mistakes can often undermine any subsequent training program and thus are critical. The chapter points out, however, that hiring has not been the subject of empirical research, and thus these decisions are often made using heuristics of unclear value. The chapter author continued in this fine tradition by providing his heuristics. There is a much-needed research agenda in hiring which the author outlines. Finally, the chapter discussed pre-doctoral and post-doctoral training opportunities, providing resources on graduate programs, consultants, certificate programs, and key readings.

References

Fisher, J.E., & O'Donohue, W. (2006). *Practitioner's guide to evidence-based psychotherapy*. New York: Springer.

O'Donohue, W., Fisher, J., & Hayes, S. (2003). *Cognitive behavior therapy*. New York: Wiley.

Effective Consultative Liaison in Primary Care

Robert E. Jackson

Introduction

All medical intervention, whether it is initiated by a health care provider or continued by the patient, has it roots in human behavior. The understanding of human behavior, how to motivate behavioral change and how it impacts medical care, is an especially valuable skill set that psychology brings to the primary care arena. And, as with any discipline, communication of that body of knowledge requires not only mastery of that area but also a keen understanding of the audience with which one is communicating. As psychologists move into the area of primary care, it becomes readily apparent that much of the consultative style that works well within traditional behavioral health care does not fit with how primary care providers (PCPs) work. This chapter will examine the key differences for psychologists working within primary care, competing approaches to patient care, and the unique consultative skills needed to adequately adapt to these differences. Finally, general guidelines will be offered regarding scheduling effective case conferences for difficult patients.

Differences Between Primary Care Consultation and Specialty Care Consultation

1. Pace: One only needs to work for a day or two within a primary care setting to realize that the work-pace is much faster than what is experienced in most behavioral health clinics. Whereas a typical community mental health clinic sees one patient per hour, most PCPs see roughly three to four patients per hour. This means that most PCPs will see as many patients in one day as a typical behavioral healthcare worker treats in an entire week. Furthermore, these patients are *unique* patients, not the same ones that return week after week. This has significant implications for the PCP as well as the behavioral health provider (BHP).

R.E. Jackson (✉)
Director, Primary Care Behavioral Health Clinics, Tripler Army Medical Center, HI, USA
e-mail: doc.jackson@yahoo.com

L.C. James, W.T. O'Donohue (eds.), *The Primary Care Toolkit*,
DOI 10.1007/978-0-387-78971-2_6, © Springer Science+Business Media, LLC 2009

Because the PCPs are seeing so many patients, it becomes harder and harder for them to know their patients in a more personal way, even when personal issues may be central to their patients' care. Many providers who feel the pressure to keep up with their schedules tend to avoid behavioral health factors because they fear they may open the Pandora's Box. For instance, if a patient begins to cry in the exam room, the PCP may not have sufficient time respond to, and thus the PCP may instinctively avoid asking the patients sensitive questions because he/she may not be prepared to handle the patient's emotional answers. Furthermore, the stress of maintaining such a rigorous schedule may also limit the PCPs' ability to stay empathically attuned. As stress increases, tolerance for ambiguity tends to decrease. Because behavioral health factors tend to involve a high degree of ambiguity, PCPs may become more easily frustrated with these factors when their stress is high.

The BHP will also experience implications due to the increased work pace. Once a PCP comes to trust and respect a psychologist or social worker who is co-located in their clinic, the number of referrals will quickly outpace what he or she could handle in traditional care. If just one PCP were to refer only 10% of his/her patients (typical estimates are that 50% of patients have behavioral health needs), that would equate to approximately 10–12 new referrals per week. If one follows a traditional model, they would be full in just two weeks of time. Furthermore, most PCP clinics have more than one provider, so it is easy to see how quickly the demand for behavioral health services increases. This requires that BHPs in primary care also adapt to the demand by shifting how they work. Seeing patients for less time (i.e. 15 and 30 minute appointment slots), group meetings, and telephone consultations are just a few of the ways behavioral care can be adapted to respond to this demand.

2. Physician Controls the Treatment: Another fundamental difference is that when a behavioral health provider works within a primary care clinic, PCPs tend to retain the lead in the care of their patients. This is the fundamental difference between a consultative relationship versus a referral relationship. When a PCP *refers* a patient to a specialty clinic, responsibility for the patient's care transfers to that specialty provider. This is true regardless of whether the referral is for behavioral health or some other specialty. However, when a PCP *consults* with a co-provider within the same clinic, he/she tends to retain "ownership" (and liability) of that patient. This can greatly affect how the counselor in a primary care setting operates. Behavioral treatment within primary care tends to be more of a "three-legged race" with the PCP setting the stride.

3. Confidentiality includes the PCP. While maintaining strict confidentiality is a key principle for establishing a safe therapeutic environment for patient care, treatment within primary care means that confidentiality is typically extended to include the PCP. This is because they are more integrally involved in the management of the patient. Many providers in traditional mental health clinics have learned to guard confidentiality fervently so that many PCPs refer to mental health referrals as "sending their patient into the black hole of mental health." Most patients are quite comfortable with this change, and it is important that they are informed of where the lines are drawn in terms of confidentiality.

4. Emphasis on public health approach. When one begins to appreciate the sheer numbers of patients empanelled to an entire primary care clinic, it is easy to see how one way to manage the needs of such a large cohort is to begin to think in terms of public health. This is in sharp contrast to the individual focus of specialty care. A public health approach in primary care means that energy and resources are often spent treating populations versus individuals. This requires some adjustment for the mindset of traditional mental health care. For instance, in primary care, it might be better to treat more people with less intensive therapies versus treating less people with more intensive therapies. Emphasis is placed on efficient, best "bang-for-the-buck" interventions that can be given to larger groups of individuals. Group therapies, psychoeducational interventions, and preventative measures are all good examples because they focus on improving the health of entire populations versus just individuals. Thus, equal importance is placed on who is and who is not receiving treatment.

Issues in Behavioral Change

Although the differences mentioned above are very easy to observe, there are still some other more subtle, yet very profound, differences in the ways that medical professionals approach behavioral change when compared to those specifically trained in behavioral science. These differences are areas actually where behavioral providers can truly shine when working in a primary care setting. Kirk Strosahl (2002) has illuminated these differences very clearly in a description of the aspects that the medical community differs in terms of their understanding of human suffering, theory of change, and on whose shoulders the burden rests. The following explores some of the differences he suggests.

Competing Theories of Human Suffering. The medical model of human suffering has a lot to do with how the physician approaches a patient and the problems the patients bring to the primary care clinic. This model tends to emphasize pathology, symptoms, and syndromes. Additionally, many syndromes share the same symptoms and respond to the same treatment. Thus, the PCPs think in terms of disease concepts and their focus centers on somatic treatments. Less weight is therefore attached to personal and environmental interactions. The context for behavior and the role of language in shaping dysfunctional behavior are de-emphasized. There is also a tendency to focus on broad treatments over time.

In contrast, behavioral health providers tend to emphasize stress-diathesis models of human suffering. This approach focuses more on the delicate balance between one's stress and one's coping responses. When treating behavioral health concerns, we know that symptoms occur when coping responses are insufficient to manage current stressors over time. Therefore, there is an emphasis on building positive coping responses and/or decreasing stress. This approach shapes interventions to be more specific to situations and in limited time.

Competing Theories of Change. The medical approach to human suffering has implications for how the PCPs see their role in change. PCPs tend to work under a theory of big change or of a "cure." People are "broken" and need to be fixed. Success is defined by the elimination of symptoms and underlying causes, which tends to be much more time-consuming. Goal setting often emphasizes large changes in behavioral, cognitive, and emotional functioning. For example, a family physician may look at a patient with diabetes with an A1c of 12 (a long-term indicator of proper management of their blood glucose) and tell that he/she needs to reduce it to a 7. Or, the physician may tell an obese patient that he/she needs to lose 100 lbs. Historically, these types of interventions may have worked well for illnesses that are mainly somatic in nature, but they tend to be very ineffective if part of the "cure" involves behavioral factors.

Behavioral interventions differ in that they tend to work under a theory of *strategic* change. This is a phenomenological approach that adopts a person–environment perspective. Small changes versus big changes are emphasized. Because evidence shows that small changes are easier to make than big changes, many behavioral interventions are aimed at "baby steps" in the hope that they have a domino-like effect, leading to even bigger changes down the road. Thus, a behavioral intervention for diabetics might be to explore small changes in their diet to reduce their A1c to a 10 or a 11. The hope is that by making this small change, a sense of "self-efficacy" will develop, and this will create momentum for further change.

Competing Theories of Agency. When discussing the health benefits of exercise, a family medicine physician was once heard saying, "if I could put exercise in a pill, I would cure half of our patients' problems." My response was, "yes, but you would still have to get them to take the pill." This interaction underscores a key difference in how many PCPs differ from behavioral health providers in their understanding of where the burden of change rests. Most PCPs emphasize change that is driven by the providers themselves. Thus, the provider assumes more responsibility for solving the patient's problems, and this places the patient in a subordinate role. Again, this approach is appropriate when behavioral factors are not influential in the outcome of the problem. As behavioral factors become more of an issue, this approach requires longer and more frequent contacts which are unsustainable by most PCPs. This approach also runs the risk of engendering dependence, passivity, low motivation for change, and non-adherence.

An alternate theory of agency involves placing the patient in the driver's seat. Responsibility for behavioral change is shifted to the patients, which places them in an active, collaborative role with the provider. The PCP then emphasizes patient education, and basic goal setting, for which the behavioral provider can provide consultation. This approach provides an opportunity for change to occur in real-life settings, not in the provider's office. It also tends to lead to greater motivation, adherence, and better delineation of "boundaries." As a result, PCPs tend to feel less "in control" which can be unnerving for some, but ultimately they find themselves less frustrated (as the burden now rests on the patient versus themselves). They also tend to become more positive about their role, especially as they see their stepping back as an effective intervention. Because many PCPs are schooled in approaching patient care from the provider-focused approach, the behavioral health provider can often round out the treatment team by working with the PCP to delineate what responsibilities the patient can take on and working with the patients to empower their sense of agency.

Skill Set for Effective Consultation

Given the difference in work environment, and approach to behavioral change, the skills of an effective behavioral health provider in primary care differ from those of traditional care. The following are seven recommended skills that will help the new behavioral health providers:

1. Be quick. The historical practice within traditional mental health has been to emphasize comprehensive evaluations in good time. It is not uncommon for some mental health professionals to take up to five sessions before they are ready to render a diagnosis. Although this diagnosis may be exceedingly accurate, as far as the PCP is concerned, the train has essentially left the station. With practice and a thorough knowledge of the DSM-IV TR, most patients can be accurately diagnosed with a reasonable degree of accuracy within the first 30 minutes of meeting them. The key is learning how to drill down to the essential information quickly and knowing how to be strategic in one's interview. For instance, one can ask a patient two questions: Have you felt sad or blue for more days than not over the past two weeks, *or* have you felt a diminished interest in pursuing any pleasurable activities? If a patient answers "no" to both, one can quickly rule out depression. If they answer "yes," then one can proceed to drill deeper into the depressive symptoms. The importance of being quick does come with an increased risk of being inaccurate in one's diagnosis. But, with practice one will find that accuracy increases as he or she gets used to the increased pace. The key to remember is that diagnoses do not have to be written in stone and can be revised as new information becomes available. Far more important is getting the data conceptualized quickly so that the PCP has something he or she can use.

2. Be definitive. Most psychological evaluations are steeped in the tradition of avoiding any definitive statements. The are filled with phrases such as "may have a tendency to...," "people who respond similarly may be prone to," or "it is possible that this person may...". As a rule, PCPs want to know simply, "is this person depressed or not ? " or "do you think this person is a good candidate for pharmacotherapy ? ". An effective behavioral health provider in primary care needs to be comfortable with saying phrases such as "Yes, this person is depressed," "No, I don't think they need to be admitted," or "The risk is high that this person will abuse his/her medications." This is the type of information that most PCPs are used to getting from other specialists (e.g. "yes, the bone is broken") and that will be most useful to them. PCPs are well aware that no one has a crystal ball and that no behavioral opinion is completely accurate. But, they will come to rely on the opinion of their behavioral health providers, if they are willing to give them information that is useful.

3. Make recommendations relevant and "doable". One common mistake that any provider receiving a referral from primary care can make is to miss the referral question altogether. Patients may come with a plethora of psychiatric issues, and they may all need attending, but be sure to first address the reason the provider referred the patient for consultation. For example, if the patient is referred for help to stop smoking, do not start treating their past abuse, unless, of course, factors of the abuse are impacting their reason for referral.

In addition to being sure that the recommendations are relevant to the reason why they referred, the real value that behavioral health providers can provide is in integrating behavioral issues into the patients' overall care plan. Behavioral health providers can apply what they know from personality dynamics to help motivate patients. For instance, a physician can be encouraged to emphasize to the hedonistic risk-taking patient what he or she is missing out on by not following the treatment plan. Similarly, the nurse practitioner can offer reassurance to the avoidant, anxious patient so that he or she can gather better clinical histories.

Finally, these recommendations need to use strategies that are relevant to the 15-minute hour. There is no use in encouraging a provider to help patient with desensitization, if it is going to take an hour. Interventions must be able to fit within the milieu of a primary care clinic. Ultimately, any recommendation must fit within the comfort level of the PCP. Some behavioral interventions might either not interest a provider or be beyond what they feel skilled to do. In these cases, it is important to decide whether the behavioral providers on-site have the resources to provide these interventions, or whether it would be more advantageous to refer to longer-term mental health care.

4. Clarifying and shaping the referral question. Although some referrals are very clear and easy (e.g. is this person depressed?), some consultations can be quite fuzzy. Often, PCPs will seek out advice or consultation from their behavioral health providers when they feel frustrated, confused, or lost about how to manage the behavioral needs of their patient. Perhaps the patient keeps forgetting to take his/her medication, or the PCP cannot get a diabetic patient to change his/her diet. Helping the PCPs to verbalize their concerns and shape their consultative concerns into a workable/answerable question will beinvaluable. This skill is not much different from the one used to help a patient create a "workable solution" within therapy. The same reflective and clarifying communication style can be put to use to help the PCPs better understand what their frustration is, what they are trying to accomplish with the patient, and where they are getting stuck. The behavioral provider can also listen reflectively to the frustrations of the PCP. This can help the PCPs get past their own blind spots, as well as model a listening style that might prove helpful to them if they were to provide the same approach to their patient. Most important in this process is helping the PCP understand what is possible within the scope of behavioral health care and what is not.

5. Be willing to make reasonable "mistakes". One of the fundamental treatment algorithms utilized in primary care is to use the least invasive intervention first and then wait and see what happens. Behavioral health providers working within primary care will learn that many can greatly benefit from interventions that seem to most as relatively benign. For instance, a depressed patient who is not suicidal might be prescribed bibliotherapy and instructed to come back in three weeks to discuss its effect on his/her mood. This may not work for all depressed patients, and it would be easy to then view this intervention as a "mistake." However, if 10–20% could benefit from this approach, then we have cut our treatment population significantly and given the patient the least necessary intervention required.

6. Know your psychopharmacology. With over 80% of psychotropic medications being prescribed by primary care providers, it is essential that any behavioral health provider working in a primary care setting have a solid understanding of these psychotropic medications. They need not possess such a commanding knowledge of these meds as if they were prescribing on their own, but the more one knows, the better. There are essentially four areas of behavioral health where PCPs tend to prescribe medicines most frequently:.depression, anxiety, sleep, and attention. Other areas, such as bipolar, schizophrenia, etc., are typically referred out to specialty clinics. This leaves the knowledge-base much narrower for the behavioral health provider. Essential to effective practice is knowledge of the most common medications in these four areas, their side effects, and the typical dosage ranges. If one wishes to dig even deeper, it is advantageous to also understand common drug interactions (e.g. Prozac after taking a TCA), contra-indications, and titration strategies. But, this information is ultimately the responsibility of the PCP and not of the non prescribing behavioral health provider.

7. Pathophysiology for dummies. Another useful tip for consulting within primary care clinics is a basic understanding of human pathophysiology and laboratory tests. One only needs to purchase a textbook from a pathophysiology course at a local university (books geared for nurse practitioners may be more easily understood) and start reading. These textbooks will provide useful information to help bridge the gap between the medical sciences and what is more germane to behavioral health. Its usefulness is in being sure that you understand how certain medical problems impact behavioral health problems. For instance, it is important to understand how thyroid function might affect mood, or how certain medications might impact attention or concentration.

When to Schedule Case Conference/Treatment Team Meeting

One of the great advantages of having a behavioral health care provider integrated into the primary care clinic is that providers from various disciplines can now work together in a way that was just not possible with traditional separate clinics. This type of integration holds new promise for many disorders that have previously been so difficult to treat. Chronic diseases such as diabetes, hypertension, hyperlipidemia, recurrent depression, substance dependence, and eating disorders can now be treated with a multi-disciplinary approach that was typically available only in expensive inpatient treatment programs. The following points outline some recommendations that will help to increase the likelihood that these "team" meetings actually achieve what they are set out to accomplish.

1. Inviting key players. Case conferences can be very effective in mobilizing and coordinating the efforts of those involved in a patient's care. It is important to make sure that before a case conference is scheduled, the organizer carefully consider who are the key players to be invited. One can err in this endeavor not only by inviting those who need not be there, but also by failing to invite players who may have a powerful impact upon the patient. The "all-inclusive" error can be problematic for several reasons. First, everyone's time is valuable, and time spent in case conference is time *not* spent in some other productive area (e.g. patient care). Furthermore, if people who don't belong are invited they run the risk of making things less efficient ("too many cooks in the kitchen").

For more common, though, is that organizers of case conferences fail to invite people who might have a very instrumental role. For instance, nurses, nurse's aids, clinical pharmacists (if available), home care givers, teachers, family members (patient privacy issues permitting) may all be influential in shaping the outcome of a patient's treatment goals. These individuals often have additional knowledge that the physician or psychologist may not have access to. For instance, a patient may mention how nervous he/she gets around doctors causing him/her to clam up. Perhaps they share with their pharmacist that they are not really taking a certain medication despite their physician's impression that they are taking it. The important point is that "patient care" starts long before they interact with their PCP. When deciding how to organize a conference meeting, some good questions to ask include

1. What specialists are currently involved in this patient's care?
2. Are these specialists' skill areas relevant to the current treatment goals?
3. What ancillary staff may have impact (nurses, physical therapists, pharmacists)?
4. Are there friends, family members, or, perhaps, clergy that could be useful?
5. Will inviting these additional players be practical in terms of coordinating schedules?

2. Delineating roles. Once a team has been organized, it is also very important to map out each participant's role in providing care. A nurse educator, physician, clinical pharmacist, and behavioral health provider can all contribute to medication adherence, but unless they coordinate what each person's role will be toward that end, it is likely that each will end up getting in the way of what the other is trying to accomplish. For instance, a diabetic patient may not be doing well in remembering to take his/her medication. Different disciplines may approach this problem differently and confusion could result. Perhaps the physician tries to "scare" the patient into what will happen if he/she does not comply, while the psychologist is trying to emphasize personal agency as a tool toward motivation. Instead, a proper delineation of roles might be ensuring that the nurse educator checks in with the patient to see whether he/she understands how to take the medication; the physician looks for possible alternative medications if the patient is perhaps not tolerating the current regime; the clinical pharmacist might help with options; and the psychologist might explore behavioral issues (e.g. denial of illness) that might be impacting the patient's behavior. By establishing what each person's role will be, the right specialists can work in their area of expertise without another provider arbitrarily working against them.

3. Prioritizing treatment goals. Along with delineating roles of each provider, it is imperative that the team also prioritize the treatment goals. Imagine the problems that could arise if the PCP is trying to aggressively control a female patient's hypertension while the psychologist decides to drill down into a patient's past history of sexual abuse, or address her chronic marital problems ? Or, what if a physician decides to prescribe an anti-depressant that has historically caused sexual dysfunction in a patient who is currently having marital problems ? As treatment goals are discussed, it is important that everyone on the team address every issue he/she believes is salient and then look for a sensible order to approach the goals (i.e. control hypertension first with meds and stress reduction strategies and *then* address marital strain).

4. Developing mindset of coordinated "team" approach. When one is part of a team, each has a role that is essential. They feel a general sense each member contributes something that would be missed if he/she were not part of the team. Developing this mindset is essential for making a case conference worthwhile. Many case conferences have been stymied by flaky attendance, non-participation by certain members, or a frustration experienced by some who feel that the meeting is a waste of time. This is typically due to the "Team" mindset not being developed. Although it is not uncommon for the PCP to take the lead in these conferences, the behavioral health providers can utilize their understanding of group dynamics to help foster a group identity that supports a team approach. This may come in the form of role and goal clarification, or simply communicating appreciation of other members' contributions.

5. Other common mistakes in case conferences. As long as the coordinator of a case conference adheres to the recommendations above, there is a strong chance that case conferences can develop into a rhythm that feeds an atmosphere to cohesion, improved patient care, and resulting increase in job-satisfaction of the providers. There are some other "minor" mistakes that can also sabotage what could otherwise be a great way to practice effective patient care.

A. Intimidation of the physician. Many behavioral health providers have difficulty believing that their skills are on par with that of the physician's. This "white coat" phenomenon that affects some patient's blood pressure can also affect a team member who feels intimidated to disagree with the perspectives of the physician. This may occur even with the most humble physician out there. It is important to remember the skill set that one brings to the team and to be ready to apply those skills effectively for the sake of the patient.

B. Not asking for clarification. Areas of expertise are broad and deep, and it is easy to forget that others possibly do not understand all the jargon of each respective discipline. It is important to understand the basic physiological issues going on with the patient being discussed. If there are particulars one does not understand, he/she should speak up and ask. Likewise, one should not hesitate to educate the group on behavioral issues that pertain to the subject at hand. This sharing of knowledge is the whole purpose of these conferences.

C. Group thinking. This occurs when group cohesion is emphasized over critical analysis or proper evaluation of opposing ideas. To counter this possibility, leaders can assign each person in turn the role of "critical evaluator" or assign someone the role of "devil's advocate" to make sure ideas are critically analyzed. It is recommended that this role be shifted to different people over time.

D. Allowing case conference to become stage for office politics. Any group is subject to group dynamics and can become the stage for dysfunctional patterns. Spending time getting to know your office staff and providers can give the behavioral health provider a unique awareness of how these group dynamics may play out and how to intervene if it does. If these dynamics start affecting the group's ability to best manage a patient, then it might be good to explore ways to diffuse the difficulties. The wise behavioral health provider should also remember that he or she is not immune to becoming part of this dysfunction as well.

E. Getting sidetracked by extraneous issues. If the group does not tend to have difficulties mentioned above, an opposite problem may exist. Case conferences can get hijacked and trail off into areas that are not productive. This might satisfy the impulses of the group at the moment, but result in a feeling of not being very helpful. The impact is felt at the next case conference when no one shows up.

F. Making them too long. People have places to be and patients to see, and time is money. Save socializing for other times unless this is needed to pull members in from the periphery. Lengthy meetings are another way to reduce attendance at the next meeting.

G. Forgetting to involve patient and/or family. Some of the most effective case conferences involve the patient and/or family themselves. This approach models much of what has been discussed above. Including patients in their own case conference can encourage a collaborative environment, increase their sense of agency, and have a powerful "intervention" effect on their treatment.

Summary

The primary care environment offers an exciting arena for behavioral health to make effective improvements in how medicine is practiced. The key to being an effective member of the primary care team involves recognizing how this environment differs from what is typical in mental health clinics. More importantly, it involves learning how to adapt to these differences in ways that are palatable to those providers already established in primary care and the patients who are being treated.

References

Strosahl, K. (2002). *Integrating behavioral health and primary care: a compass and a horizon*. Presentation conducted at Tripler Army Medical Center. Department of Psychology, Honolulu, HI.

Cultural Competency in the Primary Care Setting

Melanie P. Duckworth, Tony Iezzi, Aditi Vijay, and Erika Gerber

Culturally competent health care provision necessarily requires recognition of the range of cultural factors that are present and active in the context of health care delivery (Duckworth & Iezzi, 2005). Although health care providers commonly deal with patients of different cultures, they often neglect to focus on the effects of cultural influences on health care provision. In an idealistic spirit of "we are all the same," some health care providers purposefully ignore the myriad of cultural factors that are relevant to effective patient care. The aims of the current chapter are (1) to assist health care providers in identifying cultural factors, present in both providers and patients, that have the potential to influence providers' delivery of care and patients' implementation of health care recommendations; (2) to identify strategies through which providers may evaluate the influence of cultural biases and preconceptions on their provision of health care to culturally diverse patients; and (3) to assist health care providers in acquiring skills that will ensure effective and culturally competent delivery of health care to culturally diverse patients.

Before discussing cultural influences on health status and health care delivery, a review of definitions of culture and related terms is indicated. Hays (1996) provides one of the most comprehensive definitions of culture, describing culture as "all the learned behaviors, beliefs, norms, and values that are held by a group of people passed on from older members to newer members, at least, in part to preserve the group" (p. 333). Here, the interpersonal and social aspects of culture are emphasized, rather than physical similarities. Ethnic identity refers to the historical and cultural patterns and collective identities shared by groups of people from a specific geographical region of the world (Betancourt & Lopez, 1993). In a face-valid fashion, ethnicity provides more insight into a patient's heritage and value system than race (Atkinson et al., 1993). Human diversity refers to group-specific factors salient for the patient (Roysircar, 2004). These include gender, socioeconomic status, age, religion, race, ethnicity, regional/national origin, sexual orientation, and ability status. All these factors serve to shape the identity, world-view, attitudes, values, and beliefs of patients *and* health care providers. It should be

M.P. Duckworth (✉)
Department of Psychology/MS298, University of Nevada, Reno, MS298, Reno, NV 89577, USA

L.C. James, W.T. O'Donohue (eds.), *The Primary Care Toolkit*,
DOI 10.1007/978-0-387-78971-2_7, © Springer Science+Business Media, LLC 2009

understood that culture, race, ethnicity, and diversity are terms that are used somewhat interchangeably. This sometimes makes it difficult to establish common reference points when using these terms. In addition, these terms are emotion-laden and can create awkwardness or discomfort in health care providers and patients. Overall, when compared to race, ethnicity, and similar terms (e.g. minority group), culture is conceptualized as better capturing race, ethnicity, and other group influences that contribute to the attitudes, beliefs, behaviors, and goals held by a given individual.

Much of the credit for recognizing and valuing cultural competence in health care delivery goes to Stanley Sue. In a seminal position paper, Sue (1998) indicated that the ingredients for culturally competent health care provision include being scientifically minded, having skills in "dynamic sizing;" and acquiring knowledge about a cultural group. Scientifically minded health care providers are individuals who apply the scientific method to the health care process. Instead of making premature conclusions based on biases or assumptions about cultural factors, these health care providers form hypotheses, develop ways to test these hypotheses, and try to provide services consistent with the obtained data. Of course, most health care providers are versed in the scientific method, but they sometimes forget to apply this in the clinical context, especially when cultural factors are present. Sue defines dynamic sizing as the ability to know when to generalize and be inclusive and when to individualize and be exclusive. Sue recognizes that health care providers' perceptions of patients are influenced by stereotypes, and that these stereotypes can take away from specific characteristics in culturally different patients. In other words, dynamic sizing helps the therapist to avoid applying stereotypes to members of a particular cultural group, while appreciating the importance of the cultural group. Finally, Sue emphasizes the need for therapists to acquire knowledge that is relevant to the cultural group of interest. This includes seeking information from the literature, colleagues, community representatives (e.g. translators), and patients.

The increasing recognition of cultural influences in the context of health care delivery is a reflection of the increasing diversity of the US population. According to data compiled by the United States Census Bureau (2001), Caucasian Americans comprise the largest proportion (69%) of the US population, followed by African Americans (12.71) and Hispanic Americans (12.6%). By the year 2050, the United States Census Bureau Projects that the Caucasian American population will decrease by approximately 19% and that the Hispanic American and Asian American populations will at least double in size. A slight increase of several percentage points for the African American population is expected.

As the US population becomes more diverse, it is logical that there will be corresponding increase in the heterogeneity of patients seeking treatment in primary care settings. The extant literature suggests that by 2015 over 50% of the population seeking primary care services will be individuals from ethnically diverse populations (Eiser & Ellis, 2007). Currently, the number of culturally diverse mental health professionals available to provide health care to members of culturally diverse populations is less than optimal. There are 101 American Indian and Alaskan Native mental health professionals available per 100,000 American

Indians and Alaskan Natives; 70 Asian American and Pacific Islander mental health professionals available per 100,000 Asian Americans and Pacific Islanders; and 29 Hispanic Americans mental health professionals available per 100,000 Hispanic Americans (US Department of Health and Human Services, 2001). African Americans are reported to account for only 2% of psychiatrists, 2% of psychologists, and 4% of social workers. When combined, the changing US sociodemographic trends and the paucity of health care providers who are of culturally diverse backgrounds increase the likelihood that the culturally diverse patients will encounter Caucasian providers in attempting to obtain health care and underscore the need for providers who are culturally competent in their delivery of health care.

The importance of culturally competent practice in the primary care setting is made most evident through consideration of the disparities in health status and health care provision that exists across diverse groups of human beings (Duckworth, 2005). Physical health and disease vary significantly by racial and ethnic groups. Based on the selective review of behavioral medicine research addressing sociodemographically diverse populations performed by Whitfield et al. (2002), data pertaining to morbidity and mortality rates and health-risk behaviors among persons of diverse racial and ethnic backgrounds are presented. The age- and gender-adjusted death rate from all causes of mortality is 60% higher among African Americans as a group when compared with Caucasians as a group. Mortality data reveal excess overall mortality among American Indians/Alaskan Natives, as well as excesses for specific causes of death, including accidents, diabetes, liver disease, pneumonia/influenza, suicide, homicide, and tuberculosis. Asian and Pacific Islanders have one of the best health profiles in the United States. Heart disease and cancer are leading causes of death among adult Asians and Pacific Islanders. There may be lost health benefits for Asian Americans who opt to change to mainstream American diets rather than adhere to more traditional Asian diets. Hispanic Americans have lower mortality rates than Caucasians. However, acculturation appears to have a significant influence on mortality rates among certain cohorts of Hispanic Americans. Among persons aged 25 to 44, all Hispanic origin groups have mortality rates *higher* than that of Caucasians.

It is commonly recognized and lamented that culturally diverse individuals are likely to suffer greater physical and mental disability consequent to receiving less health care and poorer quality health care (US Department of Health and Human Services, 2000; New Freedom Commission on Mental Health, 2003). Persons of culturally diverse backgrounds are disproportionately represented among individuals for whom access to health care is limited. They are less likely to have access to mental health services, less likely to receive needed mental health care, and more likely to receive health care that is of poorer quality (US Department of Health and Human Services, 2001). In the context of pain, Tait and Chibnall (2005) have made a significant contribution by examining racial and ethnic disparities. They note that pain is the most common medical symptom that requires patients to seek medical care. The authors note that pain often presents with psychosocial sequelae and requires psychological care. In one study, 580 African Americans were compared with 892 non-Hispanic Caucasians who had filed an occupational claim with Workers' Compensation in Missouri and had settled the claim over an 18-month period (Taitet al., 2004). Data related to diagnoses, legal representation, demographics, and socioeconomic status were collected via phone interview. The investigators were also able to obtain information from the Missouri Workers' Compensation Board related to medical and temporary disability expenditures, claim duration, final disability ratings, and settlement awards. The results indicated that African American claimants and claimants of lower socioeconomic status incurred lower treatment costs, fewer compensated work absences, shorter claim periods, lower disability ratings, and smaller settlements. The results held even after controlling for both injury and socioeconomic status. Even the injury variables yielded disparate racial effects; African Americans were much less likely to be diagnosed with a disc injury and to undergo surgery. The authors concluded that the results may reflect sociocultural biases in disability management among health care providers. These data were further supported and extended in a follow-up study in which African American pain patients and lower socioeconomic claimants reported poorer mental health and more pain, catastrophizing, disability, and financial strain than Caucasians pain patients (Chibnall et al., 2005).

Based on their own studies and other literature, Tait and Chibnall (2005) outline a number of conclusions related to racial and ethnic disparities in health care delivery. First, the standard care for racially and ethnically diverse groups is inferior to Caucasians. Second, racially and ethnically diverse groups were twice as likely to view racism as a major issue in health care. Third, racially and ethnically diverse groups were more likely to believe that they would receive a lower quality of care than Caucasians. Fourth, pain symptoms in general tend to be easily dismissed by physicians, but racially and ethnically diverse groups are at even greater risk for having their pain symptoms minimized.

Screening and Assessment of Cultural Competence in the Primary Care Setting

Despite findings that attest to disparities in health care access and health care provided to persons from ethnically diverse backgrounds, Caucasian health care providers persist in believing that such biases and discriminatory practices are infrequent across health care settings in general and are absent from their practice of health care. Daniel et al. (2004) note that health care providers residing in the United States are likely to be exposed to different stereotypes that could lead to biases and unwarranted assumptions about culturally diverse patients. These authors astutely point out that therapists are likely to subscribe to cultural stereotypes, consciously or unconsciously. It is particularly at the unconscious level that health care providers are most vulnerable to their biases and assumptions regarding patients who are culturally different from them.

Attempts have been made to formalize health care providers' exposure to, knowledge of, and practice with cultural skills that are more likely to result in culturally competent practice. Medical school curricula now incorporate a "cultural competence" component, typically in the form of a required course offering (Genao et al., 2003; Taylor, 2003). While most would agree that these courses are a useful component of a multimethod approach to cultural competency training, courses in cultural competence are not sufficient to ensure culturally competent practice. The health care provider's self-awareness is viewed as essential to establishing effective relationships with culturally diverse patients. To avoid the possibility of bias in health care delivery, it is essential that health care providers conduct a self-assessment with the aim of identifying any cultural biases that they may hold and recognizing the potential impact of such biases on their delivery of health care to persons from culturally diverse backgrounds. Roysircar (2004) encourages the health care provider to become aware of his/her respective cultural influences, explore his/her own cultural heritage, and appreciate this in relation to understanding the cultural influences that are relevant to patients.

Self-assessment results in a heightened awareness of (1) all the cultural factors present in both the provider and the patient that may be of relevance to health care; and (2) all the cultural assumptions and biases that are present but outside of the awareness of the health care provider and that have the potential to influence provider interactions with culturally diverse patients. Hays (1996) developed a helpful approach for becoming aware of the many cultural factors that may influence provider–patient interactions and that may serve as potential sources of bias in providing health care to culturally diverse patients. This approach is designed to aid providers in organizing and systematically recognizing the influence of complex cultural factors on the provider–patient relationship. Hays employed the acronym ADRESSING to capture nine cultural factors including age, disability, religion, ethnicity, social status, sexual orientation, indigenous heritage, national origin, and gender. The ADRESSING model does not cover all possible cultural influences, but it does focus on variables recognized by the American Psychological Association and other organizations as important to effective health care delivery (Hays, 1996). The model can be used not only to examine a therapist's bias but also for the patient's self-assessment of cultural identity. The model recognizes that no therapist can possibly have an insider's view on all cultural influences. Hays suggests that beginning with these basic indicators can help to make a health care provider more aware of cultural influences on the psychotherapy relationship.

Hays' ADRESSING model may be viewed as a quick and easy metric for identifying cultural factors that are of potential relevance to health care delivery. Sue et al. (2007) provide an equally accessible listing of cultural insensitivities that are repeatedly suffered by persons from ethnically diverse backgrounds and that are perpetrated by some of the most well-intentioned. Sue and colleagues define racial microaggressions as those "brief and commonplace daily verbal, behavioral, or environmental indignities, whether intentional or unintentional, that communicate hostile, derogatory, or negative racial slights and insults toward people of color" (p. 271). Microaggressions are said to occur in three forms: as microassaults which are defined as "explicit racial derogation characterized primarily by a verbal or nonverbal attack meant to hurt the intended victim through name-calling, avoidant behavior, or purposeful discriminatory actions;" as microinsults which are characterized by "communications that convey rudeness and insensitivity and demean a person's racial heritage or identity;" and as microinvalidations which are characterized by "communications that exclude, negate, or nullify the psychological thoughts, feelings, or experiential reality of a person of color" (p. 274).

Because these microaggressions are often engaged in without awareness, Sue et al. (2007) point to these microaggressions as the form of ethnic and racial discrimination that is most likely to occur in the context of health care delivery. The therapeutic importance of identifying microaggressions lies in the proposed influence of microaggressions on the overall health and well-being of persons from ethnically and racially diverse backgrounds and on the rates of health care utilization and treatment outcomes experienced by persons from ethnically and racially diverse backgrounds. The unintentional use of such microaggressions by health care providers is thought to create an impasse for culturally diverse patients and may partially explain the well-documented patterns of underutilization and premature termination of therapy among such patients (Burkard & Knox, 2004; Kearney et al., 2005).

Together, the self-awareness and cultural-awareness recommendations put forward by Hays (1996), Roysircar (2004), Daniel et al. (2004), and Sue et al. (2007) serve as excellent practice guides for health care providers who are committed to culturally competent health care delivery. Other self-awareness exercises have been identified, including the use of self-report measures of multicultural knowledge and sensitivity (Sodowsky et al., 1994), journaling, and the review of clinical notes and critical incidents. Daniel et al. (2004) also recommends seeking feedback from patients, peers, supervisors, supervisees, and professional and community experts as a means of increasing self-awareness, cultural knowledge, and cultural sensitivity.

It should be understood that no health care provider, no matter how skilled, knows everything that there is to know about every culture and cultural influence. However, there are a number of strategies that a skilled clinician can rely on to improve cultural competence in practice with patients of backgrounds. Given that health care providers are genuinely invested in the provision of effective health care to all patients, health care providers are motivated to acquire cultural knowledge and skills that will ensure culturally competent health care delivery. S. Sue (2006) identifies 10 steps that health care providers can take to better ensure effectiveness in treating culturally diverse patients. In addition to steps that are designed to ensure provider self-awareness and the objective assessment of patients' presenting symptoms, Sue suggests that providers work to enhance their credibility by demonstrating an understanding of and appreciation for the patient's culture; to understand the nature of their discomfort in dealing with culturally diverse patients; to understand the patient's perspective; to explore culture-specific explanations for patient resistance without blaming the patient or the patient's culture; to engage in ongoing assessment of cultural sensitivity, treatment effectiveness, and patient and provider satisfaction with treatment outcomes; and to consult cultural experts when necessary.

There are no simple rules about when and how to address cultural differences in the context of health care provision. However, 10 clinical considerations in addressing cultural differences have been recommended by La Roche and Maxie (2003). The 10 recommendations are summarized as follows:

1. Providers need to recognize that cultural differences are subjective, complex, and dynamic. The interpretation of cultural differences of patients usually is based on subjective appraisals. The complexity of these subjective appraisals of cultural differences is also magnified by the perception of other variables including gender, age, sexual orientation, and education level. The perception of these cultural differences by the patient and provider should be viewed as dynamic over the process of treatment rather than fixed over time.

2. The most obvious cultural differences between provider and patient should be addressed first whether it be a difference in race, age, gender, etc.

3. As part of providing a culturally safe therapeutic environment, cultural similarities should be addressed before addressing cultural differences.

4. It needs to be recognized that discussion of cultural differences is easier to have with an emotionally stable and grounded patient. A very emotionally distressed and unstable patient is less likely to benefit from a discussion of cultural differences. In fact, this kind of discussion can frustrate and upset a patient even more when what is being sought is a solution to an overwhelming problem or symptom complaint. Thus, the type and amount of psychological distress can dictate when to have a discussion on cultural differences.

5. Although patients of diverse cultural background have experienced their differences as deficits, cultural differences in patients should be viewed and conceptualized as strengths, which can help move the therapeutic process.

6. Providers need to incorporate the patient's cultural history and racial identity development when assessing and conceptualizing presenting problems and outlining treatment goals.

7. It should be recognized that meaning and saliency of cultural differences are also influenced by ongoing issues that are part of the therapeutic process. The provider must remain alert for concerns related to potential cultural differences when dealing with other issues that superficially might not appear to be related

8. Providers also need to recognize that the therapeutic relationship is embedded in a broader cultural context (events that occur outside therapy like a potential first African-American president) that can influence the therapeutic process.

9. Without a doubt, cultural competence in the provider will have an impact on how cultural differences will be addressed in therapy. The more culturally competent a provider is the more likely the discussion of cultural differences will be successful.

10. Successful dialogues about cultural differences between providers and patients will also have an effect on patients' cultural context, most likely a positive effect. In other words, discussions of cultural differences in therapy can empower patients in addressing issues related to cultural differences in the outside-world context.

In addition to the clinical considerations put forward by La Roche and Maxie (2003), Cardemil and Battle (2003) have proposed a number of general recommendations for discussing race and ethnicity in the context of health care delivery. Cardemil and Battle encourage therapists to suspend conclusions about the racial and ethnic identity of clients and clients' family members until confirmed by clients. Making assumptions about race and ethnicity without verification could lead to potential pitfalls in psychotherapy. For example, a client may prefer to be described as an African-American person rather than a Black person. When in doubt about the importance of race and ethnicity in treatment, Cardemil and Battle encourage directly asking the client ("How would you describe your racial background?"). The authors encourage therapists to recognize that clients may be quite different from other members of their race and ethnic group. As noted by others (Roysircar, 2004; Sue, 1998), this reduces the likelihood of stereotyping clients. Therapists also need to consider how differences in race and ethnicity between therapist and client might affect psychotherapy. For example, cultural differences between a therapist and client could lead to differences in perception of physical space (e.g. distance between therapist and client) and verbal (e.g. directive versus nondirective statements) and nonverbal (e.g. smiling, hand shaking, or eye contact) behavior. Mismatches in perceptions can lead to awkwardness in the psychotherapeutic relationship. Finally, Cardemil and Battle recommend that Caucasian therapists acknowledge that power, privilege, and racism might affect the therapeutic relationship. Therapists have to recognize that being part of a majority culture has provided them greater power and privilege. This magnifies the power differential already inherent in the therapeutic relationship (i.e. client seeking help from therapist). Again, therapists are encouraged to openly and nondefensively discuss these issues as they come up in therapy or at least to look for opportunitiesto manage potential barriers to effective therapy.

Cultural Competency Resources for Primary Care Providers and Behavioral Health Consultants

Practicing in Primary Care

A good starting point for ensuring culturally competent practice is becoming familiar with the existing guidelines for clinical practice and research involving culturally diverse persons. The American Psychological Association has sponsored a number of reports on culture, ethnicity, age, gender, and sexual orientation: The Guidelines for Multicultural Training, Research, Practice, and Organizational Change for Psychologists (American Psychological Association, 2003a); Guidelines for Providers of Psychological Services to Ethnic, Linguistic, and Culturally Diverse Populations (American Psychological Association, 1993); Guidelines for Psychological Practice with Older Adults (American Psychological Association, 2003b); and Guidelines for Psychotherapy with Lesbian, Gay, and Bisexual Patients

(American Psychological Association, 2000). The Council of National Psychological Association for the Advancement of Ethnic Minority Issues has published relevant documents related to ethnic minorities: Guidelines for Research in Ethnic Minority Communities (2000) and Psychological Treatment of Ethnic Minority Communities (2003). Being familiar with these guidelines will not only assist with recognizing biases and assumptions therapists might have about culturally diverse patients, but will also result in clinical practices that are in keeping with the American Psychological Association and other regulatory bodies.

Books

- Carter, R. T. (Ed.). (2004). *Handbook of Racial-Cultural Psychology and Counseling, Training and Practice.* Hoboken, NJ: Wiley.
  This is a two-volume handbook that provides an overview of cultural compe tency concerns and requirements for clinical and counseling psychologists. The first volume reviews the theoretical models and empirical research related to acculturation, social class, and language and culture. In the second volume, cultural competency is addressed in the contexts of clinical training and clinical practice, with emphasis placed on culturally competent assessment and testing, supervision, practice, and continuing education
- Chun, K.M., Organista, P.B., & Marin, G. (Eds.). (2003). *Acculturation: Advances in Theory, Measurement and Applied Research.* Washington, DC: American Psychological Association.
  This book provides a comprehensive review of the most recent developments related to acculturation. The strength of the book rests with its emphasis on theoretical models of acculturation and the use of established measures to evaluate acculturation across African Americans, Asian Americans, Hispanic Americans and Native Americans. The authors also review research related to the impact of acculturation on health status, addictions, mental health, and family relations. This volume is considered an asset to both clinicians and researchers working with ethnically diverse groups.
- Constantine, M. G., & Sue, D. W. (Eds.). (2005). *Strategies for Building Multicultural Competence in Mental Health and Educational Settings.* Hoboken, NJ: Wiley.
  This handbook summarizes the APA's Multicultural Guidelines and discusses strategies for building multicultural competence in mental health and educational settings. The authors discuss the guidelines' relevance to individual and group counseling, couples and family counseling, career counseling with people of color, independent practice settings, multicultural consultations and organizational change, academic mental health training settings, clinical and hospital settings, college counseling center settings, and elementary and secondary school settings. This handbook also discusses building multicultural competence around indigenous healing practices, clinical supervision contexts, and in culturally sensitive research.

- Helms, J. E., & Cook, D. A. (1999). *Using Race and Culture in Counseling and Psychotherapy: Theory and Process*. Boston, MA: Allyn & Bacon.

  Although this volume might appear to be dated, it is still considered as seminal in its influence on our understanding of the issues of race and culture in the therapeutic context. The focus on race and culture within a sociopolitical framework provides clinicians with an opportunity to increase their cultural competence. The book not only reviews theoretical treatment models but provides a number of practical suggestions regarding the handling of racial and cultural issues. In this respect, the book is a valuable resource to all clinical practitioners engaged in the assessment and management of racially and ethnically diverse groups.

- Ponterotto, J. G., Casas, J. M., Suzuki, L. A., & Alexander, C. N. (Eds.) (2001). *Handbook of Multicultural Counseling* (2nd ed.). Thousand Oaks, CA: Sage.

  This book is the updated edition to the highly influential handbook that was first introduced in 1995. At almost 1000 pages in length, the book is very comprehensive scientific analysis of multicultural counseling. This second edition of the handbook includes a number of new contributors who provide updated perspectives on key issues related to multicultural counseling. Like other well-conceived and well-written books that examine issues related to cultural diversity, this volume provides a review of those sociopolitical factors that influence mental health and mental health care, emphasizing the power of social justice in rectifying sociocultural insensitivities and wrongs. This volume is steeped in reviewing sociopolitical influences as well as emphasizing the power of social justice.

- Pope-Davis, D. B., Coleman, H. L. K., Liu, W. M., & Toporek, R. L. (Eds.). (2003). *Handbook of Multicultural Competencies in Counseling and Psychology*. Thousand Oaks, CA: Sage.

  This book is geared toward psychologists, social workers, school counselors, and teachers. The book provides a review of the theories, training requirements, and practice strategies that contribute to multicultural competence. The handbook reviews some of the established measures of multicultural competency, analyzes the attention paid to multicultural competency by some of the more empirically supported treatments, and imparts information relevant to multicultural competency and program accreditation, teaching, and ethical practice.

- Suzuki, L. A., Ponterotto, J. G., & Miller, P. J. (Eds.). (2007). *Handbook of Multicultural Assessment: Clinical, Psychological, and Education Applications* (3rd ed.). San Francisco, CA: Jossey-Bass.

  The book represents the most current and comprehensive text on the assessment of racially and ethnically diverse groups. New and innovative testing practices are reviewed. The book also focuses on professional ethics and ethical dilemmas often encountered in the context of multicultural assessment. The book includes many case examples demonstrating culturally sensitive procedures and comparisons of different assessment protocols. Both clinicians and researchers will consider this handbook a "must have" for their reference library.

Journals

- *Academic Medicine*
- *Cultural Diversity and Ethnic Minority Psychology*
- *Journal of Counseling and Development*
- *Journal of Cross-Cultural Psychology*
- *Journal of Multicultural Counseling and Development*
- *Professional Psychology: Research and Practice*

Journal Publications

- Bernal, G., & Sáez –Santiago, E. (2006). Culturally centered psychosocial interventions. *Journal of Community Psychology*, *34*, 121–132.
- Chan, K. K. (2005). Treating outside the box: the top ten lists for treating co-morbid addictive behaviors in Indigenous, African, Hispanic, and Asian American groups. *The Behavior Therapist, 28*, 113–115.
- Daniel, J. H., Roysircar, G., & Abeles, N. (2004). Individual and cultural-diversity competency: Focus on the therapist. *Journal of Clinical Psychology*, *60*, 755–770.
- Erickson, C. D., & Al-Timimi, N. R. (2001). Providing mental health services to Arab Americans: Recommendations and considerations. *Cultural Diversity and Ethnic Minority Psychology, 7*, 308–327.
- Fuertes, J. N., Potere, J. C., & Ramirez, K. Y., (2002). Effects of speech accents on interpersonal evaluations: implications for counseling practice and research. *Cultural Diversity and Ethnic Minority Psychology, 8*, 346–356.
- Kim, B. S. K., Atkinson, D. R., & Umemoto, D. (2001). Asian cultural values and the counseling process: Current knowledge and directions for future research. *Counseling Psychologist, 29*, 570–603.
- Kim, B. S. K., Yang, P. H., & Atkinson, D. R. (2001). Cultural value similarities and differences among Asian American ethnic groups. *Cultural Diversity and Ethnic Minority Psychology, 7*, 343–361.
- La Roche, M. J. (2002). Psychotherapeutic considerations in treating Latinos *Harvard Review of Psychiatry, 10*, 115–122.
- Leong, F. T. L., & Lau, A. S. L. (2001). Barriers to providing effective mental health services to Asian Americans. *Mental Health Services Research, 3*, 201–214.
- Nagayama-Hall, G. C., & Maramba, G. G. (2001). In search of cultural diversity: Recent literature in cross-cultural and ethnic minority psychology. *Cultural Diversity and Ethnic Minority Psychology, 7*, 12–26.
- Roysircar, G. (2004). Cultural self-awareness assessment: Practice examples from psychology training. *Professional Psychology: Research and Practice, 35*, 658–666.
- Sue. S. (2006). Cultural competency: From philosophy to research and practice. *Journal of Community Psychology, 34*, 237–245.

- Whitfield, K.E., Weidner, G., Clark, R., & Anderson, N.B. (2002). Sociodemographic diversity and behavioral medicine. *Journal of Consulting and Clinical Psychology, 70,* 463–481.

Websites

- http://www.omhrc.gov/assets/pdf/checked/toolkit.pdf
- http://Diversityrx.org
- http://www.apa.org/pi/multiculturalguidelines/homepage.html
- http://www.culturalcompetence2.com/
- http://psychosocial.com/
- http://www.nmpa.com/displaycommon.cfm?an=1&subarticlenbr=33
- http://www.apa.org/apags/edtrain/achcucom.html
- http://www11.georgetown.edu/research/gucchd/nccc/ (NCCC)

Conclusions

Regardless of the degree of cultural match between health care providers and patients, all interactions between health care providers and patients are subject to cultural influences. Consistent with this reality, health care providers need to recognize and directly address those cultural influences that are determined to be exerting an influence on health care delivery. For health care providers, the ability to engage in culturally competent health care delivery is intimately tied to the provider's knowledge of the array of cultural factors that are of clinical import; the provider's awareness of the cultural assumptions, beliefs, and biases that may be influence interactions with culturally diverse patients; and the providers willingness to communicate openly with patients about sensitive cultural issues. The health care provider who is culturally knowledgeable, self-aware, and skilled ensures maximally positive outcomes for both the provider and the patient. Increased cultural competency in the primary care setting will result in positive experiences for both providers and patients. Increased cultural competency requires increased knowledge about cultural influences; increased self-awareness about cultural biases, assumptions, and beliefs; and open communication about sensitive issues related to culture.

References

American Psychological Association (1993). Guidelines for providers of psychological services to ethnic, linguistic, and culturally diverse populations. *American Psychologist, 48* 45–48.

American Psychological Association (2000). Guidelines for psychotherapy with lesbian, gay, and bi-sexual clients. *American Psychologist, 55,* 1440–1451.

American Psychological Association (2003a). Guidelines and multicultural education, training, research, practice, and organizational change for psychologists. *American Psychologist, 58,* 377–402.

American Psychological Association (2003b). Guidelines for psychological practice with older adults. *Guidelines for Psychological Practice with Older Adults.* Washington, DC: Author.

Atkinson, D. R., Morten, G., & Sue, D. W. (1993). *Counseling American minorities: A cross-cultural perspective.* Dubuque, IA: William C. Brown.

Betancourt, H., & Lopez, S. R. (1993). The study of culture, ethnicity, and race in American psychology. *American Psychologist, 48,* 629–637.

Burkard, A. W., & Knox, S. (2004) Effect of therapist color-blindness on empathy and attributions in cross-cultural counseling. *Journal of Counseling Psychology, 51,* 387–397.

Cardemil, E. C., & Battle, C. L. (2003). Guess who's coming to therapy? Getting comfortable with conversations about race and ethnicity in psychotherapy. *Professional Psychology: Research and Practice, 34,* 278–286.

Chibnall, J. T., Tait, R. C., Andresen, E. M., & Hadler, N. M. (2005). Race and socioeconomic differences in post-settlement outcomes for African American and Caucasian Workers' Compensation claimants with low back pain. *Pain, 114,* 462–472.

Council of National Psychological Associations for the Advancement of Ethnic Minority Issues (2000). *Guidelines for Research in Ethnic Minority Communities.* Washington, DC: American Psychological Association.

Council of National Psychological Associations for the Advancement of Ethnic Minority Interests (2003). *Psychological Treatment of Ethnic Minority Populations.* Washington, DC: Association of Black Psychologists.

Daniel, J. H., Roysircar, G., & Abeles, N. (2004). Individual and cultural-diversity competency: Focus on the therapist. *Journal of Clinical Psychology, 60,* 755–770.

Duckworth, M. P. (2005). Behavioral health policy and eliminating disparities through cultural competency. In N. A. Cummings, W. T. O'Donohue, & M. A. Cucciare (Eds,), *Universal Healthcare: Readings for Mental Health Professionals.* Reno, NV: Context Press.

Duckworth, M. P., & Iezzi, T. (2005). Recognizing and dealing with cultural influences in psychotherapy. In W. T. O'Donohue (Ed.), *Clinical Strategies for Becoming a Master Psychotherapist.* Boston, MA: Elsevier.

Eiser, A. R., & Ellis, G. (2007). Cultural competence and the African American experience with healthcare: The case for specific content in cross-cultural education. *Academic Medicine, 82,* 176–183.

Genao, I., Bussey-Jones, J., Brady, D., Branch, W. T., & Corbie-Smith, G. (2003). Building the case of cultural competence. *The Academic Journal of the Medical Sciences, 326,* 136–140.

Hays, P. A. (1996). Addressing the complexities of culture and gender in counseling. *Journal of Counseling & Development, 74,* 332–338.

Kearney L. K., Draper, M., & Barón, A. (2005). Counseling utilization by ethnic minority college students. *Cultural Diversity and Ethnic Minority Psychology, 11,* 272–85

La Roche, M. J., & Maxie, A. (2003). Ten considerations in addressing cultural differences in psychotherapy. *Professional Psychology: Research and Practice, 34,* 180–186

New Freedom Commission on Mental Health (2003). *Achieving the promise: Transforming mental health care in America.* Washington, DC: Author. Retrieved from http://www.mentalhealthcommission.gov/reports/FinalReport/downloads/FinalReport.pdf

Roysircar, G. (2004). Cultural self-awareness assessment: Practice examples from psychology training. *Professional Psychology: Research and Practice, 35,* 658–666.

Sodowsky, G. R., Taffe, R. C., Gutkin, T. B., & Wise, S. L. (1994). Development of the Multicultural Counseling Inventory: A self-report measure of multicultural competencies. *Journal of Counseling Psychology, 41,* 137–148.

Sue, S. (1998). In search of cultural competence in psychotherapy and counseling. *American Psychologist, 53,* 440–448.

Sue, S. (2006). Cultural competency: From philosophy to research and practice. *Journal of Community Psychology, 34,* 237–245.

Sue, D. W., Capodilupo, C. M., Torino, G. C., Bucceri, J. M., Holder, A. M. B., Nadal, K. L. et al. (2007). Racial microaggressions in everyday life: Implications for clinical practice. *American Psychologist, 62,* 271–286.

Tait, R. C., Chibnall, J. T., Andresen, E. M., & Hadler, N. M. (2004). Management of occupational back injuries: Differences among African Americans and Caucasians. *Pain, 112*, 389–396.

Tait, R. C., & Chibnall, J. T. (2005). Racial and ethnic disparities in the evaluation and treatment of pain: psychological perspectives. *Professional Psychology: Research and Practice, 36*, 595–601.

Taylor, J. S. (2003). Confronting "culture" in medicine's culture of no culture. *Academic Medicine, 78*, 555–559.

U.S. Census Bureau. (2001). *Profiles of general demographic characteristics 2000: 2000 Census of Population and Housing: United States.* Washington, DC: Author. Retrieved from http://www.census.gov/ipc/www/usinterimproj/.

U.S. Department of Health and Human Services. (2000). *Healthy People 2010: Understanding and Improving Health* (2nd ed.) Washington, DC: U.S. Government Printing Office. Retrieved from http://www.healthypeople.gov/Publications/

U.S. Department of Health and Human Services. (2001). *Mental Health: Culture, Race, and Ethnicity—A Supplement to Mental Health: A Report of the Surgeon General.* Rockville, MD: U.S. Department of Health and Human Services, Substance Abuse and Mental Health Services Administration, Center for Mental Health Services.

Whitfield, K. E., Weidner, G., Clark, R., & Anderson, N. B. (2002). Sociodemographic diversity and behavioral medicine. *Journal of Consulting and Clinical Psychology, 70*, 463–481.

The Primary Care Consultant Toolkit: Tools for Behavioral Medicine Training for PCPs in Integrated Care

Jason Satterfield and Simone K. Madan

Medical education is in the midst of major changes. Over 50% of US medical schools are currently revising their curricula, and nearly all residency programs are evolving to meet new skill-based competency requirements (Jones, Higgs, de Angelis, & Prideaux, 2001). In large part, these changes reflect an awareness of the evolving health care needs of an increasingly diverse and aging population. Now, more than ever, physicians must understand and utilize social and behavioral factors in health and health care. Unfortunately, practicing providers may find themselves "behind the curve" in both biomedical science and in the more integrative and interdisciplinary ways of thinking about health and disease (IOM, 2004).

Training primary care providers in integrated behavioral health can be a rewarding, challenging, and frustrating experience full of important possibilities. To teach successfully requires a meaningful understanding of trends in medical education and the evolving medical culture and a passionate, evidence-based belief in the value of behavioral science in medical education. This chapter first reviews the importance of understanding the role of behavior in health and how integrated behavioral health interventions benefit both health care providers and patients. Second, a brief description of the medical culture provides the context needed to design effective educational programs matching prevailing medical attitudes and including "evidence-based teaching." Finally, both process and content examples of select core competencies and teaching strategies demonstrate how essential attitudes, knowledge, and skills can be taught to a primary care team. Each section is followed by a listing of teaching tools and resources for further skill development.

Behavior in Medicine

Training in integrated behavioral health has become essential for several important reasons. First, changes in the leading causes of death point to the significant role

Jason Satterfield, PhD (✉)
Director, Behavioral Medicine, Associate Professor of Clinical Medicine, University of California,
400 Parnassus Ave, A405, San Francisco, CA 94143-0320
e-mail: jsatter@medicine.ucsf.edu

L.C. James, W.T. O'Donohue (eds.), *The Primary Care Toolkit*,
DOI 10.1007/978-0-387-78971-2_8, © Springer Science+Business Media, LLC 2009

of behavior in the treatment and prevention of chronic diseases including heart disease, cancer, cerebrovascular disease, chronic obstructive pulmonary disease, and diabetes. McGinnis and Foege (1993) analyzed the leading distal causes of death, finding that nearly half of preventable deaths occur due to behavioral factors. The primary culprits are tobacco use, diet and activity patterns, alcohol misuse, preventable exposure to microbial agents (e.g. failure to get an immunization, not washing one's hands), exposure to toxic agents, misuse of firearms, sexual behavior, motor vehicles, and illicit use of drugs. Second, the changing racial, ethnic, and age composition of the public highlight a growing need for improved communication skills and sensitivity to culture, language, aging, and other social-contextual factors. Third, a growing understanding of the physiology of stress and other psychosocial factors (e.g. social relationships) has created an irrefutable link between "soft" social factors and "hard" medical outcomes. The time is clearly ripe for consultants with behavioral and social expertise to join with medical educators and medical providers to usher in the next wave of medicine (IOM, 2004; Satterfield, Mitteness, Tervalon, & Adler, 2004).

Western medicine currently uses two competing models to explain health and illness: the biomedical model and the biopsychosocial model. The more traditional biomedical model argues that all illness can be explained as a result of some aberrant somatic process such as a biochemical imbalance or physiological abnormality. Regardless of the symptom, presentation, or diagnosis, one looks for a biomedical explanation and most likely prescribes a biomedical treatment. The biomedical model has been tremendously successful over the past century as evidenced by the dramatic shifts in the causes of death and the substantial increase in life expectancy. However, the biomedical model is unable to account for the roles of behavior and society in health and disease and thus misses many opportunities for meaningful treatment and prevention.

The biopsychosocial (BPS) model has been growing in popularity since the term was coined in 1977 (Engel 1977, 1980). Conceptualizing illness with the BPS model requires a multidimensional analysis of three different yet dynamically interdependent areas: biology, psychology, and socio-cultural factors. Biology includes genetics, biochemistry, physiology, and other usual biomedical variables. Psychology might include personality, cognitive style, mood, or other variables germane to health. Socio-cultural factors might include social support, community structures, ethnicity, socio-economic status, access to health care, traditional health beliefs, etc. The individual's health is thus impacted by a complex interaction of variables from all three dimensions. Almost by definition, an integrated health care team more frequently utilizes the BPS model and is better positioned to consider behavior and health. In such a model, the training of the primary care provider must be expanded beyond the biological to include teaching in psychological and social factors related to health and illness.

Teaching and the Medical Culture

In order to effectively teach and deliver integrated care in a medical setting, it is essential to be familiar with the medical culture or the set of values, norms, beliefs, attitudes, behaviors, and traditions that comprise the medical mindset. "Culturally-competent" medical education requires a familiarity with traditional medical teaching methods (e.g. grand rounds, case conferences), selecting highly practical and empirically-based content with an understanding of the appropriate depth and pacing, careful attention to medical language and terminology, and a special empathy for the stressors of medical practice that might impact learning and retention.

In general, physicians prefer concrete, action-oriented, symptom-focused teaching materials with clearly operationalized outcomes. Evidence-based practice and algorithmic thinking is strongly preferred. Exhaustive literature reviews and extensive explanations of the theoretical underpinnings of behavioral or other theories are not likely to be useful. Given the severe time-constraints placed on PCPs, anything or anyone that assists them with time-efficiency and patient care is likely to be embraced. Specific recommendations, clear treatment plans, and regular brief treatment updates are likely to be most valuable although further supportive, empirical literature should be available (Grol & Grimshaw, 1999).

The general approach to teaching in medicine is "see one, do one, teach one," meaning education is often based on observation and experiential learning. In contrast, graduate school education involves a greater reliance on synthesizing original writings and research to develop and debate different abstract theories—a very different way of thinking and learning. Optimally, integrated medical education would match the pre-existing expectations of medical education and then perhaps make slight yet important modifications. For example, when educating primary care providers about depression, the providers need to see a screening instrument being used, use it themselves, then demonstrate their grasp of the material by teaching others how to use the screening instrument. Providers need to observe smoking cessation counseling or other behavior change interventions, then actively practice, and teach those techniques. Although these interventions are experience-based, it is essential that the demonstrated skills be evidence-based whenever possible. Medical providers will rarely have the time or inclination to go back to the original evidence, but building and maintaining credibility rests on being able to prove the utility of the skills in question.

In medical education, there is substantial pressure to summarize and distill essential information. This process produces some discomfort in non-MD instructors who are wary of "spoon feeding" their learners and reinforcing memorization rather than active, good thinking. However, it is important to have an appreciation for the volume of information that daily deluges the PCP. Most medical professionals, on any given day, are like people trying to drink from a fire hose. There is no possible way to keep up with so many sources of information if that information is not summarized and distilled. This information-overload is a substantial source of stress, frustration, and insecurity and should not be amplified by overzealous teachers.

Finally, it is important to understand the workload and time pressures faced by most physicians on all levels of training. Most outpatient PCPs see 4–5 patients per hour, some of whom are of high complexity. They must meet rigorous and demanding productivity standards and often spend many unreimbursed hours per day filling out various forms, navigating insurance bureaucracies, answering phone messages, or returning pages. Most are required to be available in some capacity 24 hours per day, 7 days per week (Schroeder, 1992). Even so, there is often a lingering sense of guilt about not doing enough, doubt about whether something essential was missed, and an exaggerated sense of personal responsibility (Gabbard, 1985). Unfortunately, it is in this difficult maelstrom that most medical education must be delivered.

Designing an Educational Program

After developing the necessary understanding of the medical culture and an appreciation for the stressors of being a PCP, it is important to identify the level of the learner and targeted learning needs. Levels of medical education for physicians may range from "undergraduate" medical education (i.e. years 1–4 of medical school) to graduate medical education (i.e. internship, residency, and some fellowships) to continuing medical education programs for licensed physicians. Interdisciplinary teams of health care providers are becoming increasingly common and could create opportunities for behavioral health education with nurses, pharmacists, social workers, psychologists, counselors, and others. The level and discipline of the learner will obviously dictate the depth and pacing of any materials presented and will likely provide very different infrastructures to support any educational endeavor. Although higher levels of learners may have developed more rigid practice styles, they have also accumulated an extensive breadth of clinical experience. It is these clinical experiences that can be used as "hooks" to highlight the relevance and importance of behavioral interventions.

After targeting the level and discipline of the learner, it is imperative to identify needs and objectives. An assessment of awareness, attitudes, and needs of the learner will improve the efficiency and effectiveness of the limited teaching time available. A formal or informal needs assessment is a common way to start and can involve questionnaires, focus groups, or any other informal means of surveying provider and patient needs (Green, 2001). Any training program for any level of learner may first require changes in the awareness of the role of behavioral factors in health and disease and changes in the attitudes regarding who is responsible to address these factors. Learners at earlier levels (e.g. new medical students) may be more willing to embrace this material, while later learners (e.g. experienced clinicians) may have more difficulty in adjusting their practice style without substantial incentives or clinical "hooks."

Given the usual time and resource limitations, a good needs-assessment helps pinpoint the type of educational interventions that are likely to produce the highest yield (Hodges, Inch, & Silver, 2001). A deficit-based needs-assessment focuses on what populations or conditions are not being adequately diagnosed or treated. An epidemiology-based needs-assessment identifies the most common behavioral health conditions seen in primary care and would allocate teaching resources accordingly.Institutional priorities or special funding opportunities may also dictate the focus of a behavioral health education program.

Pedagogy

Evidence-based medicine has become a mainstay of medical practice and is gaining popularity in the field of mental health. "Evidence-based teaching" is currently gaining wider acceptance due to several decades of sound educational research. In teaching environments where resources are limited and time is short, evidence-based teaching maximizes the teaching effectiveness of each session and encourages ongoing content engagement even after the session has ended (Green, 2001; Norman, 2002). In general, the passive dissemination of information alone (e.g. the standard didactic lecture) isn't likely to have a significant impact on professional practice (Grol & Grimshaw, 1999). More effective teaching strategies use multimodal teaching methods such as discussions, videos, and small groups with active practice, and may include written, verbal, and visual media.

Effective education requires creating new training opportunities and insinuating behavioral health education into currently existing teaching forums. Teaching can take the form of didactic presentations, case conferences, grand rounds, CME training, provider and patient brochures, print media, medical student courses or rotations, behavioral medicine seminars, online resources, individual or group supervision for medical and psychiatric residents, clinic shadowing/joint patient appointments, referral and diagnostic information in reference and precepting rooms, providing free access to APA journals online with email notification of relevant articles, and making treatment guidelines easily available. Multiple other "microteaching" opportunities can be created simply by being present and participating in various medical meetings.

The "curbside consult" and precepting sessions are other important vehicles for teaching with strong and direct clinical applications (Ferenchick, Simpson, Blackman, DaRosa, & Dunnington, 1997). Residents initially see their patients alone and develop a preliminary diagnosis and plan. While the patient is left waiting in the exam room, the resident will seek out a faculty supervisor or preceptor in order to discuss the case. While this supervisor is usually another physician, it can include a behavioral health practitioner who covers specific areas of clinical competence. The preceptor's goal is not only to check the accuracy and quality of the resident's medical care, but also to assist the resident in learning the most effective and efficient process of arriving at a diagnosis and treatment. Socratic questioning is the most common method of eliciting the resident's thought processes and guiding the resident in helpful directions without simply telling him/her what to do. While biomedicine often takes precedence, these "curbside consults" or precepting sessions are often a good way to help the resident learn about mental health screening, behavior change, and doctoring skills such as communication and empathy.

Tools, Web Resources, and Readings for Medical Education:

1.   Association for Behavioral Science and Medical Education: www.absame.org
2.   Harvard Macy Institute at http://www.hms.harvard.edu/hmi/cme
3.   Health Education Assets Library at http://www.healcentral.org/
4.   Medical Education Portal (AAMC): www.aamc.org/mededportal
5.   Oakley, C. Moore D, Burford D. et al. (2005). The Montana model: integrated primary care and behavioral health in a family practice residency program. *Journal of Rural Health.* 21(4) : 351–354.
6.   Westburg J. Jason H. (1993). *Collaborative Clinical Education: The Foundation of Effective Health Care.* New York : Springer Publishing.

Teaching Evaluations

The effectiveness of educational interventions should be as rigorously evaluated as any medical or psychiatric treatment. Learner outcomes can be compared with initial learning objectives to assess the effectiveness of that educational intervention. Objectives can include changes in attitudes, knowledge, or behaviors and should be shared with learners at the beginning of any educational session. Other evaluation tools to measure changes in attitudes and knowledge can include pre–post questionnaires, short answer questions which pose clinical problems or require the learner to demonstrate integrative skills, essays, case stems which pose complex medical and psychosocial dilemmas, peer evaluations, and problem-based learning cases where students must demonstrate both knowledge of medical content and familiarity with the ideal process of collaboratively finding answers to difficult questions.

Assessing skills or other behavioral changes is more challenging but ultimately more important. Classroom-based assessments can include role-plays, stimulus videos which present clinical materials and require learner responses, live patient interviews, and viewing previously taped learner–patient clinic visits. Clinic-based assessments often include standardized patients, clinical OSCE's (objective structured clinical exams), preceptor ratings, peer ratings, and patient surveys (Epstein & Hundert, 2002). Consequent changes in patient outcomes such as utilization, adherence, disease, and symptom measures are ultimately most important but difficult to measure and often not dependent on any single educational intervention.

Teaching Examples: Content and Process

Specific teaching content and format will vary based on the outcome of the needs-assessment and the resources available. In general, PCPs in an integrated behavioral health team should be able to do the following:

1. Conceptualize health and disease using a biopsychosocial model.
2. Use effective communication and other interpersonal skills to elicit and address behavioral and social aspects of a patient's presenting complaint.

3. Understand the role of behavior as a major contributor to morbidity and mortality and be able to effectively facilitate patient behavior change.
4. Screen for and treat a wide variety of psychiatric disorders and manage the complex interactions between psychiatric disorders and medical co-morbidities.
5. Utilize and coordinate with other medical team members who can assist with behavioral and other interventions.

As a demonstration of how to promote the achievement of these competencies, this section begins with examples of general physician–patient interaction (PPI) skills. These skills may include creating a collaborative provider–patient relationship and more specific PPI skills such as agenda setting, "ask-tell-ask," and "closing the loop." General PPI skills are followed by examples of teaching behavior change strategies in the areas of smoking, weight management, and medical adherence. Finally, this section ends with sample skills needed for assessment and interventions for psychiatric disorders and stress in primary care.

Building a Relationship and Creating a Collaborative Environment

The effective management of chronic disease requires the active participation of the patient, the patient's social supports, and the health care team. While few PCPs disagree with this principle, many are concerned that collaborating will take too much time. However, data indicate that a few minutes spent learning what is important to the patient and why can increase visit effectiveness and efficiency. Most patients have experienced PCPs as hurried or abrupt, so time spent eliciting a patient's perspective not only improves effectiveness but also increases patient satisfaction and enhances the doctor–patient relationship.

Providers should remember that patients are experts too. Each patient is an expert on himself/herself, his/her behavior, his/her personal environment, and his/her experiences and values related to age, culture, and ethnic background. Successful disease management can best be achieved through the synergy of provider and patient expertise. Teachers might first present evidence on why collaboration is important (e.g. data on chronic disease self-management models) followed by specific tips, such as the following, on how to elicit patient expertise and build collaborations:

1. Ask patient to assist in setting agenda items to be covered in each visit (see below).
2. Collaboratively prioritize the agenda such as which behavior change is most important to begin with.
3. Develop rapport through active listening (e.g. use verbal and non-verbal cues to demonstrate attentiveness, ask deepening questions, use restatements or paraphrasing, use a form of "closing the loop").
4. Use open-ended and/or Socratic questioning to elicit patient perspective.
5. Collaboratively set goals including a method to assess progress over time (see below).

6. Discuss "treatment extenders" or ways in which patients and their supports can continue working on health issues between PCP visits (e.g. health education classes, specialist referrals, online readings).

Additional Tools and Resources Related to Collaboration and Communication

1. Doc.com: http://webcampus.drexelmed.edu/doccom/user/
2. American Academy on Communication in Health Care: http://www.aachonline.org/
3. Institute for Health Care Communication: http://www.healthcarecomm.org/
4. Cohen-Cole, S. (1991) *The Medical Interview: The Three Function Approach.* St. Louis: Mosby-Year Book, Inc
5. Fadiman, A (1997) *The Spirit Catches You and You Fall Down: A Hmong Child, Her American Doctors and the Collision of Two Cultures.* New York: Farrar, Straus and Giroux
6. Stewart, M et. al. (1995). *Patient-Centered medicine: Transforming the Clinical Method.* Thousand Oaks: Sage Publications.

Other PPI Skills

Agenda setting: Agenda setting is a structured and collaborative way to improve the efficiency of a brief medical encounter. In the first 1-2 minutes, the PCP guides the patient in creating a short list of priorities for that visit. This list typically includes both provider and patient preferences and, if too long, may be prioritized and carried over to the next visit. Agenda setting is also a useful strategy when a patient has to consider multiple behavior changes as in the following example.

> *Provider: Welcome. It is good to see you today, Mr. Chen.*
> *Pt: Good to see you too, doctor.*
> *Prov: With your heart disease, smoking, weight, and medication refill issues, I know we might have a lot on our plate today.*
> *Pt: Yeah, and I have a new problem with my back too. It hurts all the time.*
> *Prov: Ok. Let's create a short list of what is most important to get to today. It sounds like back pain is high on your list. Is that right*
> *Pt: Yeah. That and I need my medications refilled.*
> *Prov: Ok. So I have back pain and medication refills. Anything else*
> *Pt: Well, I did call that program about smoking cessation.*
> *Prov: Good. So we have back pain, meds, and smoking cessation. It's also time to order some basic lab work for you, so I'd like to add that to our list too. We'll keep diet and exercise on our list but will probably have to save them for later. Sounds ok?*

Ask-tell-ask: Providers are often responsible for sharing key information about health, disease, or behavior. Classically, this knowledge is imparted in a didactic and somewhat paternal manner. Patients often nod politely and appear to be listening, but it is unclear if the knowledge imparted has addressed the patient's personal concerns or questions. The "ask-tell-ask" method directly elicits a patient's concerns, assesses his/her baseline level of knowledge, and provides new or corrective information as needed. Several iterations might be needed before all of a patient's concerns are addressed. The following dialogue illustrates this method.

Provider: Ms. Slovensky, I wanted to share the results of your last blood work with you. Do you remember what we were testing for? (Ask)

Patient: Yeah. I was worried about having high cholesterol. My Mom had a heart attack and I'm worried I might be on that same path.

Prov: Well, we want to see a total cholesterol of under 200, but yours came in at 240. So, yes, according to this test, you do currently have high cholesterol. (Tell)

Pt: Oh no! That sounds really bad to me. This is awful!

Prov: Tell me what you know about high cholesterol. What worries you the most?(Ask)

Closing the loop: Although the ask-tell-ask method helps identify and correct a patient's unique concerns, it does not provide an adequate assessment of patient's comprehension or retention. Since research has shown that most patients leave their doctor's appointment with very little understanding of what was covered and what they are supposed to do, teaching providers to check comprehension before the end of a visit (or "closing the loop") is a valuable skill. After an ask-tell-ask exchange or other patient education, the provider could close the loop as shown below. Corrective information can be provided if necessary.

"Ms. Stratton, I want to make sure that I've done a good enough job in describing how and when you should use your asthma inhaler. Can you tell me how and when you will use the inhaler after you leave our visit today?"

Behavior Change

Behaviors are difficult to change and most health problems include a behavioral element. PCPs are trained to be experts who "prescribe" behavioral changes and expect patient compliance. Most patients share a concern about their health but are not ready to change their behavior. When change recommendations are provided prematurely, it usually leads to power struggles with the patient getting more attached to his/her behavior and the PCP growing more frustrated. Teachers can assist PCPs by providing a basic theoretical grounding for understanding change, concrete skills to prepare a patient for change, and meta cognitive skills that both PCP and patient can learn to use effectively (e.g. goal setting, self-monitoring). Each of these teaching opportunities is described briefly below.

Understanding behavior change: Although most practice environments are not able to support extensive teaching about behavioral theories, foundations for practical applications can be provided. The Transtheoretical Model (i.e. Stages of Change; Prochaska and Diclemente, 1994) has gained wide acceptance due to its strong face validity and direct clinical relevance. The conceptual aspects of this model are valuable because they help the PCP see change as an ongoing, dynamic process that includes setbacks and relapses. Behavior change is not seen as an all-or-none phenomenon and patients are not labeled as "resistant." This conceptual shift alters the tone of the relationship and provides new data that assist the PCP in selecting the most efficient and effective interventions. The model also provides

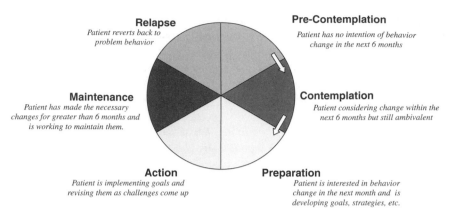

Fig. 1 Stages of change

important guidance in thinking about the processes of change or how an individual progresses in his/her level of readiness to change his/her behavior. Examples include the exploration of decisional balance (i.e. the pros and cons of the behavior and the pros and cons of changing) and the "conviction and confidence meters" (i.e. using a 1–10 scale, have the patient rate the importance of changing his/her behavior and his/her confidence in being able to do it). Teachers should remember always to follow a presentation of theoretical foundations with practical and clinically relevant applications. A sample teaching material is presented in figure 1 and table 1 below.

When teaching PCPs about the stages and processes of change, it is important to remember that PCPs may be at different stages of readiness in terms of changing their own behavior. Some PCPs may be very ready to embrace and integrate these skills, while others may be "precontemplative." One way to begin a teaching session on stages of change is to use the conviction and confidence meters on the learners as follows:

Table 1 Strategies for stages of change

Stage	Behavior Change Strategies
Pre-contemplation	Provide some education, understand and respect patient's perspective and choice, empathize, express concern
Contemplation	Discuss pros and cons of modifying/not modifying behavior, identify thought patterns that encourage problem behavior
Preparation	Goal setting for smoking reduction or smoking cessation (for example), environmental control, plan to deal with potential barriers
Action	Implement goals and deal with barriers, discuss slips and ways of dealing with them
Maintenance	Continue with goal implementation, provide positive feedback for successes
Relapse	Predict relapses, use relapses for learning, develop a plan to deal with relapses

"On a scale of 1–10, please write down how important you think it is that you learn how to use the stages and processes of change in your clinical practice. On a scale of 1–10, please write down how confident you are in your ability to use the stages and processes of change in your clinical practice."

If importance scores are low, the teacher should explore what the learners need in order to raise the level of importance—i.e. more data on behavior and disease, data on motivational interviewing, etc. If importance scores are high but confidence is low, the teacher should incorporate ways to build self-efficacy into the class—e.g. sharing success stories, providing a successful model, and providing opportunities to practice skills, etc. As with patients, the teacher needs to meet the learner where he/she is and adapt the interventions accordingly.

In teaching the above skills, it is important not to overwhelm the PCP. Mastering one or two skills at a time is a good pace for students, residents, and physicians alike. It is important to communicate that any small step is progress. The idea of planting seeds in a patient's (or PCP's) mind, one at a time with each encounter also helps the physician (or teacher) not feel overwhelmed or unduly pressured. The teacher can suggest that the physician test out these recommendations on a few patients before incorporating them on a regular basis in his/her practice. Incorporating these skills will help the physician be more effective and ultimately be more satisfied with his/her work.

Meta-Cognitive Skills

Meta-cognitive skills are conceptualized as cross-cutting abilities that assist both PCP and patient in understanding, monitoring, and facilitating behavior. These skills might include goal setting, problem solving, stimulus control, cognitive restructuring, relapse management, and self-monitoring. Teaching techniques for PCPs typically include a brief overview followed by a demonstration and active practice where PCPs attempt these skills on themselves and/or try to teach them to one another. Two examples are provided below.

Goal setting: Skillfully setting realistic goals has important implications for patient motivation, doctor–patient relationship, and eventual health outcomes. Although weight management may best highlight the importance of goal-setting skills, these skills have broad applicability for many other health-related behaviors. Goal setting can be taught to PCPs in a brief didactic form or as a paper case exercise. The following case and role-play demonstrate one such teaching exercise.

Part I: Charlie Robbins, a 35-year-old man weighing 286 lbs, complains of knee and lower back pain. Charlie considers his ideal weight to be 175. He tells you that his goal is to weigh 175 again. This means that he has to lose 111 lbs. to reach his ideal weight. He has last weighed 175 lbs when he was in high school. The sheer amount of weight loss is over-whelming and leads him to be discouraged. Charlie can easily gain 15 lbs in a year if he does not make any life style changes now. For Charlie, losing 28 lbs (10% of his body weight), or not gaining additional weight, may be more realistic and achievable outcome. However, by focusing on his goal of losing 111 lbs, he is likely to minimize any success toward meeting the target of losing 28 lbs., a more reasonable and achievable outcome. Based on the above evidence, your first task is to educate Charlie and collaborate with him on setting more realistic and achievable outcomes. The collaboration related to his goals could be achieved over the course of a few visits, but more often than not it, could take several months. You are rightfully concerned that Charlie won't receive this more realistic goal-setting information too well, so you carefully consider the best way to present this to him.

(Discussion) How would you go about setting this goal and/or presenting it to him? How would you handle his disappointment? How would you maintain a collaborative, hopeful tone?

Part II: You agree with Charlie that, you are not going to be successful in having him "lose weight" of 100 plus lbs. At the same time, you highlight that as a team, the two of you can be successful in other ways—e.g. he can initially work on stopping further weight gain and then work toward losing a more achievable 28 lbs. Charlie is likely to have several reactions such as disappointment, frustration, etc. to such suggestions and you would empathize with several of these reactions. Most likely Charlie is also going to be relieved to hear that you understand that the weight loss outcome of 100 lbs is almost impossible, and it is not a personal failure to not achieve that. In the following role-play, work with Charlie to use the following principles for defining more effective goals:

1. *Set specific goals : If Charlie defines his goals as eating better or exercising more, he is not likely to follow this through. These goals are vague—how would he know that he is being successful? Goals can be to walk for 20 minutes three times a week, play guitar (an activity incompatible with eating) three times a week in the evening to counteract the night-time cravings of food, buy healthier snacks for these cravings etc.*
2. *Set realistic goals: His attempts to eliminate all his night-time eating may be too ambitious and likely to lead to self-criticisms if he is unable to accomplish this. You also learn that Charlie has frequently set such goals related to his night-time eating which has served to decrease his self-efficacy to change this behavior.*
3. *Set proximal goals: Behavior change is more successful if goals are proximal, such as daily or weekly goals, rather than monthly or yearly. Proximal goal setting leads to more immediate feedback about successes and can keep one's commitment renewed to the goal.*
4. *Create flexible goals: The developing, revising, and meeting of goals require flex-ibility. Behavior change goals are more successful if one strives toward accom-plishing them while also being able to modify them to accommodate obstacles such as increased work or social commitments.*
5. *Ongoing and continuous review of goals: Goal setting is not a one-time process, but rather ongoing, and is informed by current progress and obstacles. Goals are individually based. Charlie's goals are based on his current situation and his willingness to increase or decrease a particular behavior.*

Self-monitoring: Self-monitoring is an important skill to establish a baseline for goal setting or to track progress toward an already established goal. There is also significant evidence that self-monitoring is an effective strategy for behavior change. By selectively directing and increasing attention, self-monitoring actually changes the behavior of interest. For example, keeping a food and exercise diary helps increase awareness of baseline behaviors, provides immediate feedback for behavior correction, yields understanding of patterns of behaviors other than desired behaviors, provides opportunity to adjust plans or goals, etc. Other examples include pain diaries, sleep logs, weight change records, mood ratings, medication adherence, etc.

Most PCPs readily understand the importance of longitudinal monitoring of clinical phenomena. However, the measurement instruments and outcomes of interest are typically set by the PCP or the medical establishment (e.g. labs or HEDIS measures). Teaching PCPs to use self-monitoring for their patients requires a shift toward more collaborative and patient-centered care. The development of personalized self-monitoring forms versus standard self-monitoring forms and ways to access these can also be discussed. Including self-monitoring of positive behaviors (e.g. the frequency of times a patient successfully curbed the desire for smoking or overeating) can serve as both a self-efficacy builder and mood enhancer. Similarly PCPs can be encouraged to keep simple logs of their adherence to new strategies they are learning to incorporate in their practices.

Since patient adherence to self-monitoring may be problematic, teaching sessions should include how to create a "differential diagnosis" of non-adherence and respond accordingly. For example, if a patient returns to a follow-up visit without her pain record, the PCP should engage in a process of inquiry to uncover the cause—e.g. the instructions may have been unclear, the rationale or need was not specified, the patient and PCP have different goals, there are new stressors in the patient's life that prevented adherence, etc.

Additional Tools and Resources Related to Behavior Change

1. Healthy People 2010: http://www.healthypeople.gov/
2. Healthier US: http://www.healthierus.gov/
3. Society of Behavioral Medicine at www.sbm.org
4. Watson D.L. Tharp R.G (1993) *Self Directed Behavior: Self Modification for Personal Adjustment*. Pacific Grove CA. Brooks/Cole
5. Prochaska J.O. Norcross J.C,. DiClemente C.C (1994). *Changing for Good*. New York: Avon Books.
6. Levinson W. et al. To change or not to change: Sounds like you have a dilemma. *Annals of Internal Medicine* 2001 135(5) 386–391

Psychiatric Disorders

Although most primary care providers will not directly deliver psychological services, many will be solely responsible for the pharmacologic treatment of their patients with psychiatric disorders. It is estimated that between 20–33% of all primary care patients have a psychiatric disorder and for half of these patients, the primary care setting is the only place they will seek help (Higgins, 1994; Leon et al., 1995). These patients also show higher health care utilization rates and greater medical morbidity and mortality hence are more expensive to treat and have poorer medical outcomes (Chiles, Lambert, & Hatch, 1999; Cummings, Cummings, & Johnson, 1997).

A large body of research has furthermore demonstrated the impact of psychiatric illness on co-morbid medical illnesses such as cardiovascular disease, diabetes, and perhaps cancer. Individuals who are depressed, anxious, or abusing substances are more likely to engage in health-compromising behaviors and less likely to adhere to needed medical treatments. Detecting and treating these psychiatric disorders thus impacts both psychiatric and medical morbidity and mortality. Educational programs for PCPs in an integrated team should therefore include the accurate detection and treatment or referral of psychiatric conditions and an understanding of how co-morbid psychiatric conditions might impact other medical diseases and health-related behaviors. Educational interventions might include the use of brief screening instruments, the use of psychopharmacology, brief behavioral interventions, or how to access local mental health resources.

PCPs should develop a heightened awareness of clues for psychiatric disorders. For example, a mental-health issue may be present if the patient has too many agenda items for each session, if the patient appears overwhelmed, or there are several psychosocial problems. Generally, an assessment for psychological problems is recommended in such cases. Providers should learn one or two brief screening questions that maximize sensitivity and specificity for each major category of psychiatric disorders. For example, two screening questions for depression would inquire about the presence of low mood or anhedonia over the past 2 weeks. If the patient is offended or denies such concerns, a physician can apologize and move on to the next agenda item. The issue can also be reframed as "stress" (which is less stigmatized) while the provider continues to look for moments when the patient is receptive. If a positive answer is elicited, the provider can move to a more in-depth assessment of the psychiatric disorder in question. If full diagnostic criteria are met, the provider can use the ask-tell-ask method to educate about the disorder. Collaborative skills can be used to develop a treatment plan and set treatment goals. Often patients are reluctant to consider mental health referrals for several reasons— stigma, cost of services, where to find services, insurance barriers, past negative experiences, distrust of mental health system etc. PCPs can be an important holding tool until mental health provers can be engaged.

Additional Tools and Resources Related to Psychiatric Disorders

1. World Health Organization Mental Health in Primary Care Guide: http://www.mentalneurologicalprimarycare.org/
2. National Library for Mental Health: http://www.library.nhs.uk/mentalhealth/
3. Clinical Practice Guidelines for Mental Health: http://medicine.ucsf.edu/resources/guidelines/guide5.html
4. American Psychosomatic Society: http://www.psychosomatic.org/ed_res/index.htm
5. Center for Anxiety and Related Disorders: http://www.bu.edu/anxiety/
6. Manning J. S., Zylstra R. G. Connor P. D. (1999) Teaching Family Physicians About Mood Disorders: A Procedure Suite for Behavioral Medicine. *Primary Care Companion to The Journal of Clinical Psychiatry.* 1(1):18–23.

Stress Management

About 70% of primary care visits are related to psychosocial stress. This stress contributes to a difficult-to-quantify, but substantial, amount of morbidity and possibly mortality (in the distal sense). Given the importance of this content area and the typical shortage of teaching hours, training PCPs about stress should receive high priority. Educational interventions can begin with basic didactic instruction on "stress processes" and their constituent elements. Useful skills to teach might include how to ask about stress, assess severity, gauge appraisals, and evaluate coping resources, and promoting more effective and protective coping responses.

"Stress" is generally used to refer to one or more of the following: (1) an aversive or threatening event or situation (i.e. a stressor), (2) an appraisal of a stressor (i.e. primary appraisal) and/or an appraisal of coping resources (i.e. secondary appraisal) and (3) a stress response that may include physiologic, emotional, cognitive, and behavioral changes--all of which may lead to or exacerbate some diseases. Stress responses include biological, emotional, cognitive, and behavioral changes. Biological stress responses involve the central nervous system and the neuroendocrine and immune systems. Much of the research on stress has focused on the hypothalamic-pituitary-adrenal (HPA) axis and stress hormones such as cortisol plus the sympathetic arousal that accompanies the "fight or flight" response. The "stress process" involves all of the above components. It emerges from a transaction of the individual and the environment.

After educating PCPs about stress processes, that knowledge should be translated into how to teach patients about stress (recall "see one, do one, teach one..."). Patients often hear from physicians, "it's stress...try not to get stressed." Patients leave with the idea, "it is in my head and I need to toughen up." Instead, physicians can normalize the stress response and educate the patient about how stress impacts the body. Stress is very much a medical phenomenon and not simply in one's head. By identifying stress (which may be a cause or effect of a disease or symptom), potential new interventions may be brought into the treatment plan.

Much as PCPs learn a set of questions to assess pain (e.g. location, intensity, quality, what makes it better/worse), PCPs could also benefit from a set of questions to assess stress and coping such as:

- *Are there any stressful things going on in your life right now? (stressors)*
- *How bad are the things you are facing? How worried are you about _____?*
  (primary appraisals)
- *Is there anyone or anything available to help you cope? What resources do you*
  have? How will you get by? (secondary appraisals)
- *How stressed do you feel right now? Physically? Mentally? Do any symptoms*
  seem worse when you are really stressed? (stress response)
- *What do you do to cope with (the stressor)? Does it help or hurt? Has anything*
  in this past week made it better or worse? (coping behaviors)
- *How can we help you cope?*

Although PCPs will not be providing ongoing stress-management training to their patients, they may offer practical advice while connecting patients to other needed supports. Practical strategies to counteract stress include rethinking primary and secondary appraisals, increasing social interactions, scheduling pleasant activities (distraction can be a useful form of emotion-focused coping when appropriate), progressive muscle relaxation, diaphragmatic breathing, meditation, or scheduling "worry times." Other strategies include journaling, which could help increase awareness, evaluation, and processing of personal stress reactions. For teachers, a commonly effective "hook" is to frame the instruction of coping strategies as a form of self-care or wellness promotion for PCPs. PCPs may be more likely to disseminate coping strategies to patients if they have personally benefited from those same interventions.

In conclusion, there are many high-yield, low-investment teaching opportunities for behavioral health practitioners in an integrated health care setting. Successful teaching requires an understanding of the culture of medical education and a flexible yet practical creativity that supports teaching tools fit for the medical milieu. Even a cursory assessment of PCP's educational and clinical needs will help guide the utilization of limited teaching resources, while building "political capital" to seek out additional teaching hours or other support. Evidence-based teaching techniques coupled with clearly relevant clinical applications will ease adoption and raise perceived value.

References

Chiles, J. A., Lambert, M. J., & Hatch, A. L. (1999). The impact of psychological interventions on medical cost offset: A meta-analytic review. *Clinical Psychology: Science and Practice, 6*(2), 204–220.

Cummings, N. A., Cummings, J. L., & Johnson, J. N. (1997). *Behavioral Health in Primary Care: A Guide for Clinical Integration*. Madison, CT: Psychosocial Press.

Engel, G. L. (1977). The need for a new medical model: A challenge for biomedicine. *Science, 196*, 129–136.

Engel, G. L. (1980). The clinical application of the biopsychosocial model. *The American Journal of Psychiatry, 137*, 535–544.

Epstein, R. M., & Hundert, E. M. (2002). Defining and assessing professional competence. *Journal of the American Medical Association, 287*(2), 226–235.

Gabbard, G. O. (1985). The role of compulsiveness in the normal physician. *JAMA, 254*, 2926–2929.

Green, M. L. (2001). Identifying, appraising, and implementing medical education curricula: A guide for medical educators. *Annals of Internal Medicine, 135*, 889–896.

Higgins, E. S. (1994). A review of unrecognized mental illness in primary care; Prevalence, natural history, and efforts to change the course. *Archives of Family Medicine, 3*, 908–917.

Hodges, B., Inch, C., & Silver, I. (2001). Improving the psychiatric knowledge, skills, and attitudes of primary care physicians, 1950–2000: A review. *The American Journal of Psychiatry, 158*, 1579– 1586.

Institute of Medicine. (2004). Improving medical education: enhancing the social and behavioral science content of medical school curricula. Washington DC: National Academy Press.

Ferenchick, G., Simpson, D., Blackman, J., DaRosa, D., & Dunnington, G. (1997). Strategies for efficient and effective teaching in the ambulatory care setting. *Academic Medicine, 72*(4), 277–280.

Grol R., & Grimshaw J. (1999). Evidence-based implementation of evidence-based medicine. *Journal on Quality Improvement, 25*, 503–513.

Jones, R., Higgs, R., de Angelis, C., & Prideaux, D. (2001). Changing face of medical curricula. *Lancet, 357*, 699–703.

Leon, A. C., Olfson, M., Broadhead, W. E., Barrett, J. E., Blacklow, R. S., Martin, B. K., et al. (1995). Prevalence of mental disorders in primary care: Implications for screening. *Archives of Family Medicine, 4*, 857–861.

McGinnis M., & Foege W. (1993). Actual causes of death. *Journal of the American Medical Association, 270*, 2207–2212.

Norman G. (2002). Research in medical education: Three decades of progress. *British Medical Journal, 324*, 1560–1562.

Satterfield J. M., Mitteness L., Tervalon M., & Adler N. (2004). Integrating the social and behavioral sciences in an undergraduate medical curriculum: The UCSF essential core. *Academic Medicine, 79*, 6–15.

Schroeder S. A. (1992). The troubled profession: is medicine's glass half full or half empty? *Annals of Internal Medicine, 116*, 583–592.

Quality Improvement in the Integrated Health Care Setting

Ranilo Laygo and Rachelle Sorci

A Brief History of Quality Improvement

W. Edwards Deming (1990–1993) is widely recognized as the originator of the quality improvement movement. Although the movement began with his early work in the 1940s in the United States, the roots of the movement are perhaps more firmly planted in his work in the post-war reconstruction of Japan's industry (Aguayo, 1990). With the later adoption of Deming's principles by US-based automobile manufacturers, the movement had finally "come home" and has proliferated in the United States ever since (Gabor, 1990).

As the consumer base has become more educated, active, and demanding, indicators of quality across a variety of fields have become widely known. Examples include the JD Power and Associates[1] quality awards in the automotive industry, the Joint Commission on Accreditation of Healthcare Organizations[2] for hospitals and other health care organizations; and the Malcolm Baldrige National Quality Award[3] in the business, education, health care, and nonprofit arenas. Consumers have even created grassroots movements to establish minimum service delivery standards where none previously existed, like the "Flyers Bill of Rights"[4].

Quality Improvement in an Integrated Care Setting

Quality improvement for behavioral health care organizations, settings, and services, however, is less expected than in other service industries. One may question why, then, should a quality improvement process be implemented in these settings.

R. Laygo (✉)
Assistant Professor, Center on Disability Studies, Honolulu, HI 96822, USA
e-mail: ranilo@hawaii.edu

[1] J.D. Power and Associates, 2625 Townsgate Road, Westlake Village, CA 91361

[2] The Joint Commission, One Renaissance Boulevard, Oakbrook Terrace, IL 60181

[3] Baldrige National Quality Program, NIST, 100 Bureau Drive Stop 1020, Gaithersburg, MD 20899–1020

[4] http://www.flyersrights.com/index.html

L.C. James, W.T. O'Donohue (eds.), *The Primary Care Toolkit*,
DOI 10.1007/978-0-387-78971-2_9, © Springer Science+Business Media, LLC 2009

- First, behavioral health care is becoming more empirically driven (Kazdin & Weisz, 2003).
- Second, the integrated care clinician may be practicing within a setting that expects quality improvement metrics to be gathered; for example, an integrated care clinician practicing within a Joint Commission accredited hospital.
- Third, quality improvement data can be used to leverage administrators to implement or expand integrated health care services.
- Finally, as postulated by Deming (2000) and proven in a variety of settings, the introduction of a quality improvement process reduces costs and improves productivity. This is particularly relevant in the primary care setting where overhead costs are increasing and insurance reimbursement rates are decreasing.

Ingredients for Creating a Quality Improvement Process

The Setting

Unlike the quality improvement efforts in other industries, quality improvement in the integrated care setting is staff and clinician driven. In other words, an outside team of surveyors, using instruments that are divorced from the integrated care setting, questioning participants weeks or even months after their purchase of services are not employed in this model. Instead, all efforts are made to seamlessly integrate the quality improvement process with the standard of practice employed in the delivery of services. When implemented correctly, the patient should be unaware that there is a separate quality improvement process operating.

Measurement in the Integrated Care Setting

The integrated care setting is a complex system allowing for a large number of metrics to be used in the quality improvement process. Discussed below are but a few domains that have been utilized in previous examinations of quality in the integrated care setting (Laygo et al., 2003).

Disease Specific

Physical Health

One of the best applications of the integrated care model is in disease and life style management. The use of biometrics as quality improvement measures with these patients is a natural choice and offers several advantages: the collection of these data is routine, if not expected, (e.g. weight, blood pressure, blood glucose levels, etc.); there are empirically derived norms or standards for these measures; and it provides a specific outcome measure that coincides with the focused intervention. Plus, the data are easily tracked and outcomes easily understood by patients.

Mental Health

On the other hand, for the many patients seeking mental health treatment in the primary care setting (Lechnyr, 1993), pen and paper measures may be more appropriate. However, because of the uniqueness of the integrated care setting, most instruments used in mental health research and practice are not well-suited for use in the integrated care setting.

Traditional psychological instruments may be quite lengthy and often yield constructs that are not meaningful within the immediate clinical setting. In the integrated care setting, patients do not complete instruments unless they provide immediate, useful information to the clinician. In addition, the instruments are brief, so that patients can fill them out just prior to or after seeing the integrated care clinician. Finally, a separate appointment with a specialist for completing the quality control metrics should not be necessary. This detracts from the integrated health care model. These and other differences are noted in Table 1.

Regardless, there are several very brief measures which would be appropriate for use in the integrated care setting such as the Beck Depression Inventory for Primary Care (Beck, Guth, Steer, & Ball, 1997) or the Beck Anxiety Inventory (Beck & Steer, 1993). Alternatively, integrated care clinicians can use subject units of distress scales (SUDS) pre-prepared for the types of problems they encounter (e.g. anxiety, depression, pain). Examples of SUDS sheets for anxiety and depression appear in Appendix A and B, respectively.

Table 1 Characteristics of traditional psychological instruments versus those used in an integrated care setting

Traditional Instruments	Instruments Used in the Primary Care Setting
Lengthy (e.g., MMPI-2[1], CBCL[2])	Brief
Yield constructs that are not helpful in delivering brief, very focused interventions (e.g., Masculinity–Femininity Scale)	Provide meaningful information that can immediately inform patient care
Need special scoring software or templates	Easy to interpret
Cannot produce scores on demand	Can be used immediately in the current session
Require special training or equipment to administer (e.g., CAFAS[3])	No special training or equipment needed
Must be administered at a time point too distant from the meeting with the behavioral health clinician	Can be administered immediately prior to or after the patient visit

[1]Hathaway, S., & McKinley, J. (1989). *MMPI-2 manual for administration and scoring.* Minneapolis, MN: University of Minnesota Press.
[2]Achenbach, T. M., & Rescorla, L. A. (2001). *Manual for the ASEBA school-age forms and profiles.* Burlington, VT: University of Vermont, Research Centre for Children, Youth and Families.
[3]Hodges, K. (1990, 1994 revision). *Child and Adolescent Functional Assessment Scale.* Ypsilanti, MI: Eastern Michigan University, Department of Psychology.

Non-Disease-Specific

Given the breadth of problems that integrated care patients present with, perhaps what is most useful for quality improvement efforts is to have a brief, general measure of both physical and mental health status. One such measure is the SF-12v2™ Health Survey Acute Recall (Ware, Kosinski, Turner-Bowker, & Gandek, 2002), which appears in Appendix C.[5] Although automated scoring is needed to calculate the two global scales on the instrument (Physical Component Score and Mental Component Score), along with the eight subscales (Physical Functioning, Role-Physical, Bodily Pain, General Health Perceptions, Vitality, Social Functioning, Role-Emotional, and Mental Health), the items are worded such that the information provided can be used to inform the immediate patient session. Also, once produced, the norm-based scores are easily interpreted and make progress-tracking quite easy.

General Functioning

Often times the impetus for patients to seek help is a decline in social, school, or vocational functioning. Measuring changes in patient functioning on these domains provide important feedback for the integrated care clinician. An example of a general measure of functioning appears in Appendix D.

Quality of Life

General satisfaction with life is a useful global measure of progress for patients treated in an integrated care model. Conveniently, there is an immense number of such scales available (Salek, 1998) which can be used with a wide range of patients, ranging from healthy individuals (Burckhardt & Anderson, 2003) to those suffering from chronic mental illness or specific medical problems (Lehman, 1992). These instruments also have the advantage of being cost-efficient and easy to administer, score, and interpret.

Consumer Satisfaction

The integrated care model is unique in that the integrated care clinician has two concurrent sets of consumers to satisfy, each with equal value in the model: the primary care providers who make referrals to the integrated care clinician and receive some direct services in the form of consultations, and the patients who receive direct services. Both sets of consumers are crucial to the success of the integrated care clinician's practice. Thus, it is very important to continually monitor the satisfaction of both sets of consumers and respond to their feedback.

---

[5] Copyright 2000 by QualityMetric Incorporated. Reprinted with permission.

Provider Satisfaction

Interestingly, while primary care providers are often the subject of satisfaction surveys, they are rarely the respondents. This state of affairs limits both the literature on the topic and the availability of instruments. One example, however, appears in Appendix E[6]

Patient Satisfaction

Patient satisfaction is more widely accepted as a quality assurance measure; thus, there is a wealth of literature and instruments that address the topic. However, in the interest of making a thorough investigation of patient satisfaction it is helpful to use an instrument with adequate psychometric properties. One example which has been used in a variety of studies is the Client Satisfaction Questionnaire—8 (Larsen, Attkisson, Hargreaves, & Nguyen 1979) which appears in Appendix F[7]

Utilization of Medical Services

Patients with mental health problems tend to tax the medical system with their overusage (Lechnyr, 1992; Cummings, Dorken, Pallak, & Henke, 1990; Borus & Olendzki, 1985). One positive effect of having an integrated care clinician is that these high-utilizing patients are diverted to the integrated care clinician, thus freeing up the primary care provider to service a greater number of more appropriate patients. Another benefit, of course, is that the high-utilizing patient receives the behavioral health service they need. Consequently this decreases their medical utilization and its associated cost. This increase in provider productivity and decrease in patient medical utilization is more difficult to examine; however, with proper tracking it is possible.

The Process

The process for tying these elements together is depicted in Fig. 1. Note, however, that the exact configuration of any process will depend on a number of factors including the number and types of providers that will make referrals to the integrated care clinician, the number of integrated care clinicians servicing these providers, available office space, information technology resources, number of support staff, etc.

Ideally, when the patient arrives at the primary care setting to meet with the integrated care clinician, they will complete any necessary administrative paperwork. With new patients in particular, there are usually insurance forms and other paperwork to complete. If any pen and paper instruments are to be administered, they

---

[6] Copyright (2005) by Rachelle Sorci, Ph.D. Reprinted with permission.

[7] Copyright (1979, 1989, 1990, 2006) by Clifford Attkisson, Ph.D. Reprinted with permission.

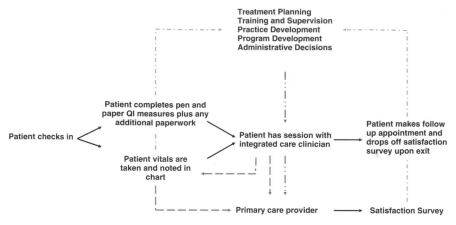

Fig. 1 The quality improvement process in an integrated care setting

should be administered at this time. Patients not used to the integrated care setting may have questions about why they are completing the pen and paper instruments. It is essential that staff explain that the instruments will be used to inform their work with the integrated care clinician and track their progress. It is helpful to reference the medical model and explain that these instruments will be completed prior to each visit with the integrated clinician, just as the patient's temperature, weight, and pulse are taken prior to visiting with their primary care provider.

Depending on the setting's standard of practice, patient vitals may be taken prior to seeing the integrated care clinician, even if the patient will not be seeing the primary care provider on that visit. If biometrics are being addressed as part of the patient's work with the integrated care clinician, it is essential that they be measured prior to the meeting with the integrated care clinician and noted in the chart. Results of any off-site testing such as blood glucose level or lipid profile should already be in the chart.

Using the methods described above, patient information makes its way to the integrated care clinician via two routes: the patients bring completed instruments with them to the session and the biometric data is recorded in the chart. This information is used to guide the patient session. Depending upon the standard of practice, the integrated care clinician's notes may be placed in the patient's medical file or kept in a separate file. Following the session, the patient is given a satisfaction form to complete. A lock box for the satisfaction forms is kept at the front desk and/or the main exit so that the patients can drop off the satisfaction form conveniently while scheduling a follow-up visit or on their way out.

Feedback to the referring physician can take two forms. Ideally, the integrated care clinician's notes are contained within the patient's medical file. In this manner, the referring physician remains continually abreast of the patient's progress. If the setting does not allow this arrangement, the integrated care clinician can update the physician in whatever convenient manner the setting allows. This could be via face-to-face meetings, team meetings, or internal memos.

As noted above, providers in the setting should be surveyed periodically to assess whether they are satisfied with the integrated care clinician'(s') services, and whether there is any feedback for improvement. A convenient method for executing this is to survey the providers regularly during staff meetings. Paper and pen surveys can be administered during the meeting, with providers asked to drop their completed surveys in the same lock box(es) that the patients use.

Using the Data

Individual-Level Data

The quality improvement data gathered are used at various levels. As noted above, patient data (lab results and pen and paper instruments) are used immediately in the session. They are also tracked over time for the purpose of treatment planning. Since the referring physician also has access to this data, it can be used to inform their treatment plans as well.

Hypothetical patient data presented below help illustrate how these data may be used[8].

Patient A

In the first example, the patient's blood pressure did not improve during the first two visits. Being aware of this lack of progress, the integrated care clinician asks the patient to keep a food diary and bring it to their next session. The integrated care clinician explains that this information will be used to further fine-tune his treatment regimen.

During the third visit, the integrated care clinician reviews the causes of hypertension with his patient, noting how the patient's lack of exercise and poor eating habits affects his blood pressure. Examples of the latter are pulled from the food diary. The integrated care clinician, with the help of the patient, develops a diet and exercise plan. One of the main goals of the diet is to reduce the notable amount of salt and caffeine the patient is ingesting.

In addition, an anxiety SUDS completed by the patient just prior to the visit indicates that the patient is under a moderate to severe amount of stress. Further probing reveals that the patient is in danger of losing his job if his sales team does not significantly improve its first quarter sales figures. The integrated care clinician teaches the patient some relaxation techniques for him to use when he felt "stressed out" at or about work.

---

[8] All data presented are fictional and are used for illustration purposes only.

Finally, the integrated care clinician flags the patient's chart for review by the referring physician, to see whether the patient is healthy enough for the proposed exercise regimen and whether blood pressure medication is warranted at this time. The physician indicates that the patient is healthy enough to engage in the outlined exercise routine and would hold off on prescribing any medication to see if diet and exercise alone could improve the patient's health status.

At the fourth visit, there is some positive change in the patient's blood pressure (Fig. 2). The patient and integrated care clinician reviews the treatment plan again and make minor changes based on the patient's feedback (e.g. patient will use an elliptical trainer rather than a treadmill due to a minor knee pain) and schedule a follow-up appointment in two weeks. Upon review, the referring physician decides not to prescribe any blood pressure medication at this point since the patient still has room to improve on his own (e.g. lose weight).

Patient B

In the second example, the patient was making good progress on his goal of losing weight. By their fourth visit, he had already lost 25 pounds. At their fifth visit, however, the integrated care clinician noted a significant *increase* in weight (Fig. 3). The patient's depression SUDS indicated that the patient was experiencing moderate to severe depression during the preceding two weeks. During their visit, the

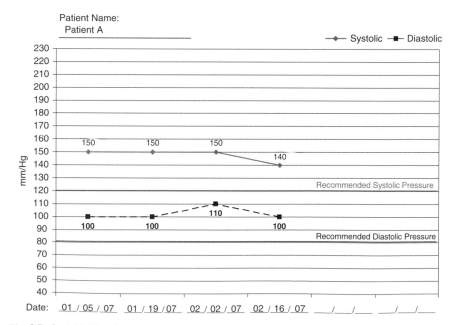

Fig. 2 Patient A's blood pressure data over time

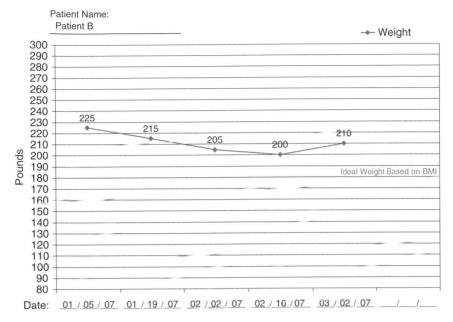

Fig. 3 Patient B's weight over time

integrated care clinician discovered that the first anniversary of the patient's divorce was approaching and the patient was overeating as a way of coping with the depression. Together, the integrated care clinician and patient agree to a brief course of cognitive-behavioral therapy with the goals of helping the patient work through his unresolved feelings around his divorce and developing health coping mechanisms for the patient to use when confronted by similar feelings of depression. They also reviewed what aspects of the treatment plan helped him lose weight with the understanding that he would restart his efforts to lose weight.

Providers

The satisfaction data from the patient surveys can be used by the integrated care clinician for practice development and understanding what additional training and supervision they may need. Surveying the primary care providers throughout the year allows the integrated care clinician an opportunity to see patterns in their satisfaction data. In a setting with a great deal of provider turnover, it allows the integrated care clinician to have many different perspectives on their services.

To illustrate, fictitious provider satisfaction data are presented in Fig. 4. A response pattern like the one seen seems to indicate that overall the integrated care clinician is doing a fine job servicing the providers in his/her clinic. Two areas for improvement, however, stand out. First, the data indicate that the integrated care

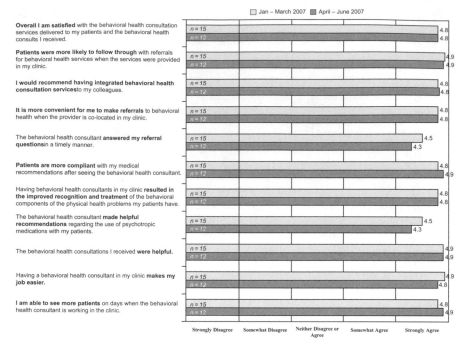

Fig. 4 Results from provider satisfaction survey over time

clinician needs to address referral questions in a more timely manner. The second area for improvement is in that of psychotropics. Perhaps the integrated care clinician needs to learn more about up-to-date uses of psychotropic medications.

System-Level Data

At the simplest level of analysis, results from patient and provider satisfaction surveys can determine whether the two sets of consumers are satisfied with the integrated care clinician's services. Aggregate data from clinical outcome measures such as the SF-12v2™ Health Survey Acute Recall (Ware, Kosinski, Turner-Bowker, & Gandek, 2002) can help determine whether the integrated care clinician's interventions are having an impact on the organization's patient population. A hypothetical example of these data is plotted out in Fig. 5. These data indicate improvements in the mental and physical health status of the 350 patients who were served in this sample.

More complex analyses, however, can help administrators make informed decisions at the system level. For example, does hiring an integrated care clinician increase physician billing? Does having an integrated care clinician increase provider satisfaction and consequently retention? Is there an organizational need for special

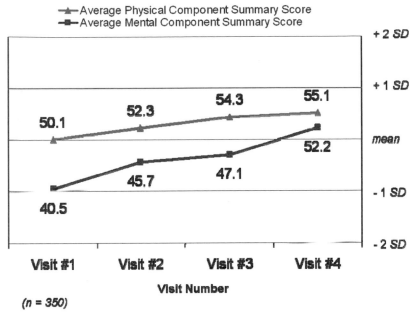

Fig. 5 Patient data from the SF-12v2[TM] health survey acute recall over time

programs? Could these be profitable? As noted above, these analyses are more sophisticated, but can be completed with adequate data.

Challenges to Consider When Implementing a Quality Improvement Process

The final section of this chapter identifies the most common challenges encountered when trying to implement a quality improvement process within an integrated health care setting. In addition, solutions to these challenges are proposed based on the authors' experiences conducting quality improvement efforts for a variety of entities including the Department of Defense (DoD), community health centers, and the National Health Service.

Overcoming Resistance to Implementation: Cultural Sensitivity in Quality Improvement

Challenge: Suspiciousness of the Quality Improvement Process

It is important to be culturally sensitive to the setting, patient population, and providers being evaluated. It is common for quality improvement efforts to be greeted with some resistance, especially by providers who are not used to having their services evaluated. It is also important to consider organizational and ethnic/cultural factors that may reinforce this resistance.

For example, while conducting an integrated health care project in rural and Native Hawaiian Health Centers, the evaluator initially faced resistance to implementing a quality improvement process because the providers were wary of how the results would be used. This wariness was due to the fact that there was a precedence of outsiders conducting research within Native Hawaiian communities promising that the data would be used to better the community, when unfortunately, sometimes the results led to inaccurate interpretations and reinforcement of negative stereotypes of Native Hawaiians.

In a separate DoD project, a military integrated health care provider was concerned about how patients' symptom survey data would be reflected in the service members' medical charts. Medical charts of active duty service members can be reviewed by their command and potentially impact their career. This provider discussed the likelihood that active duty military personnel would under-report symptoms with a "faking good" response style. Inaccurate baseline and follow-up of symptom measures would be clinically useless and invalidate outcome results.

Solutions: Sensitivity to Cultural Values as Necessary for Success

In both of these examples, potential obstacles to gathering accurate data were rooted in the concern that quality improvement data may potentially be used to harm the population that was utilizing the integrated behavioral health services. Ensuring the anonymity of all results and implementing written data-use agreements were two solutions utilized to minimize these concerns.

When working with the Native Hawaiian health system, data-use agreements explicitly defined how data would be gathered, analyzed, and used by the health centers for the specific purpose of quality improvement. In the DoD project, clinicians decided to review the symptom outcome measures as part of their clinical work, but agreed that all data would be reported by randomly assigned identification numbers that would de-identify the specific service member. Recognizing and remaining sensitive to ethnic and organizational culture, in this case assuring confidentiality and proper use of results, was essential for the successful implementation of a quality improvement process and accurate reporting of results.

Overcoming Resource Limitations: Creative Solutions for Project Sustainability

Concern: Integrated Health Care Programs Do Not Have Time or Expertise to Implement a Quality Improvement Process

In previous projects, the authors have noted that maintaining the quality improvement component of the integrated health care model has sometimes been difficult—for a variety of reasons. In post-project focus groups, providers identified several reasons for integrated health care programs discontinuing the quality improvement portion of the program. The first and most obvious reason was that administrators reported that the quality improvement process served its purpose and established that the integrated health care model "worked" and therefore was no longer a required component of service. Other reasons identified by providers, who were also held responsible for managing their own quality improvement data, included the lack of time to input data and unfamiliarity with the required statistical analysis to produce the results that were previously provided by the quality improvement coordinator. Finally, in the often fast-paced clinical setting of the integrated health care provider, the quality improvement process was perceived as too time-consuming to maintain. What program directors failed to recognize was that the same initial quality improvement data used to justify initiating the integrated health care program was also essential for maintaining and advocating for expansion of services.

Solutions: Secure Buy-In from All Levels of Your Organizational Hierarchy

In the authors' experiences, the quality improvement component of the integrated health care model is sustained mainly in settings where all members of the health care organization have an investment in the results. In such settings, both health care leadership and providers were able to utilize results from the quality improvement process to address their specific concerns and agenda, in addition to improving patient care. Long-term maintenance of the quality improvement process has to be viewed as a required service component by medical and psychological providers, and by health care leadership. For example, in one health center results from the quality improvement process were used in a variety of ways. The Chief Executive Officer (CEO) of the organization used the results to develop a "Behavioral Health Report Card" that enabled him to showcase the progress and development of the integrated health care services to his Board of Directors. Quarterly results, which provided customer satisfaction and treatment outcome data, were made available to the Board of Directors. The additional visibility of the integrated health care program at the highest level of the organization only served to grow the program even faster. The CEO reported that the accountability of the report card gave him an "at a glance" understanding of the services being provided by their integrated health care staff. He also reported that this accountability demonstrated good stewardship of resources to his Board of Directors and calmed any initial fears regarding the integration of behavioral health services with their medical services. The Chief Financial Officer (CFO) of another health center utilized analyses from the quality improvement process to develop a model for sustaining the integrated health care department. The CEO also used the analyses to strategically plan for program expansion. In a health care system with dramatically increasing costs, now approximately 15% of the United States' gross national product, competition for health care resources is increasing (Pear, 2004). The CFO was able to present quality improvement data that justified expansion of the integrated health care services versus hiring another medical or dental provider. The CFO also developed incentive programs for the integrated health care provider. The CFO tied incentives to patient and provider satisfaction as well as to the treatment outcomes.

The authors of this chapter have been approached by clinical providers that are interested in initiating a more comprehensive quality improvement component to their integrated health care service, but lack time and the financial resources for hiring a consultant. It has been said that "necessity is the mother of invention." For these providers we propose several solutions with the emphasis on starting with what is available until you can demonstrate, with data, what is possible for integrated health care programming. The most common questions that we have heard from providers include the following:

Question:

I am a clinical provider and not a statistician. I haven't used statistical software since graduate school. Analysis of quality improvement data just seems intimidating for me to complete. How do I even start ?

Response:

The integrated health care provider is a highly skilled and trained specialty provider. When quality improvement services are not funded through their department, it is often left to the chief integrated care provider to develop and maintain the quality improvement process. Clinical providers with rusty research skills may consult with their local university or professional school of psychology. Many university programs offer consultation services for a reduced price. Doctoral candidates in Industrial/Organization Psychology can often provide assistance with setting up the quality improvement infrastructure (i.e. instrument selection and conducting the analysis). Bachelors or Masters level students can assist in the ongoing gathering and entering of data. Seeking student assistance at your local university may prove to be beneficial for both providers and students seeking real-world experience.

Question:

As an integrated health care provider, I am so busy with the clinical responsibilities of the job that I just don't have the time to implement a quality improvement program. How have other providers in similar situations addressed the lack of time?

Response:

As stated in the previous section, in order for quality improvement services to be maintained over time all members of the health care organization must understand how the data will advance their individual agendas, while also improving patient care. Introducing quality improvement as essential for success and assisting your leadership in identifying ways they can utilize the data is the first step in initiating or expanding quality improvement services.

In one case, we have seen health care leadership allow providers to set aside time (typically 10% of their work week) to engage in quality improvement activities. This scenario would not cost the health center any additional dollars while providing time for the integrated health care provider to establish a quality improvement process.

These examples are just some of the obstacles faced by and solutions proposed for integrated health care programs when initiating and implementing quality improvement components into their programming. Each organization, undoubtedly, will have its own set of challenges.

Summary

Quality improvement may not be the first thing that comes to mind when thinking of behavioral health; however, it is essential to the integrated health care model. Patient data help guide treatment planning on the consumer side of the equation and may indicate areas for improvement on the provider side. Feedback from the primary care provider may help the integrated care clinician recognize gaps in knowledge or areas for improvement. At the aggregate level, longitudinal data can help make system-level decisions—such as simple hiring/firing decisions—as well as important financial decisions, such as whether employing the integrated health care model can increase revenue or open new practice areas. Finally, while implementing a quality improvement process in an integrated health care setting is challenging and requires an investment of time and money, once all stakeholders in the health care setting understand how they can reap the benefits of that investment, the process will begin to sustain itself.

Appendix A: Anxiety Subjective Units of Distress Scale

Date: _____/_____/_____

Clinician Instructions: For each item, please read the appropriate question based on whether this is a baseline administration or follow-up. Please record patient's responses in the area provided.

Baseline Questions: In the past two weeks how many days did you feel anxious?

_____

On average, when you felt anxious, how would you rate your level of anxiety? _____

Follow-up Questions: Since your last visit approximately (prompt) days ago, how many days did you feel anxious? _____

On average, when you were anxious, how would you rate your level of anxiety? _____

10 Extreme anxiety; could not function at all

9

8

7 Severe anxiety; had serious difficulty functioning

6

5 Moderate anxiety; anxiety present but manageable; moderate difficulty functioning, but I could function if I pushed myself

4

3 Mild anxiety; some problems in functioning

2

1 Minimal anxiety; only mild and occasional problems in functioning, but barely noticeable

0 No anxiety; no problems functioning at all

Appendix B: Depression Subjective Units of Distress Scale

Date: ____/____/____

Clinician Instructions: For each item, please read the appropriate question based on whether this is a baseline administration or follow-up. Please record patient's responses in the area provided.

Baseline Questions: In the past two weeks how many days did you feel depressed?

____

On average, when you felt depressed, how would you rate your level of depression? ____

Follow-up Questions: Since your last visit approximately (prompt) days ago, how many days did you feel depressed? ____

On average, when you were depressed, how would you rate your level of depression? ____

10 **Extreme depression**; could not function at all

9

8

7 **Severe depression**; had serious difficulty functioning

6

5 **Moderate depression**; depression present but manageable; moderate difficulty functioning, but I could function if I pushed myself

4

3 **Mild depression**; some problems in functioning

2

1 **Minimal depression**; only mild and occasional problems in functioning, but barely noticeable

0 **No depression**; no problems functioning at all

Appendix C: SF-12v2™ Health Survey Acute Recall

Your Health and Well-Being

This survey asks for your views about your health. This information will
help keep track of how you feel and how well you are able to do your usual
activities. *Thank you for completing this survey!*

For each of the following questions, please mark an ⊠ in the one box that
best describes your answer.

1. **In general, would you say your health is:**

Excellent	Very good	Good	Fair	Poor
▼	▼	▼	▼	▼
☐ 1	☐ 2	☐ 3	☐ 4	☐ 5

2. **The following questions are about activities you might do during a
   typical day. Does <u>your health now limit you</u> in these activities? If so,
   how much?**

	Yes, limited a lot	Yes, limited a little	No, not limited <u>at all</u>
	▼	▼	▼
(a) <u>Moderate activities</u>, such as moving a table, pushing a vacuum cleaner, bowling, or playing golf..	☐ 1	☐ 2	☐ 3
(b) Climbing <u>several</u> flights of stairs	☐ 1	☐ 2	☐ 3

---

3. **During the <u>past week</u>, how much of the time have you had any of the following problems with your work or other regular daily activities <u>as a result of your physical health</u>?**

	All of the time	Most of the time	Some of the time	A little of the time	None of the time
	▼	▼	▼	▼	▼
(a) <u>Accomplished less</u> than you would like..	☐1	☐2	☐3	☐4	☐5
(b) Were limited in the <u>kind</u> of work or other activities	☐1	☐2	☐3	☐4	☐5

4. **During the <u>past week</u>, how much of the time have you had any of the following problems with your work or other regular daily activities <u>as a result of any emotional problems</u> (such as feeling depressed or anxious)?**

	All of the time	Most of the time	Some of the time	A little of the time	None of the time
	▼	▼	▼	▼	▼
a <u>Accomplished less</u> than you would like..	☐1	☐2	☐3	☐4	☐5
b Did work or other activities <u>less carefully than usual</u>	☐1	☐2	☐3	☐4	☐5

5. **During the <u>past week</u>, how much did <u>pain</u> interfere with your normal work (including both work outside the home and housework)?**

Not at all	A little bit	Moderately	Quite a bit	Extremely
▼	▼	▼	▼	▼
☐1	☐2	☐3	☐4	☐5

6. **These questions are about how you feel and how things have been with you <u>during the past week</u>. For each question, please give the one answer that comes closest to the way you have been feeling. How much of the time during the <u>past week</u>...**

	All of the time	Most of the time	Some of the time	A little of the time	None of the time
	▼	▼	▼	▼	▼
a Have you felt calm and peaceful?	☐1	☐2	☐3	☐4	☐5
b Did you have a lot of energy?	☐1	☐2	☐3	☐4	☐5
c Have you felt downhearted and depressed?	☐1	☐2	☐3	☐4	☐5

7. **During the <u>past week</u>, how much of the time has your <u>physical health or emotional problems</u> interfered with your social activities (like visiting friends, relatives, etc.)?**

All of the time	Most of the time	Some of the time	A little of the time	None of the time
▼	▼	▼	▼	▼
☐1	☐2	☐3	☐4	☐5

Thank you for completing these questions!

Appendix D: Adult Daily Functioning Form

Date: ____/____/____

The following questions concern the behavioral health consultation services you have received and your daily functioning since *the last time* you met with the behavioral health consultant. Please read each statement and indicate the degree to which you disagree or agree with the statement.

The services I received from the behavioral health consultant helped me . . .	Strongly Disagree	Somewhat Disagree	Neither Disagree or Agree	Somewhat Agree	Strongly Agree	NA
find a job that pays (including self-employment).						
earn more income.						
work more hours.						
work more days.						
miss fewer days of work.						
work more productively during the time I was at work.						
reduce the number of disruptions to my regular daily activities, routines, and responsibilities.						
reduce the use of medical services such as seeing the doctor, having medical tests, or using urgent or emergency medical facilities.						
reduce the amount of over-the-counter and prescriptions drugs I use.						

Appendix E: Primary Care Provider Satisfaction Survey

Introduction

Thank you for taking the time to answer these questions. Your opinion is very important to us. All of your responses will be kept confidential and used solely for the purpose of improving the behavioral health consultation services offered in your clinic.

Please click "Next" to get started with the survey. If you'd like to leave the survey at any time, just click "Exit this survey". Your answers will be saved.

Today's Date

Please Enter Today's Date

	MM	DD	YYYY
Date	☐ /	☐ /	☐

Provider and Location Info

What type of provider are you?

☐ Medical Doctor
☐ Resident
☐ Intern
☐ Nurse
☐ Other (please specify)

Utilization of Behavioral Health Consultation Services

During the months of January, February, and March 2007, did you refer any patients to the Behavioral Health Consultant in your clinic?

○ Yes
○ No

Reasons for Not Referring

Why not?

- [ ] I did not work at the clinic during those months.
- [ ] I did not know there was a Behavioral Health Consultant working in my clinic during those months.
- [ ] I did not know how to make a referal to the Behavioral Health Consultant.
- [ ] I did not have time to make any referrals during those months.
- [ ] I did not see any patients during those months that were appropriate for referral.
- [ ] I do not believe behavioral health services are necessary or effective for my patients' problems.
- [ ] I do not believe behavioral health services should be offered in my clinic.

Satisfaction Questions

Please read each of the following statements carefully and mark your response to each item in the columns next to the statement. Please base your responses on the experiences you've had with the behavioral health consultant within the months of January, February, and March 2007. If you did not have the interaction with behavioral health consultant described in the item, please respond "NA".

	Strongly Disagree	Somewhat Disagree	Neither Disagree nor Agree	Somewhat Agree	Strongly Agree	N/A
Overall I am satisfied with the behavioral health consultation services delivered to my patients and the behavioral health consults I received.	○	○	○	○	○	○
Patients were more likely to follow through with referrals for behavioral health services when the services were provided in my clinic.	○	○	○	○	○	○
I would recommend having integrated behavioral health consultation services to my colleagues.	○	○	○	○	○	○
It is more convenient for me to make referrals to behavioral health when the provider is co-located in my clinic.	○	○	○	○	○	○
The behavioral health consultant answered my referral questions in a timely manner.	○	○	○	○	○	○
Patients are more compliant with my medical recommendations after seeing the behavioral health consultant.	○	○	○	○	○	○
Having behavioral health consultants in my clinic resulted in the improved recognition and treatment of the behavioral components of the physical health problems my patients have.	○	○	○	○	○	○
The behavioral health consultant made helpful recommendations regarding the use of psychotropic medications with my patients.	○	○	○	○	○	○
The behavioral health consultations I received were helpful.	○	○	○	○	○	○

| Having a behavioral health consultant in my clinic makes my job easier. | ○ | ○ | ○ | ○ | ○ | ○ |
| I am able to see more patients on days when the behavioral health consultant is working in the clinic. | ○ | ○ | ○ | ○ | ○ | ○ |

What can behavioral health consultants do to improve their services?

Appendix F

CSQ-8 English

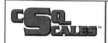 **CLIENT SATISFACTION QUESTIONNAIRE**
CSQ-8

Please help us improve our program by answering some questions about the services you have received. We are interested in your honest opinions, whether they are positive or negative. *Please answer all of the questions.* We also welcome your comments and suggestions. Thank you very much. We appreciate your help.

CIRCLE YOUR ANSWERS

1. How would you rate the quality of service you received?

4 Excellent	3 Good	2 Fair	1 Poor

2. Did you get the kind of service you wanted?

1 No, definitely not	2 No, not really	3 Yes, generally	4 Yes, definitely

3. To what extent has our program met your needs?

4 Almost all of my needs have been met	3 Most of my needs have been met	2 Only a few of my needs have been met	1 None of my needs have been met

4. If a friend were in need of similar help, would you recommend our program to him or her?

1 No, definitely not	2 No, I don't think so	3 Yes, I think so	4 Yes, definitely

5. How satisfied are you with the amount of help you received?

1 Quite dissatisfied	2 Indifferent or mildly dissatisfied	3 Mostly satisfied	4 Very satisfied

6. Have the services you received helped you to deal more effectively with your problems?

4 Yes, they helped a great deal	3 Yes, they helped somewhat	2 No, they really didn't help	1 No, they seemed to make things worse

7. In an overall, general sense, how satisfied are you with the service you received?

4 Very satisfied	3 Mostly satisfied	2 Indifferent or mildly dissatisfied	1 Quite dissatisfied

8. If you were to seek help again, would you come back to our program?

1 No, definitely not	2 No, I don't think so	3 Yes, I think so	4 Yes, definitely

References

Aguayo, R. (1990). *Dr. Deming: The American Who Taught the Japanese About Quality*. New York, NY: Fireside.

Gabor, A. (1990). *The Man Who Discovered Quality: How W. Edwards Deming Brought the Quality Revolution to America—The Stories of Ford, Xerox, and GM*. New York: Times Books.

Kazdin, A. E., & Weisz, J. R. (Eds.). (2003). *Evidence-based Psychotherapies for Children and Adolescents*. New York: Guilford Press.

Deming, W. E. (2000). *Out of the crisis*. Cambridge, MA: MIT Press.

Laygo, R., O'Donohue, W., Hall, S., Kaplan, A., Wood, R., Cummings, J., et al. (2003). Preliminary results from the Hawaii Integrated Healthcare Project II. In Cummings, N., O'Donohue, W., & Ferguson, K. (Eds.), *Behavioral health as primary care: Beyond efficacy to effectiveness* (pp. 111 – 143). Reno, NV: Context Press.

Lechnyr, R. (1993). The cost savings of mental health services. *EAP Digest, 22*, 23.

Beck, A. T., & Steer, R. A. (1993). *Beck Anxiety Inventory Manual*. San Antonio, TX: Psychological Corporation.

Ware, J. E., Kosinski, M., Turner-Bowker, D. M., & Gandek, B. (2002). *User's manual for the SF-12v2™ Health Survey (with a supplement documenting SF-12® Health Survey)*. Lincoln, RI: QualityMetric Incorporated.

Salek S. (1998). *Compendium of Quality of Life Instruments*. (5 vols.). Chichester, West Sussex: Wiley.

Burckhardt, C. S., & Anderson, K. L. (2003). The Quality of Life Scale (QOLS): Reliability, Validity, and Utilization. *Health and Quality of Life Outcomes, 1*, 60. Retrieved November 23, 2007, from http://www.hqlo.com/content/1/1/60#refs.

Lehman, A. F. (1983). The well-being of chronic mental patients: assessing their quality of life. *Archives of General Psychiatry, 40*, 369–373.

Larsen, D. L., Attkisson, C. C., Hargreaves, W. A., & Nguyen, T. D. (1979). Assessment of client/patient satisfaction: Development of a general scale. *Evaluation and Program Planning, 2*, 197–207.

Lechnyr, R. (1992). Cost savings and effectiveness of mental health services. *Journal of the Oregon Psychological Association, 38*, 8–12.

Cummings, N. A., Dorken, H., Pallak, M. S., & Henke, C. (1990). *The impact of psychological intervention on healthcare utilization and costs*. South San Francisco: The Biodyne Institute.

Borus, J. F., & Olendzki, M. C. (1985). The offset effect of mental health treatment on ambulatory medical care utilization and charges. *Archives of General Psychiatry, 42*, 573–580.

Ware, J. E., Kosinski, M., Turner-Bowker, D. M., & Gandek, B. (2002). *User's manual for the SF-12v2™ Health Survey (with a supplement documenting SF-12® Health Survey)*. Lincoln, RI: QualityMetric Incorporated.

Pear, R. (2004). U.S. Health Care Spending Reaches All-Time High: 15% of GDP. The New York Times, 9 January 2004, 3.

Behavioral Screening in Adult Primary Care

Michelle R. Byrd and Kevin N. Alschuler

The Importance of Screening in Integrated Care

From the moment patient are seen by a nurse in the primary care setting, they are placed on a multifaceted decision tree designed to screen for myriad medical diagnoses ranging from minor annoyances to life-threatening illnesses. Unfortunately, it is typically only when medical etiologies have been ruled out that the decision tree branches sufficiently to include psychological concerns and disorders. The integrated care setting invites the opportunity to screen for psychological problems *while* screening for medical etiologies. However, in doing so, the complexity of the already daunting task of identifying the likely causes of a patient's distress increases exponentially.

Despite the inherent challenge, the value of screening for behavioral issues at (apparently) the same time as the physically based complaints cannot be overstated. As the growing body of literature on integrated care has shown, neglecting behavioral issues ultimately also means ineffectively treating physical complaints. Attending to behavioral and physical concerns communicates to patients that health care providers are interested in them as whole people, body and mind. Furthermore, routine screening in primary care visits leads to a change in the medical culture, and, ultimately, the culture at large, by reducing the stigma associated with mental health. Without adequate screening, several of the primary goals of integrated care cannot possibly be reached, namely detecting psychological problems that are not readily apparent and having the opportunity to prevent exacerbation of symptoms which are not yet clinically significant.

We know of three studies which have empirically examined the utility of screening in primary care settings. However, none of these studies were conducted in integrated care settings, so their applicability is limited; but as no similar empirical studies of screening in integrated care have yet been published, these data provide

M.R. Byrd (✉)
Department of Psychology, Eastern Michigan University, 537 Mark Jefferson, Ypsilanti, MI 48197, USA
e-mail: mbyrd@emich.edu

L.C. James, W.T. O'Donohue (eds.), *The Primary Care Toolkit*,
DOI 10.1007/978-0-387-78971-2_10, © Springer Science+Business Media, LLC 2009

our best evidence for screening in integrated settings. In the first study, Cowan and Morewitz (1995) found that the use of a questionnaire about psychosocial concerns increased the likelihood that college-aged patients and their physician could talk about behavioral issues contributing to their health concerns. Referring to patients' medical charts, the researchers found that 36% of the 200 patients who received a screening questionnaire had severe psychosocial problems (e.g. substance abuse, clinical depression) recorded, statistically significantly higher than the 8% recorded in the charts before the study. The authors also noted that physicians cited the utility of the questionnaire in many of their reports, leading to the belief that the use of the screening was valuable to their practice.

Similarly, in a second study examining college health centers (n = 200), Alschuler, Hoodin, and Byrd (2008) found that screening for behavioral concerns resulted in statistically significantly higher rates of discussion of behavioral concerns between patient and provider and prescription of psychotropic medications, but not in referrals for follow-up behavioral care. Of the 109 patients randomly assigned to be screened, 28% met full diagnostic criteria for a psychological disorder as measured by self-report. Furthermore, patients and providers in the experimental condition indicated a strong desire to continue using the screening instrument in future visits.

In a study of screening in pediatric care, Byrd and O'Donohue (in progress) found that the majority of parents who were randomly assigned to complete the screener (78%) indicated that they had a least one concern regarding their child's behavior, their parenting, and/or following medical directions. In this vein, a little more than half of the parents surveyed indicated that screening made it easier for them to remember and initiate discussions about their children's behavioral concerns. Correspondingly, parents in the experimental condition had higher satisfaction with their primary care visit than did parents who did not participate in screening, and about half of parents reported that they would approve of their pediatrician screening at every visit.

The Purpose of This Chapter

A review of the literature quickly demonstrates that of the essential elements of integrated care, screening has not been written about a great deal nor has it been well-researched. More attention has been given to screening in pediatric primary care settings, where well-baby and well-child visits are routine, and providers have established repertoires with regard to developmental and, therefore, behavioral concerns. However, there has been no standard established for screening for behavioral health problems in adult primary care. Indeed, integrated care itself is still at the frontier of clinical science and practice. Although several titles are forthcoming, at the time this chapter was written there has been only one exhaustive text devoted to the issues inherent in assessment in primary care, *Handbook of Psychological Assessment in Primary Care Settings* (Maruish, 2000), which includes one chapter (pp. 115–152; Derogaitis & Lynn, 2000) on the particular issues inherent in screening, although several other chapters are somewhat relevant. We highly recommend these readings to clinicians undertaking an integrated care practice; however, these resources do not address the very practical concerns of developing a screening protocol.

Given that the purpose of this volume is to function as a "toolkit," we will attempt to focus on more practical considerations involved in screening rather than a more scholarly review of available measures, etc., particularly as the latter is greatly dependent on the particular practice in question and such reviews are available in the literature mentioned above and elsewhere. We write this chapter from our perspective as researchers having conducted studies examining the utility of screening for behavioral problems in medical settings and as clinicians having provided direct care in both primary as well as specialty medical care centers. The purpose of this chapter is to discuss issues we consider relevant to the task of screening in medical settings and to make some preliminary recommendations with regard to the implementation of screening procedures; however, we are doing so with full acknowledgment that our comments are without the benefit of sufficient empirical study.

Defining Screening

First and foremost in the discussion of screening in primary care is the necessity of distinguishing between screening and assessment. The nature of screening is to attempt to examine a broad population of people with the intention of detecting those who are most likely to meet diagnostic criterion for a particular problem either now or in the near future (The American Heritage Medical Dictionary, 2007). Screening is intended to be an initial attempt at determining the probability of a person meeting the criterion for a diagnosis, the broadest part of the funnel, and, therefore, is highly susceptible to error. Screening in and of itself cannot, by definition, result in a diagnosis being made. Psychological assessment and diagnosis are clinical activities typically conducted at the level of the individual and with specific hypotheses to be tested with the end goal of establishing a definitive diagnosis(es). By design, screening should be far less time- and labor-intensive than assessment and, as a result, will likely be less precise. It is expected that effective screens will make specificity errors (false positives), but should not make sensitivity errors (false negatives). Assessment devices should not make either kind of error.

While the distinction between screening and assessment may appear academic or semantic, this distinction is important both from a practice and from a legal standpoint. A concern of many medical providers with regard to integrating care is that screening will result in the identification of too many patients with too many concerns than can be further evaluated or treated, the proverbial Pandora's Box, resulting in needs being unmet, the potential of decreased patient (and provider) satisfaction with the provision of care, and even increased risk of malpractice. Differentiating screening and assessment speaks to this concern in several ways.

First, as suggested above, the fact that a person has a positive screen for a particular problem or global level of distress does not constitute meeting diagnostic criterion for a disorder and does not necessarily even compel additional assessment. The provider has exactly the same legal and ethical obligations to treat a person who has been screened as one who has not, as screening does not constitute competent, thorough assessment. Screening simply provides the clinicians with additional data about their patient's functioning that may or may not be pursued in the service of diagnosis and treatment planning.

In fact, even if a patient disclosed a potential concern during screening, it does not even necessarily mean that they would consent to additional assessment or treatment. It may well be the case that a provider might track a potential problem via screening for an extended period of time before the patient progresses to a stage of change corresponding to being willing to pursue the matter further, and neither party (provider or patient) should be compelled by the procedure of screening to deviate from standard clinical care, if they are either not willing or not able to do so. In our respective work, in fact, upwards of 30–50% of patients who indicate a behavioral concern upon screening do not wish to pursue the matter further with their provider at that particular visit. A positive screen might lead to additional assessment, but a determination may be made by the provider whether the assessment should occur during that visit, be scheduled for a future visit, or be referred out to a specialist. Likewise, if the result of the screening is of sufficient concern such that treatment should be initiated, the provider and patient would have the same options: treating within the visit presuming sufficient provider expertise and time for both parties are available, scheduling a new visit for the purpose of initiating treatment, or referring the patient out for treatment and follow-up. Ideally, in a fully integrated setting, the medical provider should be able to make an instant referral to the on-site behavioral health care specialist for collaborative treatment and follow-up of the patient's behavioral concerns. Even if a site is not fully-integrated, the introduction of a behavioral screening procedure should never compel a medical provider to practice outside of his/her scope, although it may well cause them to admit to themselves and their patients that they have limited knowledge of behavioral treatment options and to increase their familiarity with locally available behavioral health resources if co-located services are not available.

In addition, there is considerable evidence in the behavioral medicine literature to suggest that screening for behavioral problems might actually be a powerful first step toward understanding and resolving existing clinical presentations, rather than *opening* a Pandora's Box in primary care and unfurling new and difficult-to-manage concerns within the context of a supposedly circumscribed visit. Therefore, with minimal investment of time or effort, screening offers the opportunity to extend the primary care diagnostic decision tree with little risk and the possibility of great gain for patients and providers. Optimization of this risk to benefit ratio is consistent with the current trend in medicine to reduce medical errors by decreasing the probability of missing a diagnosis that should have been made.

Characteristics of Screening in Primary Care

Mental health professionals are trained to conduct assessments with great care. While the process of screening should also be undertaken carefully, the rigors of the primary care setting necessitate deviations in traditional expectations in several domains.

Primary care screening may take a variety of forms. Screening in integrated care typically involves either the completion of a brief paper and pencil questionnaire or clinical interview, though not uncommonly both are employed. Some practices have moved to technically savvy procedures such as having patients complete screening instruments online prior to their scheduled visit and then e-mailing their responses back for scoring. Of course, this model is only appropriate for particular populations for whom access to and comfort with the Internet are reasonable assumptions to make. Other offices we have seen have a similar procedure, but have patients complete the screening instruments via an electronic kiosk located in a more private corner of the waiting room, thereby eliminating the need for Internet access at home, and with the added bonuses of making the patient's time spent waiting useful and ensuring (or at least increasing the probability that) the patient completes the screener. Despite the availability of high-tech options, most practices employing a behavioral screener are using a paper and pencil questionnaire, so this chapter will make that assumption as well and make suggestions accordingly.

Regardless of how it is administered, it is critical that a screening instrument designed for primary care be easy to administer, complete, and score. While it is the case that the average primary care visit is less than five minutes, it is also the case that there is tremendous variability both between and within medical practices with regard to how long patients wait to be seen.

Timing is Everything

Patients wait an average of 20 minutes to see their doctor (American Medical Association, 2003). Practices vary, however, on where the wait occurs: is it in the waiting room or the exam room itself, and whether the wait happens after the patient has been triaged (vitals, history or complaint taken, etc.) or before. In designing a screening protocol for a particular practice, it is critically important to understand the flow of that practice, being mindful that even providers practicing under the same roof sometimes vary with regard to efficiency and wait times. Furthermore, many practices experience weekly and seasonal fluctuations in their practice patterns, creating changes in their wait times and physician availability. For example, Monday mornings are notoriously busy in most primary care practices, but wait times on Friday afternoons may be equally long because of provider shortages heading into the weekend. It is advised that before implementing screening that a study of patient flow be conducted within the practice for at least a week to determine when and where patients wait to see their primary provider.

The findings from this time-study should then dictate when and where patients should complete screenings, with two primary goals in mind. First, for screening to be successful, patients should not feel that their time is being wasted or their visit lengthened because of being screened. Patients should also feel that ,along with their time, their confidentiality is being respected, and screening should occur in a manner and a context that provides for this need (Robinson & Strosahl, 2000). For example, even if screening is done in the waiting room via questionnaire, confidentiality could be improved by having a cover sheet on top of the screener to hide the patient's responses.

The second goal related to time management in screening is that providers need to have adequate time to score and interpret screenings prior to seeing the patient, as most providers report feeling uncomfortable and inefficient completing those tasks in the exam room. Because of the demands of the primary care setting, it is important to choose a method of screening that is easily scored, ideally via minimal arithmetic and/or visual inspection, and does not demand comparison with norm charts or other ancillary documents in order to be interpreted. In our conversations with providers, regardless of the demonstrated utility of an instrument, if it cannot be administered in less than three minutes and scored/interpreted in less than two minutes, it will not routinely be used in practice unless another multidisciplinary team member (such as a behavioral health specialist) assumes full responsibility for screening.

With these goals in mind, practices may then make strategic decisions with regard to which patients should be screened and how frequently. Depending on the needs and resources of the clinic at a given time, it might be desirable to have a different level of screening. For example, for a clinic that boasts of a full-time co-located behavioral health specialist, both the breadth (more problems) and depth (including problems of lesser severity) of screening could be greater than those in less-equipped settings. For a clinic with few behavioral resources, management might opt for yearly behavioral health screenings or screenings only at physicals and not at sick visits.

Clinics also need to make decisions about which patients will be screened, regardless of behavioral resources. Commonly, clinics will screen patients before they are seen for service and independent of the reason for their visit; however, some opt to screen only when there is either no known medical etiology for the patient's complaint or when the patient's symptoms do not remit as expected, more strongly suggesting a psychological driver. Similarly, clinics may choose to screen at minimum only their highest utilizers, as the data would suggest that they may be more likely to be experiencing anxiety and/or depression (Katon et al., 1990; Von Korff & Simon, 1996). Many clinics do not screen when patients are being seen for follow-up from a previously diagnosed illness, though this practice might be questionable given that patients might be more forthcoming once the acute crisis of their illness has abated. Accordingly, many clinics waive screening when a patient's physical illness is so severe that completing a screen would be arduous; however, clinics vary on whether or not they allow patients to self-select when and whether they complete behavioral screenings, with some practices asserting that obtaining behavioral information is essential to competent clinical care.

Recommended Screening Instruments

In their classic 1989 study, Kroenke and Mangelsdorff first demonstrated that the majority of primary care visits are actually psychosocial in nature, citing that approximately 90% of the ten most common primary care complaints have no known medical etiology. These data, to a large extent, have been supported by subsequent research (e.g. Fries, Bloch, Harrington, Richardson, & Beck, 1993) and provide a basic guideline for what should be screened for in primary care. Based on all available estimates, the most prevalent behavioral problems presented in primary care are anxiety (14% of visits), depression (14% of visits), pain/somatization (18% of visits), and stress/adjustment issues (35% of visits). Accordingly, we suggest that, at minimum, adult primary care clinics screen for these highly prevalent problems. Given that most clinics at least initially integrate care using only a paper and pencil screener, we provide two suggestions for broad-based screening instruments that are designed for and well-tested in primary care settings: The Patient Health Questionnaire (PHQ; Spitzer, Kroenke, & Williams, 1999) and the DUKE (Parkerson, Broadhead, & Tse, 1990).

Patient Health Questionnaire (PHQ). The PHQ was derived from the Primary Care Evaluation of Mental Disorders (PRIME-MD) (Hahn, Kroenke, Williams, & Spitzer, 2000), a screening and diagnosis instrument designed to be administered by primary care physicians. In designing the instrument, the developers of the PRIME-MD (Hahn et al., 2000) determined that a particular domain had to meet several criteria in order to be included. They included behavioral problems that were highly prevalent and could cause impairment in health-related quality of life. Second, they included problems that could be screened for accurately yet within an acceptable level of cost. Third, they focused on problems for which early detection would likely improve treatment outcome. Finally, they included only problems for which an acceptable and effective treatment is available at the time of identification. The PRIME-MD measures five domains: physical symptoms, disordered eating, mood disturbance, anxiety, and substance abuse.

A validation study of the PRIME-MD on 1,000 patients found that nearly half of the patients who screened positive on the PRIME-MD had not been previously recognized by the physician as having a behavioral problem (Spitzer et al., 1994). Furthermore, the PRIME-MD has been shown to have good validity and utility with a sensitivity of 83%, specificity of 88%, and overall accuracy of 86% in comparison to the diagnoses of mental healthcare providers (Hahn et al., 2000). Despite the utility of the PRIME-MD, it was underutilized because of the time required for providers to complete the screening (which included a structured clinical interview), leading to the development of the Patient Health Questionnaire.

The PHQ was developed with the intention of taking the burden of the application time of the screening instrument off the physician and putting it on the patient (Spitzer et al., 1999). The PHQ was constructed with specific identifying questions and skip-outs when criteria are not met. It contains 15 items, many of which have follow-up questions. The PHQ measures the following domains: somatization, major depression, panic, anxiety, bulimia, binge eating, and alcohol abuse.

The PHQ has been found to be equally valid and more time-efficient than the original PRIME-MD (Spitzer et al., 1999). The PHQ has been validated on a sample of 3,000 adult patients (Spitzer et al., 1999). A comparison analysis showed that, in general, the PHQ is less sensitive than the original instrument for broad categories (e.g. "any mood disorder;" p. 1740) but has the tendency to be more sensitive for specific disorders (e.g. "major depressive disorder;" p. 1740). The validation study reported overall accuracy of 85%, sensitivity of 75%, and specificity of 90% when the PHQ results were compared to the diagnoses made by mental health professionals on the basis of a clinical interview. Additionally, the PHQ was found to be comparable to the original clinician-administered PRIME-MD in terms of diagnostic validity. Importantly, comparison of time taken to review the PHQ and the PRIME-MD showed that the PHQ took less than 3 minutes to complete 85% of the time, whereas the PRIME-MD took less than 3 minutes only 16% of the time.

DUKE Health Profile (DUKE; Parkerson et al., 1990). The DUKE is a brief screening questionnaire that has evolved from the Duke-UNC Health Profile (DUHP; Parkerson et al., 1981). Like the PRIME-MD, the original DUHP was criticized for being too cumbersome for the primary care setting. The 17-item DUKE was developed in an effort to better measure health outcomes while respecting the brevity necessary for assessment in the primary care setting (Parkerson et al., 1990).The three domains of the DUKE reflect the recommendation of the World Health Organization (WHO) with regard to dimensions inherent to quality of life: physical, mental, and social health (Parkerson et al., 1990). Aside from the domain scores, the DUKE also produces a general health score, perceived health score, self-esteem score, and individual scores for anxiety, depression, pain, and disability.

A validation study of the DUKE demonstrated sound reliability and validity (Parkerson et al., 1990). More specifically, criterion validity was established with appropriate comparator measures (e.g. Sickness Impact Profile), and discriminative validity established between patient scores across a variety of medical conditions, indicating sensitivity to differences that could be expected between those conditions (e.g. pain patients indicated worse physical health, while mental health patients indicated worse mental health). Further research has identified the anxiety and depression sections of the DUKE (DUKE-AD) as comparable psychometrically, but shorter in length, and therefore preferred for primary care, than the combination of the State Trait Anxiety Inventory (STAI) (Spielberger, Gorsuch, & Lushene. 1970) and the Center for Epidemiologic Studies Depression Scale (CES-D; Radloff, 1977), gold-standard measures of anxiety and depression (Parkerson, Broadhead, & Tse, 1996).

Notably, the DUKE has also been used in the development of predictive models of treatment outcomes for primary care patients. Parkerson, Harrell, Hammond, and Wang, (2001) utilized the DUKE along with an estimate of severity of illness and diagnosis to accurately predict one-year medical outcomes. Further research produced similar results by employing the DUKE alongside age and gender in a predictive model (Parkerson, Hammond, Michener, Yarnall, & Johnson, 2005). Significant implications stem from these studies, as they indicate that the DUKE could be employed as a powerful aid in the identification and treatment of patients who are at a high risk of poorer future health outcomes.

Other Screeners

While the PHQ and the DUKE are highly recommended for general adult outpatient populations, it may well be the case due to physician specialty or the demographic characteristics of a particular patient population that specialty screening instruments should be employed to better detect highly prevalent behavioral problems within that population. For example, a clinic serving a primarily geriatric patient population would be well advised to tailor its screening to include measures of cognitive func tioning. The parameters of this chapter do not permit exploration of screening issues and instruments for particular patient populations; however, these recommendations are more readily gleaned from the extant literature than the more broad-based and practical discussion herein.

Summary and Conclusions

The necessity of screening in developing an integrated care practice is paramount. However, if the screening protocol is not carefully constructed such as to minimize effort and discomfort for both provider and patient, not only will the screening procedures fail to be implemented and relevant behavioral concerns fail to be detected, but the overall attempt at integrating behavioral care will likely fail as well. Simply stated, if problems cannot be detected, they cannot be treated.

That said, there is some limited evidence to suggest that with consideration to setting, timing, and instrumentation, screening can lead to statistically and clinically significant improvements in the detection of behavioral problems and preliminary discussion of those problems with the primary care provider. Additional study is greatly needed to investigate how the presence of a co-located behavioral health specialist could improve upon current models of screening and related treatment, ultimately leading to the establishment of accepted practice standards in the area of integrated care.

As a first step in establishing screening standards, we should first develop standardized and empirically supported screening protocols for specialty care clinics where diagnosis-based psychosocial correlates have already been established, and behavioral support services are more likely to be offered as part of a multidisciplinary team. To that end, the authors have several ongoing research projects examining the utility of screening procedures in outpatient college health centers, and in orthopedic and pediatric primary care settings.

References

Alschuler, K. N., Hoodin, F., & Byrd, M. (2008). Integrated care in a college health center: A preliminary investigation. *Health Psychology, 27*(3), 288–393.

American Heritage Medical Dictionary (2007). Boston: Houghton Mifflin.

American Medical Association (2003). Physician Socioeconomic Statistics, 2003. Chicago: AMA.

Byrd, M. R., & O'Donohue, W. T. (In progress). *Assessing behavioral problems in the primary care setting: The development and preliminary evaluation of the pediatric screening inventory.*

Cowan, P. F., & Morewitz, S. J. (1995). Encouraging discussion of psychosocial issues at student health visits. *Journal of American College Health, 43*, 197–200.

Derogaitis, L. R., & Lynn, L. L. (2000). Screening and monitoring psychiatric disorder in primary care populations. In Maruish, M. (Ed.) Introduction, *Handbook of psychological assessment in primary care settings* (pp. 3–42). Mahwah, NJ: Lawrence Erlbaum Associates.

Fries, J. F., Bloch, D. A., Harrington, H., Richardson, N., & Beck, R. (1993). Two-year results of a randomized controlled trial of a health promotion program in a retiree population: The Bank of America study. *The American Journal of Medicine, 94*, 455–462.

Hahn, S. R., Kroenke, K., Williams, J. B. W., & Spitzer, R. L. (2000). Evaluation of mental disorders with the PRIME-MD. In M. Maruish (Ed.), *Handbook of psychological assessment in primary care settings* (pp. 191–254). Mahwah, NJ: Lawrence Erlbaum Associates.

Katon, W., Von Korff, M., Lin, E., Lipscomb, P., Russo, J., Wagner, E., et al. (1990). Distressed high utilizers of medical care. DSM-III-R diagnoses and treatment needs. *General Hospital Psychiatry*, Nov 12(6), 355–62.

Kroenke, K., & Mandelsdorff, A. D. (1989). Common symptoms in ambulatory care: Incidence, evaluation, therapy, and outcome. *American Journal of Medicine, 86*, 262–266.

Maruish, M. (2000). Introduction. In M. Maruish (Ed.), *Handbook of psychological assessment in primary care settings* (pp. 3–42). Mahwah, NJ: Lawrence Erlbaum Associates.

Parkerson. G. R., Broadhead, W. E., & Tse, C. K. J. (1990). The Duke health profile: A 17-item measure of health and dysfunction. *Medical Care, 28*, 1056–1072.

Parkerson. G. R., Broadhead, W. E., & Tse, C. K. J. (1996). anxiety and depressive symptom identification using the duke health profile. *Journal of Clinical Epidemiology, 49*, 85–93.

Parkerson, G. R., Gehlbach, S. H., Wagner, E. H., James, S. A., Clapp, N. E., & Muhlbaier, L. H. (1981). The Duke –UNC Health Profile: An adult health status instrument for primary care. *Medical Care, 19*, 806–828.

Parkerson, G. R., Hammond, W. E., Michener, J. L., Yarnall, K. S. H., & Johnson, J. L. (2005). Risk classification of adult primary care patients by self-reported quality of life. *Medical Care, 43*, 189–193.

Parkerson, G. R., Harrell, F. E., Hammond, W. E., & Wang, X. Q. (2001). Characteristics of adult primary care patients as predictors of future health services charges. *Medical Care, 39*, 1170–1181.

Radloff, L. (1977). The CES-D scale: A self-report depression scale for research in the general population. *Applied Psychological Measurement, 1*, 385–401.

Robinson, P., & Strosahl, K. (2000). Improving care for a primary care population: Depression as an example. In M. Maruish (Ed.), *Handbook of Psychological Assessment in Primary Care Settings* (pp. 687–711). Mahwah, NJ: Lawrence Erlbaum Associates.

Spielberger, C. D., Gorsuch, R. C., & Lushene, R. E. (1970). *Manual for the State Trait Anxiety Inventory*. Palo Alto, CA: Consulting Psychologists Press

Spitzer, R. L., Kroenke, K., & Williams, J. B. W. (1999). Validation and utility of a self-report version of PRIME-MD: The PHQ Primary Care Study. *Journal of the American Medical Association, 282*, 1737– 1744.

Spitzer, R. L., Williams, J. B. W., Kroenke, K., Linzer, M., deGruy, F. V., Hahn, S. R., et al. (1994). Utility of a new procedure for diagnosing mental disorders in primary care: The PRIME-MD 1000 Study. *Journal of the American Medical Association, 272*, 1749– 1756.

von Korff, M. & Simon, G. (1996). The relationship between pain and depression. *British Journal of Psychiatry, 30*, Suppl, 101–108.

Part II
Toolbox for Integrated
Consultation-Liaison Services:
Guidelines and Handouts

The Primary Care Consultant Toolkit: Tools for Behavioral Medicine

Erica M. Jarrett

Basic Facts About Depression in Primary Care

Depression is one of the most common disorders seen in primary medical care clinics, and more patients are treated for depression by primary care providers than by mental health specialists (Katon, 1987; Regier et al., 1993). Research indicates that the general medical practitioner exclusively delivers half of all the formal mental health care in the United States (Narrow et al., 1993). Primary care providers are the sole contacts for more than 50% of patients with mental illness and have thus been described as the defacto system of treatment for mental health (Callahan et al., 1996). Reliable estimates suggest that symptoms consistent with depression are present in nearly 70% of patients who visit primary care providers. Approximately 35% of patients who are seen in primary care meet criteria for being diagnosed with some form of depression, with 10% of patients suffering from major depression. The prevalence of major depression is 2 to 3 times higher in primary care patients than in the overall population, because depressed persons use health care more frequently (Regier et al., 1993).

In outpatient primary care settings, the incidence of depression by type breaks down as the following: major depression, 4.8–8.6%; dysthymia, 2.1–3.7%; and minor depression, 8.4–9.7% (Katon & Schulberg, 1992).Thus, the total for all types of depression comes to 15.3–22% of all patients seen in primary care offices. These numbers are supported by findings of site studies, in which investigators administered depression self-rating scales, combined with structured psychiatric interviews, to all primary care patients during office visits for any reason (Katon & Schulberg, 1992).

Despite the high prevalence of depression in primary care settings, it is estimated that only one-third of the patients with depressive symptoms are properly diagnosed by primary care physicians (Budman & Butler, 1997; Munoz, Hollon, McGrath,

E.M. Jarrett (✉)
Chief, Primary Care Psychology Service, Department of Internal Medicine, Walter Reed Army Medical Center, Washington, DC, USA
e-mail: erica.jarrett@amedd.army.mil

L.C. James, W.T. O'Donohue (eds.), *The Primary Care Toolkit*,
DOI 10.1007/978-0-387-78971-2_11, © Springer Science+Business Media, LLC 2009

Rhem, & VandenBos, 1994) and as many as 50% are incorrectly identified as depressed by primary care doctors (Perez-Stable, Miranada, Munoz, & Ying, 1990). Even fewer patients who are incorrectly identified as clinically depressed receive treatment (Kupfer, & Freedman, 1986). Studies show that primary care physicians who provide usual care fail to recognize depressive symptoms in 30–50% of patients with depression (Katon & Schulberg, 1992). What is being missed is not a small problem here and there, but a range of disorders, some of which—such as major depression—occur frequently and can be quite severe.

Physicians may have a challenging time recognizing depression in primary care, because patients, especially men, rarely describe emotional difficulties spontaneously. On the contrary, patients with depression who present themselves to a primary care physician often describe somatic symptoms such as fatigue, sleep problems, pain, or multiple vague symptoms (Sharp, Martin, & Lipsky 2002). In primary care, presenting complaints for psychological problems are more likely to be somatic than psychological. Back pain, chest pain, problems with sleep or appetite, and fatigue are among the most frequent presenting symptoms (Hirschfeld, 2001).

If unrecognized and undiagnosed, depression can contribute to high medical utilization in the primary care setting. Twenty-four percent of high utilizers (the top 10%) have been found to suffer from current major depression (Katon,Von Korff, & Lin 1990). The clinical implications of elevated rates of depression in primary care settings are important and multifaceted. These implications include: (1) increased health care costs, (2) impaired quality of life, and (3) adverse progression of co-morbid diseases. (Simon, Revicki, & Heilgenstein, 2000; McQuaid, Stein, Laffaye, & MCCahill, 1999).

Multiple reasons may account for the under-diagnosis/under-treatment of depression, including (1) physician under-estimation of adverse effects of depression on medical condition; (2) the somatic presentation of depression in the primary setting; (3) time constraints associated with assessment in primary care setting; or (4) lack of awareness of treatment options (Kop, 2001). The prevalence of depressive disorders, coupled with the inaccuracy of identification and lack of effective care provision, indicates a clear need for psychologists to address the problems of assessment and treatment of depression in primary care practice settings.

The integration of behavioral health care specialists as part of the treatment team in the primary care setting is integral in treating depression in primary care. Psychologists contribute to the care of patients in primary care by providing assessment, treatment, consultative and educational services (Freedland, Carney, & Skala, 2004). The integration of behavioral health assessments and services into primary care setting is an excellent mechanism both for providing quality care and for improving the health of a population. As a primary care consultant integrated into primary care, one will be able to (1) improve the recognition of behavioral health needs, (2) improve collaborative care and management of patients with psychosocial issues in primary care, (3) serve as an internal resource for primary care providers to address behavioral and mental health concerns, (4) provide immediate access to a consultation with rapid feedback, and (5) prevent more serious mental disorders through early recognition and intervention.

How to Effectively Screen and Assess for Depression in Primary Care

The need to assess for depressive symptoms in primary care has been documented. More specifically, in 2002 the US Preventive Service Task Force endorsed screening for depression in primary care settings, particularly when screening is coupled with a system that helps ensure adequate treatment and follow-up (Pignone, Gaynes, Rushton et al., 2002). Research has shown that successful screening, diagnosis, and management of patients with depression is best achieved through a multifaceted approach, with the use of standardized screening and assessment tools, and in most cases a combination of medication and counseling with close ongoing cooperation between primary care and mental health professionals (Pignone, Gaynes, Rushton et al., 2002). Moreover, the capacity to sustain successful diagnosis and treatment approaches often include integration of clinical and economic systems at multiple levels and engagement of multiple stakeholders including patients, providers, practices, health plans, and purchasers (Robinson & Reiter, 2007). It is vital that we address these challenges to improve care for persons with depression. A critical first step is to assist primary care physicians and psychologists in using the most efficient and effective approaches to screening, diagnosis, and care for patients with depression in the primary care setting.

Self-report measures can be important for a variety of reasons. Brief measures can be used to help detect behavioral problems that might otherwise go unnoticed. They can also be useful for planning individualized interventions and evaluating the impact of the interventions in follow-up (Robinson & Reiter, 2007). There are numerous assessment tools for identifying and tracking depressive symptoms. According to a review by Schade, Jones, and Wittlin (1998), the most extensively studied questionnaires are the Geriatric Depression Scale (Yesavage et al., 1982), the Beck Depression Inventory (Beck, Ward, Mendelson, Mock, & Erbaugh, 1961), the General Health Questionnarie (Goldberg & Blackwell, 1970), the Zung Depression Scale (Zung, 1965) and the Center for Epidemiological Studies Depression Scale (CES-D) (Radloff, 1977). Some of these are used in the context of making formal research diagnosis, while others are tailored to different theoretical models for depression.

However, it is important to note that patients in the primary setting tend to present differently than patients in the outpatient mental health, for which most of these previous instruments were developed. Therefore it is important to use measures that not only have been validated in primary care, but can also be used at follow-up visits to evaluate effectiveness of treatment. Additionally, it is also important to choose an instrument that best fits the patient population served and the practice setting.

Robinson & Reiter (2007) offer the following characteristics that are most desirable when selecting a measure to be used in primary care:

- *Brevity.* Both psychologist and primary care physician visit require brief measures. Questionnaires with more than 20 items are probably too lengthy.
- *High quality.* Psychologists are trained to be very selective in the assessment instruments they use, and for good reason. In the primary care clinic, measures

chosen will be completed by thousands of patients, and they will often play a central role in treatment planning. Be sure to examine carefully the psychometrics of all measures being considered for use.

- *Appropriate reading level.* A widely used measure should probably require a maximum of eighth-grade reading skills. Patients who are unable to read may not convey this to the psychologist, choosing instead to answer randomly or only selected questions.
- *Easy to score.* This is related to the brevity concept in that measures requiring a lot of time to score are not usually feasible in primary care.
- *Available for free or at a low cost.* Owing to the volume of patients seen, clinics will burn through copies of the measures in quick time. For this reason, measures available free of cost publicly, such as via download from the Internet, are suggested.

Developing a Team Approach to Utilizing a Depression Screening Tool

Primary care clinics rely on smooth running—teamwork. Physicians, nurses, medical technicians, other health care providers, office managers, and receptionists all perform interrelated duties to ensure quality care for patients (Gatchel & Oordt, 2002). Due to the collaborative nature of primary care, a team approach to depression screening may be warranted. Successful planning for a primary care-based screening may require a check-list that relies on clear answers to who, when, where, how, and how much time with regard to the logistics of depression screening. Robinson & Reiter (2007) have provided excellent questions a psychologist may want to answer prior to implementing depression screening in primary care.

1. *Who will ask the screening or assessment questions?* Support staff selected for this task (often medical/nursing assistants) should be trained in utilizing the screening tool, and be responsible for maintaining the supply of measures and keeping them well-organized.
2. *When will the screening or assessment occur?* Should it be done as needed, when a problem is suspected or identified? Or could it be done routinely, which is most workable for the clinic?
3. *Where will screening occur, and where will any paper measures be stored?* Completion of measures usually occurs in exam rooms, but it could be done it the waiting room or as part of the vital-sign screening.
4. *How will screening and assessment results be scored, communicated to providers, and entered into the medical records?* Clinics using electronic measures may want to build room for screener scores in provider templates or even have the patient complete the screener on the computer in the waiting room.
5. *How much time will screening and assessment require?* Measurement activities for PCP visits, including administration, scoring, and documentation should require less than 5 minutes to meet the PCP feasibility criteria.

Once these questions are answered, then it will be important to identify a system that helps ensure adequate treatment and follow-up of those individuals who are screened positive for symptoms of depression. For example, General Internal Medicine at WRAMC has developed a team approach with the Primary Care Psychology Service utilizing a depression screening tool. Patients are routinely screened for depression when they present to the nurse or LPN to have their vital signs recorded during their office visit; the patient's emotional health is considered the "eighth vital sign" and therefore incorporates the biopsychosocial model of health.

Patients are screened utilizing a standardized primary care depression screening tool; the PHQ-2. A physician is notified if the patient scores positive on the screen for depression. The patient is offered a same-day appointment with a psychologist for further evaluation of his/her symptoms. If the patient is amenable to a same-day evaluation, a behavioral health consultation is conducted. The psychologist submits his/her findings in the patient's electronic medical chart and then provides face to face feed back to the physician; a collaborative plan is discussed and implemented to effectively manage the patient's depressive symptoms.

Depression Screening Measures

Depression screening measures do not diagnose depression, but they do provide an indication of the severity of symptoms, and assess the severity within a given period of time (e.g. 7 to 14 days). Once there is a clinical suspicion that depression plays a role in a particular patient's problem, it is important to identify reliable, accurate ways of confirming the diagnosis and monitoring the patient's progress over time. Identifying psychometrically sound user-friendly tools that give clinically useful information for a variety of patients and settings when administered by different clinicians (i.e. either physician or psychologist) is imperative. The primary objective is to use a standardized instrument that will quantify and document future progress, and allow different disciplines to effectively communicate their findings to one another while they collaborate to effectively address the depressive symptoms.

Four depression screening measures, PHQ-2, PHQ-9, BDI-2, and GDS, are recommended based on their validation in a primary setting and utility in follow-up care. These depression screening tools can be easily incorporated into primary care, despite a clinician's busy schedule, or into a psychologist's evaluation/collaborative care.

The PHQ-2 is an abbreviated version of the PHQ-9. It is characterized as the sum of the anhedonia and mood items of the PHQ-9 and can be used as a very brief depression screening tool in primary care. The use of the following two screening questions alone have shown a sensitivity and specificity of 97% and 67%, respectively, when tested in a primary care setting on patients not receiving psychotropic drugs (Aroll, Khin, & Kerse, 2003).

1. Have you been bothered by little interest or pleasure in doing things?
2. Have you been feeling down, depressed, or hopeless in the last month?

If a patient responds positively to these two questions, only four follow-up questions—on sleep disturbance, appetite change, low self-esteem, and anhedonia—are needed to confirm a diagnosis of depression. If a patient has a positive response on at least two of these four questions, the specificity of a positive test increases to 94%. The PHQ-2 also performed quite well as a depression-screening tool with nearly identical performance to the PHQ-9 in identifying subjects with any form of depression.

The PHQ-9 has been validated for screening, diagnosis, evaluation of severity, monitoring response to therapy, and determining remission. Adult patients with grade 4 English literacy skills can complete the form in less than 3 minutes (Griever, Anderson, & Baumgarten, 2005). Clinicians can score it quickly and easily and can then use the answers to direct the course of the consultation. The sensitivity and specificity of the PHQ-9 compare favorably with a structured psychiatric interview. Compared with the HAM-D7, the PHQ-9 is much faster and easier for physicians to administer and is, therefore, more likely to be adopted in busy primary care practices (Griever, Anderson, & Baumgarten, 2005). The PHQ-9 also offers a severity score for each symptom, and hence can also be used to follow outcome.

The BDI-II is a 21-item self-report measure of the severity of depressive symptoms of depression. It has high sensitivity and specificity and is valid and reliable in assessing the severity of the symptoms. Among its shortcomings are its high item difficulty and poor discriminant validity against anxiety.

The Geriatric Depression Scale (GDS) is a self-report measure designed to minimize the impact of somatic symptoms associated with aging and illness. It has a yes/no format, and the 15-item version, using a cutoff of five, has good sensitivity and positive predictive values for diagnosis of major depression (Anderson, Michalak, & Lam, 2002).

On a day-to-day basis, use of the two PRIME-MD PHQ-2 screening questions followed by either the rest of the clinician-administered PRIME-MD or the self-report PHQ-9, remains the briefest, simplest, and the most accurate way to diagnose major depression in an adult population (Sharp, Martin, & Lipsky 2002). Using the self-report BDI or the PHQ-9 to follow scores at baseline and designated follow-up intervals is an accurate and reliable strategy that allows to identify those individuals who are unresponsive to treatment and/or require further intervention or consultation. Consistent use of this systematic approach to depression management can improve diagnostic accuracy, save time, help choose appropriate treatment interventions, and effectively monitor outcomes. This approach should also allow further reduction of the significant burden associated with depression in primary care.

Diagnostic Issues of Depression in Primary Care (Medical or Pharmacological Factors at Play?)

Psychologists in primary care must be prepared to see mood disorders ranging from mild adjustment reactions to severe forms of depression, both in otherwise healthy and medically ill patients (Freedland, Carney, & Skala,2004). Additionally, a psychologist practicing in a primary care setting needs to be aware of the close link between physical disease and depression. Therefore, it is paramount that a psychologist in primary care is able to make a gross distinction between physical disease illnesses that may have a psychological component and those that are entirely psychological in nature (Robinson & James, 2002).

A range of medical conditions are associated with depression, highlighting the importance of thorough physical examinations and basic investigations. The more common conditions associated with depression include endocrine disorders (hypothyroidism, hyperthyroidism, Cushing's disease and Addison's disease), infections (infectious mononucleosis, influenza, tertiary syphilis and AIDS), neurological disorders (multiple sclerosis, Parkinson's disease), and cerebrovascular disorders (Ellen, Norman, & Burrows, 1998). Underlying malignancies should also be considered. Alternatively, depression may be a direct consequence of the physical illness. Both Cushing's disease and hypothyroidism are well-known examples of endocrinopathies for which depression may be the first manifestation.

Medications may cause symptoms (also known as adverse reactions or side effects), and at times these symptoms may be psychological, behavioral, or emotional (Gunning, 2004). In addition to directly causing psychological symptoms, medications may produce symptoms in several other ways by unmasking an underlying disorder, by interacting with other medications, when overdosed, or when discontinued (Gunning, 2004). It is therefore essential that a careful medication history is elicited.

The list of drugs suspected of causing depression is long. The patient's medication history should be reviewed thoroughly for classes of agents known to cause depression, such as interferon, isotretinoin, benzodiapines, B-blockers and sleep aids containing diphenhydramine (Baron, 2003). Additionally, drugs commonly associated with depression are antihypertensive agents, corticosteroids, oral contraceptives, and antineoplastic agents (Ellen, Norman, & Burrows, 1998). Recreational drugs such as alcohol and amphetamines can cause depression either during intoxication or during withdrawal (Ellen, Norman, & Burrows, 1998).

Careful questioning about the timing of the drug dose in relation to the symptoms is important. A carefully taken history will dictate the next step: If symptoms preceded the start of the medication, it should probably not be the focus of subsequent management strategies (Baron, 2003). However, if mood changes appeared after the patient began taking the medication, it might be appropriate to recommend to the physician changing the dosage or switching to another agent (Baron, 2003).

What is Effective Consultation/Liasion for Depression in Primary Care?

The culture of primary care is distinct from other health care settings in which a psychologist may work. Primary care settings are marked by brief visits, frequent interruptions, and emphasis on rapid diagnosis and treatment planning (Cowley, Katon, & Veith, 2000). Psychologists working in such environments are expected to be prompt, clear, and directive in their recommendations. The approaches for providing psychological service in primary care tend to fall on a continuum. Gatchel & Oordt (2002) have described a number of models (e.g. Co-located Clinics Model, Psychologist as Provider Model, Behavioral Health Consultant Model, Faculty Advisor Model, and Combination Models) that have been used for integrated care with varying levels of medical–behavioral collaboration. Overall, each of the models highlight that psychologists who are integrated into a primary care setting will need specific skills to adapt to that setting (Gatchel & Oordt, 2002). These skills will be highlighted in the context of managing depression in primary care.

Due to the diversity of models that exist for collaborating in primary care, it is important to highlight the model for managing depression that will be discussed in this chapter. The Behavioral Health Consultant Model will be utilized in this discussion of managing depression in primary care. It is a model in which the psychologist is a member of the primary care management team and is called on to provide expertise for behavioral, emotional, and psychosocial aspects of the health care plan (Gatchel & Oordt, 2002). The behavioral health consultant sees patients for evaluation and makes recommendations to the primary care manager. The behavioral health consultant may follow the patient to monitor implementation of the recommendations, but in most cases, will limit contact to four to eight sessions over the course of one to two months. In seeing the patient for follow-up, the primary care consultant collaborates by providing psychological and behavioral interventions while maintaining communications about the patient's progress and treatment plan with the physician, who remains the primary decision-maker (Gatchel & Oordt, 2002). In situations in which more definite mental health care is needed, the behavioral health consultant makes the recommendation to the primary care manager and facilitates the referral.

When Is It Appropriate to Use the Behavioral Consultant Model to Manage Depression in Primary Care?

In the primary care setting, effective practice management skills require a primary care consultant to see 10–12 (and often more) patients in a practice day, to stay on time and to monitor clinical response in a time-efficient manner (Strosahl, 2005). The fast pace of primary care setting dictates the use of efficacious, problem focused, and efficient intervention strategies; a strong background in cognitive-behavioral approaches is essential.

It is also important to have sharp diagnostic skills to differentiate early in the consultation process patients appropriate for working in the primary care setting from those needing specialty care. (Etherage, 2005). The goal in an initial consultation visit is a quick triage analysis of the likelihood of the patient benefitting from primary behavioral health consultant services. There are a number of potential indicators which may suggest that the individual may not be appropriate for the Behavioral Health Consultant Model. Steenbarger, Greenberg, and Dewan (2004), through a review of practice, as well as research, on short-term work, have highlighted a number of factors that should be kept in mind when determining a client's appropriateness for active short-term therapy. Many elements in short-term therapy are reflective of the behavioral health consultant model. Therefore, this model can also be applied when conducting an initial evaluation. Steenbarger, Greenberg & Dewan (2004) came up with a template (DISCUS) to be used as a useful heuristic in patient selection. Some elements in this template include

- *Duration of the presenting problem*—When a problem pattern is chronic, it has been overlearned and often will require more extensive intervention than a pattern that is recent and situational.
- *Interpersonal history*—In order for therapy to proceed time-effectively, a rapid alliance between therapist and patient is a necessity. If the client's interpersonal history includes significant incidents of abuse, neglect, or violence, it may take many sessions before adequate trust and disclosures can develop.
- *Severity of the presenting problems*—A severe disorder is one that interferes with many aspects of the client's life. Such severity often also interferes with the individual's ability to actively employ therapeutic strategies between sessions, a key element in accelerating change.
- *Complexity*—A highly complex presenting concern, one that has many symptomatic manifestations, often requires more extensive intervention than highly focal problem patterns.
- *Understanding*—Brief therapy tends to be most helpful for patients who have a clear understanding of their problems and a strong motivation to address these concerns.
- *Social Support*—Many clients enter therapy for ongoing support. While social support is a necessary and legitimate end of psychotherapy, situations requiring extensive support will necessarily preclude highly abbreviated course of treatment.

These six criteria represent a useful heuristic when determining a patient's appropriateness for working in the primary care setting. The presence of multiple DISCUS criteria at consultation is almost certain to identify a situation in which treatment using a consultation model, such as the behavioral health consultant model, will raise odds of future relapse (Steenbarger, 1994). The behavioral health consultant model requires a high degree of activity for both parties. Therefore, it is of paramount importance to assess the ability and willingness of the patient to engage in hands-on effort at change.

Treatment of Depression in Primary Care

Interventions utilized by a behavioral health consultant are generally behaviorally focused and brief (Gatchel & Oordt, 2004). Therefore, a solid foundation in cognitive behavioral theory and practice as it is applied to depression, is likely to be useful.

Cognitive behavioral theory fits the existing methods of working in primary care quite closely in that problems can be defined and conceptualized in operational and functional terms (France & Robson, 1998). A typical cognitive behavior therapy (CBT) functional analysis has three components including problem specification, hypothesis generation, and identification/teaching of alternative behaviors. The concept of functional analysis tends to fit well in the behavioral health environment, where primary care physicians focus on functioning (Robinson & Reiter, 2007). It allows the primary care psychologist to offer the patient a clear plan that can be supported well by a PCP and fits the time constraints of the primary care setting (Robinson & Reiter, 2007).

The overall aim of cognitive behavior therapy in the management of depression in primary care is to help patients achieve a remission of depression by solving problems and reducing symptoms. Specifically, CBT encourages the behavioral health consultant to diagnose possible dysfunctions by assessing how a person appraises the world, solves interpersonal problems, and navigates the social environment (Clabby, 2006). It is practical, active, and problem oriented CBT aims to teach patients skills to cope more effectively (Clabby, 2006). This is achieved through a collaborative, empirical approach, which teaches patients to view reality more clearly through an examination of their central distorted cognitions (Beck & Bieling, 2004).

Traditional CBT treatments for depression typically focus on strategies to identify dysfunctional thinking, to generate alternatives to ineffective thought processes, and to have patients identify/document their thoughts so that they might eventually alter their negative cognitions (Callaghan & Gregg, 2006). CBT approaches also include teaching the patient a stepwise problems-solving strategy such as defining the problem, identifying clear goals, and brainstorming solutions. Finally, the last major goal of CBT is to behaviorally activate the patient; focusing on the patient's level of activity helps them identify and engage in actions that are more likely to reduce depression(Callaghan & Gregg, 2006). This has the simultaneous effect of raising the patient's energy level, directly countering some of their distorted thinking, providing a sense of pleasure and mastery, and reducing their sense of hopelessness (Beck & Bieling, 2004).

It is very important to note that, in managing a patient with depression in primary care, all of the CBT concepts are not expected to be utilized in a behavioral consultation. However, it is essential that a behavioral health consultant develop a menu of CBT concepts and techniques and select the simplest and most practical CBT procedures from this menu that best fit their personal style and patient population. In addition, given the short amount of time for intervention, more extensive handouts than the ones typically used in specialty mental health practices are recommended (Rowan & Runyan, 2005). Handouts used in primary care need to be like "self help literature." They need to be concise, but provide all the details necessary to do it "on your own."

Additionally, to increase the likelihood of following through on intervention recommendations, it is important that the behavioral health consultant utilizes a "behavioral prescription pad" (See Appendix 1. Behavioral Rx: Used with permission of USAF Behavioral Health Optimization Program), goal setting forms, and written relapse plans.

Elements of an Effective Primary Care Consultation

There are two basic types of consultation services in primary care: brief and continuity (US Air Force Medical Operations Agency Population Health Support Division, 2002). Brief are time-limited and usually appropriate for primary care patients who are more functional, and continuity consultations serve primary care patients who require more assistance, but are best treated in primary care versus specialty services in mental health clinic (US Air Force Medical Operations Agency Population Health Support Division, 2002). They are appropriate for patients with psychological conditions and/or medical conditions who require a continual, intermittent consultative approach (US Air Force Medical Operations Agency Population Health Support Division, 2002). Given that depression often occurs on a continuum, each of these consultation services may be applied to manage depression in primary care.

The initial consultation visits for depression are significantly shorter than the typical mental health intake. This requires the consultant to align quickly with the patient, conduct rapid appropriate diagnostic and functional assessments, limit the scope of the target problem, and select bite-sized, behaviorally oriented interventions that can be supported by any team member (Strosahl, 2005). The initial consultation visit is structured in three phases: the introduction, the assessment, and the interventions (Etherage, 2005).

Rowan & Runyan (2005) provide an excellent example of the phases of a 30-minute initial appointment.

1. Introduction of behavioral health consultation service and the provider, linking the general process to quality health care (2–5 minutes)
2. Identifying/clarifying consultation problem (10–60 seconds)
3. Conducting functional analysis of the problem (12–15 minutes)
4. Summarizing the understanding of the problem (1–2 minutes)
5. Starting a behavioral or cognitive change plan (7–10 minutes)

In primary care it is difficult and disadvantageous to separate assessment and therapy in the conventional sense owing to time constraints resulting from the fast pace. Therefore, one of the special characteristics of offering a cognitive behavioral approach in this setting is that any session will be a mixture of assessment and education in the model and treatment (France & Robson, 1998).

Assessment Phase

Initial assessment of depression involves a cognitive conceptualization of the patient's depressive episode. An accurate conceptualization helps the behavioral consultant to organize the multitude of data presented by the patient to identify the patient's most central dysfunctional cognitions and behaviors. It also allows the consultant to select key thoughts, beliefs, and behaviors to target for change (Beck & Bieling, 2004).

Often the initial contact serves to define or structure the problem into the behavioral, cognitive, and physiological components and their interactions (France & Robson, 1998). The patient should be asked to describe precisely the frequency and intensity of the depressive symptoms and give an idea of why he/she has come for help at this time. Next, the precipitating factors or the unique stressors or events that have triggered the current episode of depression should be identified (Beck & Bieling, 2004). Once a clear description has been obtained, it is worth summarizing this with the patient who will thus be able to confirm that it is correct, and will probably be reassured that his or her difficulty has been understood.

Next, a functional analysis of the depressive episode is conducted. The object is to discover the factors currently maintaining the depressive episode, in what way is it interfering with the patient's life, and also whether its persistence is serving any useful purpose for him or for others (France & Robson, 1998). The object of the functional analysis is to look at the target problem or behavior in relation to its antecedents and consequences. Each of these factors increases or decreases the behavior and makes it more likely that it will occur either externally (overtly) in the outside world or internally (covertly) in the thoughts and feelings of the patient.

Assessing the patient's strengths and skills is an important part of assessment for two reasons. First, it is useful to note how aware the patient is about his/her good points and how ready he/she is to talk about them; the discovered assets will often be used in a subsequent treatment plan. It is also useful to inquire about past activities which have now been discontinued. This often serves to demonstrate how changes in life style have contributed to the current difficulties, and the reintroduction of these or related activities will be a goal in the treatment of depression.

Psycho-Education Interventions (Treatment Rationale and Medication Use)

The rationale of how depression comes about and how it can be treated often brings hope. As mentioned previously, due to the time constraints in primary care, there is a blending of both assessment and intervention at initial contact. Therefore in that first contact an active intervention should be conducted. An active intervention such as teaching the patient about the causes of depression can be done; this may be done concomitantly with the use of a handout (See Appendix 2). For example, an explanation that depression is influenced by a number of factors (e.g. thoughts, emotions, and behaviors) and each factor can affect the others. Additionally, it should also be explained that in a depressive cycle, one's thoughts, emotions, and behaviors can lead him/her to feel worse and do less. It should be highlighted that changing any one or several of the different areas including thoughts, emotions, and behaviors can be helpful to help the person feel and function more they way they would like to.

If the patient meets criteria for major depression, suggest the use of medication as a way to help with the neurovegatative symptoms, which may, make it easier to follow-through on the behaviors and change in thinking. Most patients tend to discontinue medication owing to side effects or misconceptions about how quickly the medication should affect symptoms. Therefore, providing a handout explaining the medication and its effectiveness in the treatment, as well as, important information for people starting on antidepressant medication would be useful (See Appendix 3. Important Information for People Starting Antidepressant Medication: Used with premission of USAF Behavioral Health Optimization Program).

Behavioral Interventions

The next step to focus on in the interventional strategy is behavioral activation. Explain to the patient that as people become more depressed they generally cut out fun and enjoyable activities. Help the patient develop several fun or enjoyable activities they will start. Write them on a piece of paper and write specific days and times to start and finish. Explain that increased physical activity can play a significant role in improving concentration, sleep, and energy. Start the patient on a physical activity program. Have them pick specific days, times and what they will do (walking is usually a good activity to start with). The objective is to increase the patient's present activity level and to expand the patient's positive activities by carefully graded tasks.

Cognitive Strategy Interventions

The role of cognition can play a central role in promoting depressive symptoms. Therefore, explaining the role of thinking as it relates to depressed mood is paramount. It will be necessary to emphasize that thinking patterns and interpretation of events affect mood. Introduce the concept of self talk and highlight that what we say to ourselves about life's events and how we interpret them powerfully affect how we feel. It would also be helpful to develop a handout on cognitive factors involved in depression (See Appendix 4. Thinking and Stress: Used with premission of USAF Behavioral Health Optimization Program). Many patients get depressed because they habitually use self critical language or overgeneralize the implications of a negative event. This habit greatly increases a distressing event's emotional toxicity (Clabby, 2006). They maintain perceptions that, frankly, are just not true (e.g. " I can't stand this"), thus sinking further into the quagmire of negative emotions.

A start is then made on training the patient to identify, count, and challenge negative automatic thoughts. This again is largely between sessions but guidance as to the procedures will be necessary. The objectives are to recognize and modify negative and distorted thinking patterns and modify rigid and unhelpful life rules and assumptions.

The hallmark of CBT approach is teaching patient to avoid perceiving or judging situations as "terrible" or "awful" or "catastrophic" or "impossible to handle" (Clabby, 2006). CBT maintains that such extreme interpretations and judgments can occur quickly and can be psychologically toxic, leading a person to feel depressed. The CBT approach helps patient recognize that forming these harsh perceptions is harmful and teaches them to use more realistic and factual appraisal of events (Clabby, 2006).

There are a number of different techniques that can be used, but most revolve around four groups of questions:

1. Does the evidence support the way you think or oppose it? What objective evidence do you have to back it up? Would some one else accept that evidence?
2. What are the alternative explanations? Is there another more positive alternative?
3. What is the effect of thinking this way? Does it help the situation? Does it help you get what you want out of life or is it getting in your way? Is there a more constructive way of thinking?
4. What thinking errors are you making?

Follow-Up Visits

CBT procedures can be offered singly or in various combinations in one or several patient visits. BHC follow-ups that will be utilized are similar in structure to a typical CBT follow-up. Specifically, the appointment begins by assessing how the patient did on the task from the last appointment (Rowan & Runyan, 2005). The impacts of these efforts on his/her depressive symptoms is then determined, and the need for additional skill training is assessed. If there is a need for additional intervention, it will be conducted and the task for the next follow-up period is discussed (Rowan & Runyan, 2005).

There is compelling evidence that CBT works in primary care. The CBT techniques described here are drawn from that tradition. Although it may seem that this approach is too complex and time-consuming to be easily adaptable to the primary care setting, there are several advantages (Paykel & Priest, 1992).

1. The techniques are easily broken down for the use in very short contact sessions. For example, one thought or thinking error can be examined at a time.
2. The individual techniques can be usefully employed without a commitment to the whole package being necessary. For example, with the severely depressed, much time may have to be spent in activity recording and scheduling, whereas the cognitive elements of thought stopping and the corrections of thinking errors can often be introduced more rapidly with mildly depressed often seen in primary care.
3. Much of the work is done by the patient between sessions.

Consultation Skills

In the behavioral health consultant model, the behavioral health consultant does not retain responsibility of the patient. Therefore any assessment or intervention needs to be coordinated closely with the PCM and this is crucial in the practice of a behavioral health consultant (Etherage, 2005). Communicating back to the primary care physician is one of the primary care consultant's highest priorities (US Air Force Medical Operations Agency Population Health Support Division, 2002). In primary care, it is necessary to provide both written and oral feedback for the PCP; feed back is best given the same day the person is seen (US Air Force Medical Operations Agency Population Health Support Division, 2002). Oral feedback can take the form of a quick "curbside" consult (immediately following a patient visit) or other flexible approaches toward communication such as using e-mail (only over LAN or secure channels) or telephone contact (Cowley, Katon, & Vieth, 2000). Written feedback can be placed in the medical record as a SOAP note. In the plan section of the SOAP note, the behavioral health consultant can advise the PCP regarding specific strategies recommended during the behavioral health consultation visit (Etherage, 2005).

Other Keys To Supporting the PCP

This model is designed to increase collaboration between medical and behavioral health providers and support the delivery of specialty behavioral health care. Within that vein, there are a number of things a primary care consultant can do to help PCP succeed in this primary care team-based approach. These include teaching the PCP how to give psycho-education information about antidepressants, providing scripts on how to refer patients, and recommendations for the PCP.

Psycho-Education About Medication

Adherence to medication is alarmingly low. As many as half of all primary care patients receiving a psychoactive drug will discontinue after 30 days (Robinson, Wischman, & Del Vento, 1996). This occurs in part because patients are not provided education about the antidepressant they are prescribed. It would be helpful to train the PCP how to provide education about antidepressants in the form of a few basic brief tips to be provided to the patient regarding antidepressant medication, which include statements such as:

- Your response will be gradual, and the medication will take two to six weeks to work.
- The first week you may expect your sleep and appetite to improve. It may take a few weeks for mood and energy to improve and negative thinking to decrease.
- Take your medication every day. Based on the side effects, it may work better to take it in the morning or evening, but generally, it is best to take it about the same time each day.
- If side effects occur early, they usually improve or can be treated.
- Continue taking medication, even if you feel better.
- Do not stop taking medication before talking to your PCP.

Scripts for the PCP to refer patients

Another important element of a consultation practice is that the referred patient must understand the role of the consultant in relation to the referring medical provider. Therefore, the primary care consultant must clearly articulate the role of the consultant in relation to the referring medical provider and the primary team. It is also very important to train PCPs as to how to discuss referrals with their patients. The PCP's choice of words can influence the patient's expectation and affect the patient's willingness to be referred (Robinson & Reiter, 2007). PCPs who struggle with how to refer patients are usually less likely to do so. For these reasons, consider offering a handout with phrases for a referring PCP to use (See Appendix 5: Used with permission of USAF Behavioral Health Optimization Program). Overall, physicians need to emphasize that the referral is because of an interest in the whole person, with the recognition that all illnesses have psychological components, and that other disciplines have skills to offer that have been helpful in similar cases (Belar & Deardorff, 1996).

Tailor Recommendations to PCP

In the behavioral health consultant model the consultant does not take responsibility for treating the patient, but operates in temporary co-management role with the referring medical provider. Therefore, it is crucial that any recommendation must be tailored to fit the skills, abilities, and interest of the referring provider and be supported and understood by other primary care team members. A primary care consultant must be able to extract the core principle associated with the intervention, eliminate jargon, and simplify the operational definition of an intervention (Strosahl, 2005). Each provider has a different level of interest and skill in dealing with behavioral health. The consultant must understand and address each primary care provider within these parameters (Strosahl, 2005).

CBT techniques can be unpacked and made clear and accessible for busy physicians. For example, a recommendation to ask the patient to participate in at least three social activities weekly to decrease social isolation can easily be accomplished in a 2–3 minute discussion. Creating this kind of simplicity is implicit in helping the PCP to promote and maintain the collaborative team approach of a primary care.

Referral and Stepped Care

Stepped care provides a framework for using limited resources to the greatest effect (Gilbody & Bower, 2005). Professional care is stepped in intensity—that is, it starts with limited professional input and systematic monitoring and is then augmented for patients who do not achieve an acceptable outcome (Gilbody, 2004). Initial and subsequent treatments are selected according to a stepped algorithm in light of a patient's progress (Gilbody, 2004). The principle of increasing intensity of professional input for those who do not respond to initial management is familiar in primary care. This is a primary strategy for managing a scarce resource, in this case the primary care provider's time (Strosahl, 2005).

Organized stepped care requires the systematic monitoring of progress and higher levels of coordination between PCP and the primary care consultant. Patients with the highest level of need and severity of illness receive the most intensive forms of intervention, such as the collaborative care and case management (Bower & Gilbody, 2005). Stepped care is individualized according to each patient's preferences and progress (Von korff, Glasgow, & Sharpe, 2002). It is only when a patient fails to respond to the first level of care that a second level of care is initiated.

In primary care a stepped-care approach may be used, whereby a physician initially consults with the behavioral health consultant to formulate a behavioral treatment plan (Gatchel & Oordt, 2005). If the patient does not make the desired changes, the behavioral health consultant may then interview the patient to further assess the problem and refine the intervention (Gatchel & Oordt, 2005). If again there is no sufficient improvement, the consultant may decide to refer the patient to a specialty mental health facility so that the patient can receive a treatment protocol, with weekly therapy sessions, to increase the likelihood of change.

Summary

Integrating behavioral health into the primary care system will facilitate more effective psychological and behavioral interventions in the early treatment of depression. Evidence shows that integration is cost-effective, produces improved clinical outcomes, and is more satisfying for patients and providers alike (Groth & Elkins, 1996). There has been consistent and convincing evidence of the benefits of changing the way primary care systems are organized for the management of depression (Neumeyer – Gromen et al. 2004; Genischen et al. 2006; Craven & Bland, 2006). Findings like these underscore the probability that the evolution of health care will most likely involve the continued integration of behavioral services into the routine process of primary care medicine.

There is substantial evidence on the effectiveness of cognitive behavioral interventions in the treatment of a wide range of mental disorders, physical disorders, and psychosocial problems commonly encountered in a primary care setting (APA, 1998). Using CBT to manage depression in primary care fits the existing methods of working in primary care quite closely in that problems can be defined and conceptualized in functional terms (France & Robson, 1998). In primary care settings, efforts have focused on providing both CBT and pharmacotherapy treatments; both have been found to be effective (Schulberg, Katon, Simon, & Rush, 1999) and cost-effective (Lave, Frank, Schulberg, & Kamlet, 1998).

The prevalence of depressive disorders, coupled with the inaccuracy of identification and lack of effective care provision, indicates a clear need for psychologists to address the problems of assessment and treatment of depression in primary care practice settings using interventions that fit the population and pace of primary care.

Clinical health psychologists, who serve as primary care consultants in primary care, can serve as the central figure in the assessment and are integral in the treatment of depressive disorders. Integrating clinical health psychologists into primary care setting is an excellent mechanism for both providing quality care and improving the health of a population.

Self Help Resources for Managing Depression

The Feeling Good Handbook by David Burns
Mind over Mood by Dennis Greenberger & Christine Padesky
Overcoming Depression: Client Manual by Gary
Overcoming Depression by Paul Gilbert
Mood Gym: moodgym.anu.edu.au Information, quizzes, games, and skills training to help prevent depression

Recommended Readings for Managing Depression in Primary Care

Robinson, P., Wischman C., & Del Vento, A. (1996). *Treating Depression in Primary Care: A Manual for Primary Care and Mental Health Provider*, Reno, NV: Context Press

France, R., & Robson, M. (1998). *Cognitive Behavioural Therapy in Primary Care: A Practical Guide*. London/Philadelphia: Jesicca Kingsley Publishers.

Callaghan, G. M., & Gregg, J. A., (2006). The role of the behavioral health care specialist in the treatment of depression in primary care setting. In W. T. O'Donahue, M. R. Byrd, N. A. Cummings & D. A. Henderson (Ed.), *Behavioral Integrative Care: Treatments That Work in the Primary Care Settings* (pp. 15–52). New York. Brunner-Routledge

References

Anderson, J. E., Michalak, E. E., & Lam, R. W. (2002). Depression in primary care: Tools for screening, diagnosis, and measuring response to treatment. *British Columbia Medical Journal, 44*(8), 415–419.

Aroll, B., Khin, N., & Kerse, N. (2003). Screening for depression in primary care with two verbally asked questions: cross sectional study. *British Medical Journal, 327*, 1144–1146.

Baron, D. A. (2003). Case histories for understanding depression in primary care. *Journal of the American Osteopathic Association, 8*(4), 16–18.

Beck, A. T., Ward, C. H., Mendelson, M. Mock, J., & Erbaugh, J. (1961). An inventory for measuring depression . *Archives of General Psychiatry, 4*, 561–571.

Beck, J. S., & Bieling, P. J. (2004). Cognitive therapy: Introduction to theory & practice. In M. J. Dewan, B. N. Steenbarger, & R. P. Greenberg (Eds.), *The Art and Science of Brief Psychotherapies: A Practitioner's Guide* (pp. 1–14). Washington, DC American Psychiatric Publishing, Inc.

Belar, C. D., & Deardorff, W. (1996). *Clinical health psychology in medical settings: A practitioner's guide book*. Washington, DC: American Psychological Association.

Budman, S. H., & Butler, S. F. (1997). The lily family depression project: Primary care prevention in action. In N. A. Cummings, J. L. Cummings, J. N. Johnson & N. J. Baker (Eds.) *Behavioral health in primary care : A guide for clinical integration.* (pp. 219–238). Madison, CT: Psychosocial Press/International Universities Press, Inc.

Callahan, E. J., Bertakis, K. D., Azari, R., Robbins, J., Helms, L. J., & Miller, J. (1996). The influence of depression on physician patient interaction in primary care. *Family Medicine, 28,* 346–351.

Callaghan, G. M., & Gregg, J. A. (2006). The role of the behavioral health care specialist in the treatment of depression in primary care setting. In W. T. O'Donahue, M. R. Byrd, N. A. Cummings & D. A. Henderson (Eds.), *Behavioral integrative care: Treatments that work in the primary care settings* (pp. 15–52). New York: Brunner-Routledge

Clabby, J. F. (2006). Helping depressed adolescents: A menu of cognitive behavioral procedures for primary care. *Primary Care Companion Journal of Clinical Psychiatry, 8*(6), 131–141.

Cowley, D. S., Katon, W., & Veith, R. C. (2000). Training psychiatry residents as consultants in primary care settings. *Academic Psychiatry, 24,* 124–132.

Craven, M. & Bland, R. (2006). Better practices in collaborative mental health care: An analysis of the evidence base. *Canadian Journal of Psychiatry, 51* (Suppl 1)

Ellen, S. R., Norman, T. R., & Burrows, G. D. (1998). 3. Assessments of anxiety and depression in primary care. *Medical Journal of Australia, 167,* 328–333.

Etherage, J. E. (2005). Pediatric behavioral health consultation. In L. C. James & R. A. Folen (Ed.), *The primary care consultant: The next frontier for psychologists in hospitals and clinics* (pp. 173–190). Washington, DC: American Psychological Association.

France, R. & Robson, M. (1998). *Cognitive behavioural therapy in primary care: A practical guide.* London/Philadelphia: Jesicca Kingsley Publishers.

Freedland, K. E., Carney, R. M., & Skala, J. A. (2004). Depression and mood disorders. In L. J. Haas (Ed.) *Handbook of primary care psychology* (pp. 279–298). Oxford University Press.

Gatchel, R. J., & Oordt, M. S. (2002). *Clinical health psychology and primary care.* Prctical advice and clinical guidance for successful collaboration. Washington DC: APA.

Genisichen, J., Beyer, M., Muth, C., Gerlach, F., Von Korff, M., & Ormel, J. (2006). Case management to improve major depression in primary health care: a systematic review. *Psychological Medicine, 36*(1), 7–14.

Gilbody, S. (2004). What is the evidence on effectiveness of capacity building in primary health care professionals in the detection, management, and outcome of depression? Copenhagen, WHO Regional Office for Europe.

Gilbody, S. M., & Bower, P. (2005). Common mental health disorders in primary care – access, effectiveness and choice. In Knapp, M. D., M, Mossialos, E., Thornicroft G. (Eds.). *Mental health policy and practice across europe.* Buckingham: Open University Press.

Goldberg, D. P., & Black well, B. (1970). Psychiatric illness in general practice. A detailed study using a new method of case identification. *British Journal of Medicine, 1,* 439–443.

Griever M., Anderson E., & Baumgarten E. (2005), (January 10). Another approach to managing depression. *Canada Family Physician, 51*(1), 25–29.

Groth, G. & Elkins, G. (1996). Professional psychologists in general health care settings: A review of the financial efficacy of direct treatment interventions. *Professional Psychology: Research & Practice, 27,* 161–174.

Gunning, K. (2004). Could the symptoms be caused by the Patient's Medication? A guide to assessment. In L. J. Haas (Ed.) *Handbook of primary care psychology* (pp. 611–626). Oxford University Press.

Hirschfeld, R. M. (2001). The comorbidity of major depression and anxiety disorders: recognition and management in primary care. *Primary Care Companion Journal Clinical Psychiatry, 3*(6), 244–252.

Katon, W. (1987). The epidemiology of medical care. *International Journal of Psychiatry in Medicine, 17,* 93–112.

Katon, W., & Schulberg, H. (1992). Epidemiology of depression in primary care. *General Hospital Psychiatry, 14*, 237–247.

Katon, W., Von Korff, M., & Lin E. (1990). Distressed high utilizers of medical care: DSMIII-R diagnosis and treatment needs. *General Hospital Psychiatry, 12*, 355–362.

Kop, W. J., & Ader D. N. (2001). Assessment and treatment of depression in coronary artery disease patients. *Italian Heart Journal, 2*, 890–894.

Kupfer, D. J., & Freedman, D. X. (1986). Treatment for depression. *Archives of General Psychiatry, 43*, 509–511.

Lave, J. R., Frank, R. G., Schulberg, H. C., & Kamlet, M. S. (1998). Cost effectiveness of treatments for major depression in care practice. *Archives of General Psychiatry, 55*(7), 645–651.

McQuaid, J. R., Stien M. B., Laffaye C., & MCCahill M. E. (1999). Depression in a primary care clinic: The prevalence and impact of an unrecognized disorder. *Journal of Affective Disorder, 55*, 1–10.

Munoz, R. F., Hollon, S. D., McGrath, E., Rhem, L. P., & VandenBos, G. R. (1994). On the AHCPR depression in primary care guidelines: Further considerations for practitioners. *American Psychologist, 49*, 42–61.

Narrow, W., Reiger, D., Rae, D., Manderscheid, R., & Locke, B., (1993) . Use of services by persons with mental and addictive disorders: Findings form the national Institute of mental Health Epidemiological Catchment Area Program. *Archives of General Psychiatry, 50*, 95–107.

Paykel, E. S., & Priest, R. G. (1992). Recognition n& management of depression in general practice: Consensus statement. *British Medical Journal, 305*, 1198–1202.

Perez-Stable, E. J., Miranada, J., Munoz, R. F., & Ying , Y. W. (1990). Depression in medical outpatients. Underrecognition and misdiagnosis. *Archives of Internal Medicine, 150*, 1083–1088.

Pignone, M., Gaynes, B. N., Rushton, J. L., et al. Screening for Depression. Systematic Evidence Review No. 6 (Prepared by the Research Triangle Institute—University of North Carolina Evidence-based Practice Center under Contract No. 290-97-0011) AHRQ Publication. No. 02-S002. Rockville, MD: Agency for Healthcare Research and Quality, May 2002.

Radloff, L. S. (1977). The CES-D scale. A self report depression scale for research in the general population. *Applied Psychological Measurement, 1*, 385–401.

Regier, D. A., Narrow, W. E., Rae, D. S., Manderscheid, R. W., Locke, B. Z., & Goodwin, F. K. (1993). The defacto U.S. mental and addictive disorders service system. Epidemiologic catchment area prospective 1-year prevalence rates of disorders and services. *Archives General Psychiatry, 50*, 85–94.

Robinson, P. J., & Reiter, J. T. (2007). *Behavioral Consultation and Primary Care: A guide to Integrating Services.* New York: Springer.

Robinson, P., Wischman, C., & Del Vento, A. (1996). Treating depression in primary care: A manual for primary care and mental health provider, Reno, NV: Context Press.

Rowan, A. B., & Runyan, C. N. (2005). A primer on the consultation model of the primary care behavioral health integration. The Primary Care Consultant: The next frontier for psychologists in hospitals and clinics (pp. 9–28). Washington, DC: American Psychological Association.

Schade, C. P., Jone, E. R. J., & Wittlin, B. J. (1998). A ten year review of the validity and clinical utility of depression screening. *Psychiatric Services, 55*, 1121–1127.

Simon, G. E., Revicki, D., Heiligenstein, J., Grothaus, J., Vonkorff, M., Katon, W., & Hylan, T. (2000). Recovery from depression, work productivity, and health care cost among primary care patients. *General Hospital Psychiatry, 22*, 153–162.

Sharp, L. K.,& Lipsky, M. S. (2002). Screening for depression across the life span: A review of measures for use in primary care settings. *American Family Physician, 66*(6), 1–15.

Steenbarger B. (1994). Duration and outcome in psychotherapy: An integrative review. *Profession Psychology Research & Practice, 25*, 111–119.

Steenbarger, B. N., Greenberg, R. P., & Mantosh, J. D. (2004). Introduction. In M. J. Dewan, B. N. Steenbarger, & R.P Greenberg (Eds.), *The art and science of brief psychotherapies: A practitioner's guide* (pp. 1–14). Washington, DC: American Psychiatric Publishing, Inc.

Strosahl, K. D. (2005). Training behavioral health and primary care providers for integrated care: A core competency approach. In W. T. O'Donahue, M. R. Byrd, N. A. Cummings & D. A. Henderson (Eds.), Behavioral Integrative Care: Treatments that work in the primary care settings (pp. 15–52). New York: Brunner-Routledge.

US Air force Medical Operations Agency Population Health support Division, Office for Prevention & Health Services Assessment. 2002. Primary care behavioral health care services practice manual version 2.0. http://www.integratedprimarycare.com/Air%20Force%20 Manual/ primary%20care%20practice%20manual.pdf

Von Korff, M., Glasgow, R. E., & Sharpe, M. (2002). ABC of psychological medicine: Organizing care for chronic illness. *British Medical Journal, 325*, 92–94.

Yesavage, J. A., Brink, T. L., Rose, T. L. Lum, O., Huang, V. Adey, M. & Leier, V. (1982). Development and validation of a geriatric depression screening scale: A preliminary report. *Journal of Psychiatric Research, 17*, 37–49.

Zung, W. W. (1965). A self rating depression scale.*Archives of General Psychiatry, 12*, 63–70.

Appendix 1: Behavioral R$_x$

Erica M. Jarrett Ph.D.,
Behavioral Health Consultant, Internal Medicine Clinic, Walter Reed Army Medical Center

Behavioral R$_x$

Behavior Change Plan:

Follow-up with Dr. Jarrett scheduled for :_____

Call (202) 782 -0907 if you need to leave a message or change you appointment time.

Erica M. Jarrett, Ph.D.,
Behavioral Health Consultant, Internal Medicine Clinic, Walter Reed Army Medical Center

Behavioral R$_x$

Behavior Change Plan:

Follow-up with Dr. Jarrett scheduled for :_____

Call (202) 782 – 0907 if you need to leave a message or change you appointment time.

Used with permission of the USAF Behavioral Health Optimization Program

Appendix 2: OVERCOMING DEPRESSION

This booklet is designed to provide information about strategies for overcoming depression. It discusses a model or framework for understanding depression (the "depression spiral") and presents an overview of treatment of depression, including use of medication and strategic coping strategies. The booklet is designed to be used on your own, or with the assistance of your Primary Care Manager or Behavioral Health Consultant.

The Depression Spiral

The figure below depicts one helpful way to think about and understand depression. Our life experience (including depression) is influenced by a number of interrelated factors: our environment, biological factors, our thoughts and beliefs, our behaviors, and our emotions. Each factor can affect the others.

For example, Sue recently began working in a fast-paced, high-pressure job (*environmental factor*). She began to have thoughts such as "There's no way I can get all this work done. It's impossible. If I don't get it done, I may lose my job." As a result, she began to work longer hours, cut out all extra, fun activities, and withdraw from family and friends (*behaviors*). With this decrease in many of the positive, rewarding aspects of her life, she began to feel down, depressed, and more irritable (*emotions*). As the depression cycle started to take hold, she had more difficulty sleeping and concentrating (*biological factors*), which led to even more irritability and depression (*emotions*) and further withdrawal from activities and people (*behaviors*). At some point in the cycle, the balance of chemicals in her brain also began to alter (*biological factor*), which further deepened the spiral of depression.

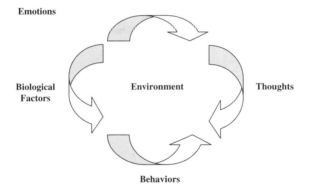

Emotions

Biological Factors   Environment   Thoughts

Behaviors

BREAKING THE DEPRESSION SPIRAL

As you can see, a variety of factors, including thoughts, behaviors, emotions, and environmental and biological factors can cause, maintain, and worsen depression. Fortunately, there are effective ways of breaking the spiral of depression. Since all the factors are interrelated (with one aspect affecting the others), even making small changes in just one or two areas can lead to significant improvements in other areas.

For example, Sue noticed her worsening moods and decided to take action to break the depression spiral. She focused first on one area that she felt would be easy to change: her behaviors. Specifically, she wanted to make changes in how she spent her time in the evenings after work. She made a goal of spending 30 minutes each evening relaxing and doing fun activities with her family (*behaviors*). After several weeks, she noticed that she was beginning to feel lower levels of stress and her sleep began to improve (*biological factor*). Feeling more rested and better able to concentrate (*biological factors*) increased her belief that she could effectively manage the demands of her new job (*thoughts*). She noticed that she had fewer days of feeling down and depressed (*emotions*).

Other people working to improve their depression may choose to focus initially on other areas. Some people benefit from starting an antidepressant medication (*biological factor*) to begin to break the depression cycle. Others focus first on increasing regular physical exercise (a *behavioral and biological factor* that may help decrease depression), recognizing and changing thought patterns that contribute to depression or worry (*thoughts*), or learning and trying out new behaviors to improve work or family situations (*behaviors*, e.g., problem-solving, effective communication, time management, etc.).

As you can see, there are a <u>variety</u> of coping methods and behavioral strategies that may be helpful in decreasing depression. It is probably not in your best interests to try <u>all</u> or <u>too many</u> strategies at any one time. Rather, keep it simple and do not overwhelm yourself. It is usually best to pick one or two strategies that sound most relevant to you, try those coping strategies for a few weeks or longer, and then move on to other coping strategies that you think may be important later on. And remember -- even if you are just working directly on one or two coping strategies, you will probably be having an indirect positive effect on other areas.

The following pages include information on how to begin four of the most effective strategies for breaking the depression spiral and decreasing depression. These are:

_____ a. **Increase the rewarding activities in my life (p. 3)**

_____ b. **Take antidepressant medication as directed (p. 7)**

_____ c. **Increase physical exercise (p.8)**

_____ d. **Increase balanced thinking (p. 10)**

INCREASING REWARDING EXPERIENCES

There is strong theory and research indicating that depression may be caused or worsened by a significant decrease in rewarding experiences and activities. Therefore, one effective strategy for reducing depression may be to increase the amount of rewarding activities in your life.

There are two types of rewarding activities: "pleasurable" activities and "mastery" activities.

- **Pleasurable activities** are those that are just plain fun.

- **Mastery activities** are those that give you a sense of accomplishment or pride.

Increasing pleasurable and mastery activities may seem difficult at first. You may feel that there is *no time* in your day for any thing else. You may also feel that you have *no interest* or *no motivation* to do anything. These are common feelings and reactions in people who are depressed. It is often necessary, therefore, to *make a plan* for increasing rewarding activities, and to *stick to the plan*, even when you don't particularly feel like it. As you begin to increase your rewarding activities, you will likely find that your motivation and interest in doing them gradually increase, as well. Use the exercise below to make improvements in this area.

Make a list any pleasurable activities that you have decreased (or quit) doing recently:

_____   _____

_____   _____

_____   _____

Make a list of any mastery activities that you have decreased (or quit) doing recently:

_____   _____

_____   _____

_____   _____

Now make a list of *additional* activities that you believe *might* be fun and pleasant, or might give you a sense of accomplishment and mastery. If you have trouble coming up with ideas, consider talking with a friend, family member, or behavioral health consultant to help generate ideas. You may also find some activities that seem to "fit" you and your life from the list on the following page.

_____   _____   _____

_____   _____   _____

_____   _____   _____

_____   _____   _____

Use your own list of pleasurable and mastery activities to make a plan to increase rewarding experiences in your life each day.

In the morning, plan at least one pleasurable and one mastery activity for the day. At the end of the day list several things you did that day that gave you a sense of pleasure and accomplishment.

The following chart may help you get started, remain motivated and "on track," and remind you of the progress you make.

Date	My pleasurable activity today will be….	My mastery activity today will be…	My most fun activities today were…	My significant accomplishments today were…

Appendix 3: <u>Important Information for People Starting Antidepressant Medication</u>

1. It may take 10-21 days before you notice any reduction in symptoms.

2. **<u>Symptom improvement</u>** is primarily seen in problem physiological symptoms like

    A) Sleep   E) Restlessness, Agitation or feeling physically slowed down
    B) Appetite   F) Feeling worse in the morning
    C) Fatigue   G) Poor Concentration
    D) Sex Drive

Many other symptoms like **<u>Depressed Mood & Low Self-Esteem</u>**, may respond only partially to medication. The medication you'll be taking is not a "happy pill", it is unlikely to totally erase feelings of sadness or emptiness.

3. The best **<u>signs that your medication is working</u>** include
    A) Improved Sleep
    B) Less Day Time Fatigue
    C) Improved Emotional Control (fewer crying spells, better frustration tolerance)

4. There may be **<u>Side Effects</u>** (see below). However, these side effects can most often be managed by dosage adjustment or by switching to another medication.
    A) **<u>Dry Mouth</u>**-drink plenty of water, chew sugarless gum, use sugarless candy
    B) **<u>Constipation</u>**-eat more fiber rich foods, take a stool softener
    C) **<u>Drowsiness</u>**-take frequent walks, take medication earlier in the evening, or if taking medication during the day ask your primary care manager if you can take it at night
    D) **<u>Wakefulness</u>**-take medications early in the day
    E) **<u>Blurred Vision</u>**-remind yourself that this is a temporary difficulty, talk with provider if it continues
    F) **<u>Headache</u>**-usually temporary and can be managed by analgesics (aspirin, acetaminophen) if needed
    G) **<u>Feeling Speeded Up</u>**-tell yourself this will go away in 3-5 days, if not, call your provider
    H) **<u>Sexual Problems</u>**-talk with your provider a change in medications may help
    I) **<u>Nausea or Appetite Loss</u>**-take medication with food

5. Length of treatment can vary widely from person to person. **Typically, it may take 4-8 weeks for the major depressive symptoms to significantly decrease. It is important not to discontinue treatment** at this point. The relapse rate can be as high as 80%. In general medication treatment goes at least 6 months beyond the point of symptom improvement. Then medication reduction under your provider's management can be started. If symptoms return during medication-reduction, the dosage should be increased and continued for another 4-6 weeks before another trial on lower doses. Occasionally, a person may need to be on long-term medication management.

6. Antidepressants are **not addictive**.

7. **Do not drink alcohol** if you are taking antidepressant medication. Alcohol can block the effects of the medication. If you desire to drink occasionally or socially (never more than 1 drink per day) discuss this with your provider.

Appendix 4.

Thinking and Stress

Your thoughts are often the source of physical and emotional problems you can experience in response to any situation. This section will provide you with some information that may help increase your understanding of the role your thoughts play in managing stress.

❖ In general, your thoughts about a situation (also called "beliefs" or "self-talk") determine your **PHYSICAL, EMOTIONAL,** and **BEHAVIORAL** responses to that situation.

Accurate vs. Distorted Beliefs

❖ **ACCURATE BELIEFS AND SELF-TALK** can enhance your ability to maintain your treatment goals and minimize the negative physical and emotional consequence of a situation.

❖ However, sometimes thoughts can be **INACCURATE**, **UNREALISTIC**, or **DISTORTED**.

❖ When your beliefs about a situation are inaccurate, unrealistic or distorted, we refer to them as **ALARMING SELF-TALK** because they result in negative impacts on our physical and emotional health.

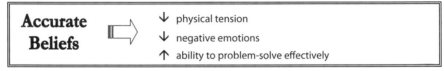

BUT...

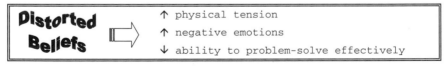

For example, imagine how you would feel if you were given a task to do and you had thoughts like:
☂ I'm never going to get this work done.
☂ I'm terrible at this kind of thing.
☂ I'm sure I'm going to just mess it up somehow.

Most people would feel `miserable` if they had these beliefs.

Used with permission of the USAF Behavioral Health Optimization Program

Changing Alarming Self-Talk

The GOOD NEWS IS...

> ➤ alarming self-talk can be changed, and
> ➤ changing alarming self-talk can be one of the most helpful changes you will make.

Unfortunately it is also one of the most difficult because it takes:

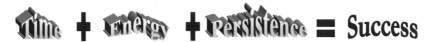

The remainder of this handout is designed to help you get moving down this path. BUT, you will need to take this information and work diligently to make the necessary changes.

Thankfully, the effort brings rapid rewards because changes in your reactions (emotional and behavioral) will begin to occur as soon as you start changing these thoughts.

A heart at peace gives life to the body, but envy rots the bones.

Proverbs 14:30

ABC's of Stress Management

Activating event:

Any potentially stressful situation.
- conflict with your boss,
- late for a special event,

Example: A project is due today, and you're not going to make the suspense.

Beliefs or self-talk

ALARMING THOUGHTS are thoughts which often lead to intense emotional responses.

Example: "My boss is going to kill me. The whole project will be delayed now. I should have got it done sooner."

REASSURING THOUGHTS lead to moderate, healthy emotional responses.

Example: "I did the best I could. I'll give my boss a head's up that it's going to be late. He probably won't chew me out. He knows I've been working hard on it and I usually meet suspenses. The project will only be delayed the 24 hours I'll need to get it done."

Consequences

Potential consequences of alarming thoughts fall into three categories:

Physical - Such as headache, stomach upset, for some, changes in glucose levels.

Emotional – Examples include anxiety, depression, frustration, and guilt.

Behavioral - These include snapping at your spouse, giving up in other areas, withdrawal from people and activities.

> **Misery is not solely caused by things (Activating Events), but by our *view* of things (Beliefs or Self-Talk).**

4 Types of Alarming Thoughts

1. Demandingness: Thoughts or beliefs in which we expect ourselves, others, or life
in general to live up to some type of *unrealistic* standard, goal, or rule which is unrealistic

☟ **Demands About Self**
> *"I should be able to manage my stress better!"*
> *"I must get my weight down to 180 pounds!"*

☟ **Demands About Others**
> *"She should treat me better!"*
> *"He should understand how hard this is!"*

☟ **Demands About the World/Conditions**
> *"My doctors should know how to fix me!"*
> *"It isn't fair that I have to deploy!"*

* Hint: Look for words such as *"Should"*, *"Must"*, *"Ought"*, and *"Have to"* in
order to detect demandingness

2. Awfulizing: Rating the quality of a person (ourselves or others) or events in
extreme terms. Often involves words such as "awful" "terrible" or "disaster."

> X   *"I can't do anything I enjoy anymore because I'm so tired!"*
> X   *"I had a bad day yesterday, this coping stuff must not be working anymore!"*

3. 'I Can't Stand It'-itis: Convincing yourself that you will not be able to tolerate
unfortunate or frustrating occurrences.

> X   *"If I don't get some relief quickly I'll go crazy!"*
> X   *"I'm so tired, how can I be expected to work today?"*
> X   *"I can't take another day at this job!"*

4. Faulty Evidence/Assumptions: You accept a belief without considering
the evidence against that belief.

> X   *"Life would be better if I could just get out of the military."*
> X   *"She won't mind if I'm late again."*
> X   *"If I just avoid him, he won't be able to yell at me."*

Reassuring Thoughts

IN ORDER TO THINK REALISTICALLY, YOU MUST...

☞ Express your thoughts as *preferences* (even strong preferences).

☞ Recognize that **most things** are preferences (i.e., things you do not **_need_** to live).

☞ Realize things might not turn out like you would prefer.

For example:

✓ "I hope today is not so stressful, but if it isn't, I'll cope okay. No reason to make myself crazy about it."

✓ "I wish my boss was more understanding, but she isn't. That's the way she is going to act."

✓ "No one can prove that my life *has to be* hassle free, and it is almost certain not to be."

✓ "I prefer that life is stress free, but it's almost certain not to be. I need to focus on managing the stress."

REASSURING THOUGHTS AVOID AWFULIZING AND I CAN'T STAND IT ITUS. You view things realistically and rationally rather than in exaggerated terms.

✓ "Having to work here is a real hassle, but it doesn't' have to ruin my life."
"I'm having trouble learning this new procedure, but I've learned this kind of thing in the past. I need to just keep at it."

REASSURING THOUGHTS CAREFULLY EXAMINE THE EVIDENCE FOR A BELIEF.

✓ "There are hassles and frustration in civilian jobs also. They are just different.

✓ "Avoiding problems is only a short term fix. I need to do something about this."

Remember, Reassuring Thoughts Are REALISTIC Thoughts. They are not unbelievable positive thoughts. Aiming for "Positive Thinking" places you at risk for constructing thoughts that are as unrealistic as alarming beliefs.

EXAMPLES OF UNREALISTIC, POSITIVE THOUGHTS:

☠ "Life is fair, I'll always get what I deserve."

☠ "People will always look out after my best interests."

☠ "Soon I'll have my glucose under control and won't have to think about this stuff anymore."

☠ "I know I'll be able to make my boss like me and then things will be better."

☠ "Good things always happen to good people."

☠ "This class will finally enable me to get my old life back."

Changing Alarming Self-Talk

GENERAL QUESTIONS TO CHALLENGE ALARMING THOUGHTS

⇨ Am I alarming myself unnecessarily? Can I see this another way?

⇨ What am I demanding *must* happen? What do I *want* rather than *need*?

⇨ Am I rating something a *catastrophe*? Is it every bit that *awful*?

⇨ Am I rating a *type of person*? What is the *action* I don't like?

⇨ What's *untrue* about my thoughts? How can I stick to the *facts*?

STRATEGIES TO CHANGE ALARMING EVALUATIONS (AWFULIZING)\

A. **LISTEN FOR THE EXTREME OR CATASTROPHIC RATING WORDS** (*horrible, terrible, disaster, awful*) of an event. For example, a thought about how things couldn't be worse and how you will not be able to survive the event.

B. Instead of using this extreme rating when it doesn't fully apply, **THINK OF THE EVENT IN TERMS OF DEGREE OF DISAPPOINTMENT OR INCONVENIENCE.** Other words might better describe the relative severity of the event, such as *annoying, nuisance, irritating, unfortunate, frustration, or problem.*

C. **LISTEN FOR THE EXTREME OR OVERLY GENERAL RATING OF A PERSON** (*loser, stupid, inconsiderate, pushy, selfish, jerk, incompetent*), something which implies that there are good and bad people in the world and this person definitely is part of the bad group while others (often including ourselves) are in the good group.

D. **FOCUS YOUR JUDGMENT MORE ON THE SPECIFIC ACTION AS THE PROBLEM** rather than what you believe is the general type of person involved. Realize that you are on shaky ground whenever you think you can fairly and without doubt categorize someone as totally fitting a particular type. It is much more relevant to think in terms of the actions which someone did that you disagree with or you see as mistakes. This pertains to your rating of yourself as well as others.

Examples:

ALARMING EVALUATIONS:	*REASSURING EVALUATIONS:*
1. I didn't get promoted. They must think I'm no good.	1. Promotions are influenced by a lot of things besides job performance. My boss has told me many times I'm doing a good job.
2. My boss is a total idiot.	2. My boss is probably as frustrated as I am with the way things are at work. But, I don't like the way he takes his frustrations out on us. I need to think about how to handle this better.
3. Things just couldn't be worse.	3. Things can always be worse. Thinking like this will just get me depressed. I need to do something I will enjoy to help myself feel better.

STRATEGIES TO CHANGE ALARMING EXPECTATIONS (DEMANDINGNESS)

❶ Pick out the element of _truth_ or the _preference_ in your alarming expectation.

❷ Remove the *absolute demand words* (must, should, need, have to) and replace them with words of *preference* (want to, would like, wish, it would be better if).

❸ Check that your preference is *reasonable* considering the cost of it to your health, convenience, relationships, or your other priorities.

Examples:

ALARMING EXPECTATIONS:	REASSURING EXPECTATIONS:
1. I need this problem to be gone now!	1. I'd like it to be gone, but I can manage it by using management skills I've been learning.
2. They've got to have a cure for this.	2. Many medical conditions are incurable, but many people have learned to manage them and enjoy life at the same time. I can too.
3. Those who really care about me will know I'm feeling stressed.	3. I can't expect them to read my mind. I need to share with them what I'm feeling. Maybe they can help me look at it a little more objectively.

STRATEGIES TO CHANGE ALARMING PREDICTIONS (I CAN'T STAND IT ITIS & FAULTY EVIDENCE/ASSUMPTIONS)

❶ Pick out what you see as the alarming scenario.

❷ Ask yourself, "***What are the odds of this entire scene taking place?***" If it is not really likely, remind yourself of the more probable events.

❸ Play out what your options could be and how you would like to respond should something like your "what if" scenario take place. Think about what you might have learned from similar situations before.

Examples:

ALARMING PREDICTIONS:	REASSURING PREDICTIONS:
1. This is more than I can bear.	1. I sometimes feel overwhelmed, but I can't expect to not have some struggles. I need to keep trying to learn how to cope, even when it's not going as well as I would like.
2. I am doing so badly adhering to my diet, I must have no self-discipline.	2. It's not just a problem of self-discipline. Problems learning to eat healthy are common and result from lots of different factors. I need to do some problem solving to see if I can get on track.
3. This will never get easier.	3. Learning new ways of responding to stressful situations is always harder at first. As these changes become a habit they will get much easier to do and stick with.

Appendix 5: Behavioral Health Consultation

The Behavioral Health Consultant (BHC) for the General Internal Medicine is Dr. Erica Jarrett.
- Her role is to assist you in addressing behavioral/emotional issues with your pts and make your job easier.
- The BHC conducts a brief assessment of problems identified in your referral question (usually a 30-minute interview) and provides recommendations you can incorporate into your treatment plan.
- The focus is on primary and secondary prevention and assisting you in managing your patients.
- You don't need to screen patients to determine if they are appropriate referrals. Consult anytime you believe it would benefit your patients or ease your treatment of them.
- However, just to get you thinking, here are some examples of complaints that often benefit from referral:

- Chronic Pain (e.g., back, pelvic, shoulder, etc.)
- Tension or Migraine Headaches
- Irritable Bowel Syndrome
- Depression
- Difficulty coping with chronic illness (e.g., diabetes, asthma)
- Anxiety
- Questions re: Psych Meds

- Non-adherence to Medical Regimens
- Fibromyalgia
- Insomnia
- Relationship Problems
- Hypertension/heart disease
- Chronic Fatigue Syndrome
- Stress
- Etc.

- Phrasing of the referral is important. Tips are provided on the back.
- How to refer: On the "BHC Consultation Request Form" check the primary concern and/or provide additional information or questions. Give to the patient and ask them to give it to the exit nurse when they book the appointment. Also provide patient with blue BHC patient brochures to educate them on the service.

Erica Jarrett, Ph. D.   Office Phone: 202/782 - 5578   Pager: 202/782-7585 *1807

Fold Here

Suggestions for Phrasing Referrals

Sample Statement	Key Points
1. "I can see you're really depressed. I've got a colleague down the hall, Dr. Jarrett our Behavioral Health Consultant, who's real good with these types of things."	Use term "Behavioral Health Consultant" Avoid MH terms (e.g., mental health, counseling, therapy) Emphasize importance of addressing emotions/behaviors for good healthcare.
2. "We've worked together on many patients and her input has been very helpful to me."	Communicate that BHC is part of team, will work together and you will be in charge of their care
3. "How about I walk you down and introduce you to Dr. Jarrett?"	When BHC is available, walking down reinforces message of team relationship and provides "warm handoff"
4. "Would you be willing to make an appointment with one of our Behavioral Health Consultants? You can usually get appointments within a few days"	When "warm handoff" not possible, encourage pt to make appointment.

Handling Resistance to Referral

Patient Statement	Sample Response
1. "I don't need to see a shrink!" or "You think I need to go to mental health?"	"They are psychologists, but they are part of the General Internal Medicine Team. They are my consultants on any issues that need to be addressed to maintain good health. Would you be willing to give it a try?"
2. "Do you mean you think this is all in my head?" or "Do you mean you think I'm crazy?"	"No. Physical and emotional health are not inseparable. Each affects the other. Therefore, we need to pay attention to both."
3. "I don't want a mental health note in my chart. It will ruin my career."	Same as #1 above. And, ask if have specific concerns and address. If unable to answer pt concerns, feel free to walk them down so we can answer their questions or offer for us to call them and answer their questions.

Assessment and Treatment of Anxiety in Primary Care

Holly Hazlett-Stevens

Anxiety is a common complaint among primary care patients. Anxiety disorders are prevalent in the general population; some of which are twice as prevalent in the primary care setting. Despite the associated high rates of health care utilization, anxiety disorders often are not detected or appropriately treated in such medical settings. Brief diagnostic assessment measures, including short clinician-administered interviews and diagnostic patient-screening questionnaires, have been developed for primary care settings. In addition, several accessible therapist treatment guides, patient workbooks, and self-help resources based on empirically supported treatment methods are commercially available. In this chapter, these resources are reviewed after a brief discussion of anxiety disorders in the primary care setting.

Basic Facts About Anxiety and Primary Care

Anxiety disorders represent a widespread mental health problem in the United States. A recent large-scale epidemiological survey investigation (National Comorbidity Survey Replication, NCS-R; Kessler et al., 2005) revealed a lifetime prevalence estimate of 28.8% for the anxiety disorders. This rate was higher than lifetime prevalence estimates obtained for mood disorders (20.8%), impulse-control disorders (24.8%), and substance use disorders (14.6%). Among the anxiety disorders, specific phobia and social phobia were most common, with lifetime prevalence estimates of 12.5% and 12.1% respectively. Post-traumatic stress disorder (6.8%), generalized anxiety disorder (5.7%), and panic disorder (4.7%) also appeared quite prevalent. NCS-R estimates of 12-month prevalence were concerning as well. Anxiety disorders again were associated with the highest prevalence rate, an estimate of more than 18% (Kessler et al., 2005). When the individual anxiety disorders were examined, 12-month prevalence estimates were 8.7% for specific phobia, 6.8%

H. Hazlett-Stevens (✉)
University of Nevada, Reno, NV, USA
e-mail: hhazlett@unr.edu

L.C. James, W.T. O'Donohue (eds.), *The Primary Care Toolkit*,
DOI 10.1007/978-0-387-78971-2_12, © Springer Science+Business Media, LLC 2009

for social phobia, 3.5% for post-traumatic stress disorder (PTSD), 3.1% for generalized anxiety disorder (GAD), and 2.7% for panic disorder. Obsessive-compulsive disorder (OCD) and agoraphobia without panic appeared the least common anxiety disorders, with lifetime prevalence estimates of 1.6% and 1.4% respectively. Likewise, 12-month prevalence estimates for these two disorders were 1.0% and 0.8% respectively.

Anxiety disorders follow a chronic course for the majority of individuals diagnosed with panic disorder with agoraphobia, GAD, and social phobia (Yonkers, Bruce, Dyck, & Keller, 2003). This large-scale, prospective longitudinal investigation, commonly referred to as the Harvard/Brown Anxiety Research Program (HARP), studied the natural course of several anxiety disorders over several years. Remission rates reported for individuals who received only a "panic disorder without agoraphobia" diagnosis were notably higher than those for other anxiety disorder groups, with 76% of women and 69% of men experiencing some remission by eight years (Yonkers et al., 2003). However, relapse was a common occurrence across the anxiety disorders, especially among women diagnosed with panic disorder without agoraphobia. Thus, anxiety disorders left untreated are unlikely to remit on their own, and when they do, relapse often follows.

Despite findings of high prevalence, less than half the NCS-R respondents diagnosed with a 12-month DSM-IV disorder received treatment within the previous year (Wang et al., 2005). Among respondents diagnosed with an anxiety disorder, only 42.2% received mental health services within the previous 12 months. Reported mental health service use was highest for panic disorder (65.4%) and lowest for specific phobia (38.2%), with PTSD (57.4%), agoraphobia without panic (52.6%), GAD (52.3%), and social phobia (45.6%) falling in between. Similar findings emerged from the HARP project. Between the years 1991 and 1995–96, the use of psychosocial treatments by individuals diagnosed with anxiety disorders either remained the same or declined (Goisman, Warshaw, & Keller, 1999). Furthermore, when such individuals did seek psychological treatment, dynamic psychotherapy was received most often. Behavioral and cognitive treatments, the types of treatment that have received the greatest amount of empirical support, were less frequently provided.

The observed discrepancy between prevalence of anxiety disorders and treatment received does not indicate a simple lack of suffering. Anxiety disorders have been linked to significant functional impairment and a poor quality of life. For example, Stein and Heimberg (2004) found that GAD was associated with low life-satisfaction and poor emotional well-being, even after comorbid major depressive disorder was taken into account. Relationships between panic disorder and impaired social and occupational functioning are well established. Reduced work productivity, compromised employment status, lost work days, increased reliance on welfare, and impairments in social relationships all have been documented among individuals with panic disorder (Edlund & Swann, 1987; Siegel, Jones, & Wilson, 1990; Markowitz, Weissman, Ouellette, Lish, J. D., & Klerman, 1989).

An additional cost of anxiety disorders can be found across primary care and specialty medical settings. Anxiety disorders, particularly panic disorder and GAD, consistently have been associated with increased health care utilization. In their review of this literature, Roy-Byrne and Wagner (2004) found that the point prevalence of GAD and of panic disorder among primary care patients were at least twice the current prevalence rates reported in epidemiological community survey research. Individuals suffering from GAD and panic disorder excessively seek medical services such as physician visits, emergency room visits, hospitalizations, and laboratory tests (Roy-Byrne & Wagner; Swinson, Cox, & Woszcyna, 1992). Individuals with anxiety disorders also over-utilize medical specialist services. Kennedy and Schwab (1997) found that individuals with panic disorder sought help from primary care physicians as well as from otolaryngologists, obstetricians-gynecologists, neurologists, and urologists more often than individuals with GAD or OCD. Individuals with GAD visited gastroenterologists more often than the other two anxiety disorder groups; dermatologists and cardiologists were seen most frequently by individuals with OCD. Although individuals with various anxiety disorders often seek treatment from their medical providers, anxiety disorder conditions are poorly recognized in such settings. Roy-Byrne and Wagner reported that a mere 23% of anxiety disorder only cases were detected in primary care settings compared to 56% of depression cases. In short, primary care and other medical providers are facing a significant service delivery problem: individuals with anxiety disorders often present for treatment, but these chronic conditions most often go undetected, untreated, or are inappropriately treated.

Individuals with anxiety disorders may be inclined to seek help from medical providers for a couple of reasons. First, the somatic nature of many anxiety-related complaints leads individuals with anxiety disorders to seek medical relief for their symptoms. For example, worry and similar negative thought intrusions appear to maintain insomnia (Harvey, 2002). Insomnia as well as other forms of sleep disturbance, physical restlessness, and excessive muscle tension commonly can be found in cases of GAD and PTSD. Furthermore, the unexpected panic attacks seen in panic disorder involve intensive physiological sensations that are often interpreted by the individual as a sign of physical harm. Individuals with anxiety disorders also may seek medical treatment because they suffer from comorbid medical conditions. Sareen and colleagues found a unique relationship between anxiety disorders and physical disorders after adjusting for comorbid mental disorders (Sareen, Cox, Clara, & Asmundson, 2005). PTSD was associated with a variety of metabolic/autoimmune, bone or joint, neurological, and other physical conditions. Panic attacks and agoraphobia were largely associated with cardiovascular conditions and, to a lesser extent, bone and joint diseases. Strong relationships also were found between social phobia and metabolic/autoimmune disorders and between specific phobia and respiratory diseases. Finally, GAD was linked only to gastrointestinal conditions, consistent other research findings linking GAD and irritable bowel syndrome (e.g. Tollefson, Tollefson, Pederson, Luxenberg, & Dunsmore, 1991).

In sum, anxiety disorders present a serious challenge to providers in primary care and other medical settings. Although individuals suffering from anxiety tend to seek treatment in such settings, medical providers often fail to detect such conditions. Effective treatment options are not provided consistently, even though anxiety disorders are characterized by a chronic course and high relapse rates. Fortunately an array of assessment instruments and treatment resources are now available to behavioral health providers working in primary care settings. Brief diagnostic screening measures, accessible treatment guides, and self-help materials may improve the dissemination of effective psychosocial anxiety treatment in primary care.

Effective Screening and Assessment in Primary Care

Brief diagnostic screening procedures are quite feasible to administer in managed care and primary care medical settings. These assessment instruments include short clinician-administered interviews and diagnostic screening questionnaires. One such instrument, the Primary Care Evaluation of Mental Disorders (PRIME-MD; Spitzer et al., 1994), was designed specifically for the primary care setting. Primary care patients first complete a brief questionnaire, the Patient Health Questionnaire (PHQ). This one-page questionnaire contains 26 items. Patients indicate whether or not they have experienced various DSM-IV psychiatric symptoms using a "yes–no" response format. The primary care clinician next administers those diagnostic modules of the interview that were endorsed on the questionnaire. Good diagnostic agreement was found between diagnosis obtained with the PRIME-MD and diagnosis obtained by an independent mental health professional evaluation, even though primary care physicians completed the interview in an average of 8.4 minutes (Spitzer et al.). A computer-administered telephone interview version of the PRIME-MD also is available (Kobak et al., 1997). This version obtains diagnostic information over the telephone using interactive voice response (IVR) technology. Kobak and colleagues found preliminary empirical support for this computer-administered version as a valid and reliable diagnostic procedure with good sensitivity and specificity. One interesting discrepancy was found between the computer-administered version and the original version of the PRIME-MD. Primary care patients reported twice as much alcohol abuse on the computer-administered version compared to the original clinician-administered version. Although the PHQ originally was designed to guide administration of the PRIME-MD interview, this questionnaire alone also may serve as a reliable and valid diagnostic screening measure (Spitzer, Kroenke, & Williams, 1999). Furthermore, 80% of the primary care physicians who participated in that investigation endorsed that routine use of the PHQ would be useful in their work setting.

The Mini International Neuropsychiatric Interview for DSM-IV, English version 5.0.0 (MINI; Sheehan & Lecrubier, 2002), provides an alternative to the PRIME-MD. This clinician-administered structured interview assesses most anxiety, mood, eating, substance use, and psychotic disorders. The MINI is comprised of specific close-ended questions. As a result of this format, administration takes approximately 15 minutes only. The MINI appears to be a valid and reliable diagnostic measure. When compared to an extensive diagnostic clinical interview, the MINI correctly identified diagnosis in 85 to 95% of the cases (Sheehan, et al., 1998). Evidence of good sensitivity, specificity, and predictive utility were found as well.

Diagnostic screening questionnaires other than the PHQ are completed by primary care patients in the absence of a clinical interview. Once patients score positive for a given mental disorder, their primary care providers simply refer them to appropriate behavioral health services. Many of the available psychiatric screening questionnaires measure only the degree of psychopathology or psychosocial impairment and do not provide diagnostic assessment results. However, the Psychiatric Diagnostic Screening Questionnaire (PDSQ; Zimmerman & Mattia, 2001a) obtains DSM-IV diagnostic information for 13 different anxiety, eating, mood, substance use, and somatoform disorders. This 126-item questionnaire was designed to be completed in the waiting room within 10 to 15 minutes. Evidence of good internal consistency, test–retest reliability, as well as evidence of discriminant and convergent validity has been reported for the PDSQ subscales (Zimmerman & Mattia, 1999; 2001a; 2001b).

Three additional diagnostic screening questionnaires were designed to detect the presence of specific anxiety disorders in large-scale research settings. The Generalized Anxiety Disorder Questionnaire-IV (GAD-Q-IV; Newman et al., 2002) is a single-page pencil-and-paper measure containing DSM-IV diagnostic criteria for GAD. The GAD-Q-IV contains "yes–no" questions about excessive and uncontrollable worry, a checklist of required somatic symptoms, and Likert rating scales to assess degree of interference and distress resulting from worry and associated anxiety symptoms. A total score is calculated according to a scoring system, and a designated cutoff score yielded 89% specificity and 83% sensitivity in initial Receiver Operating Characteristics analyses (Newman et al., 2002). Strong diagnostic reliability, test–retest reliability, and convergent and discriminant validity also were demonstrated. Instead of the dimensional scoring system, primary care providers can opt to match item responses to the respective DSM-IV diagnostic criteria.

This research group has since developed similar diagnostic screening questionnaire measures for social phobia and panic disorder. The Social Phobia Diagnostic Questionnaire (SPDQ; Newman et al., 2003) is a single-page self-report measure in which respondents answer "yes–no" questions about excessive anxiety in social situations, concern about acting in a way that could cause embarrassment or humiliation, and avoidance of social situations. Respondents also rate the degree of fear and avoidance associated with a list of common social situations, answer further questions about fear in such situations, and rate the degree of associated impairment and distress. This brief measure of social phobia produced diagnostic results with 85% specificity and 82% sensitivity that were comparable to diagnosis obtained with an extensive clinician-administered interview. Evidence of good internal consistency, good split-half and test–retest reliability, and strong convergent, discriminant, and clinical validity also were found. The Panic Disorder Self-Report (PDSR; Newman, Holmes, Zuellig, Kachin, & Behar, 2006) contains 24 questions that map directly onto DSM-IV diagnostic criteria. Items assess the presence and frequency of unexpected panic attacks, worry about future attacks and feared consequences of attacks, and behavior changes resulting from the attacks. A checklist of panic attack symptoms, ratings of impairment and distress, and exclusion questions regarding substance use effects and medical conditions follow. The PDSR demonstrated 100% specificity and 89% sensitivity as well as test–retest reliability and excellent agreement with an extensive clinician-administered diagnostic interview. Convergent, discriminant, and clinical validity for this measure also was established. Unlike the PDSQ, the GAD-Q-IV, SPDQ, and PDSR were developed with undergraduate college student samples for research purposes and have not been examined in the primary care setting. Nevertheless, the presentation of specific diagnostic criteria in a simple lay-language format might improve detection of these specific anxiety disorders among primary care patients.

These brief diagnostic assessment procedures indeed may be feasible to administer in a variety of primary care medical settings. For further information about specific primary care assessment procedures, the reader is referred to Bufka, Crawford, and Levitt (2002). Primary care patients might complete diagnostic screening questionnaires, such as the PHQ from the PRIME-MD, the PDSQ, or the GAD-Q-IV, SPDQ, and PDSR in the waiting room before an appointment. Responses to such questionnaires either could be followed up with a brief diagnostic interview or could guide referrals to a behavioral health provider. Diagnosis of anxiety disorders may be crucial to treatment planning because most empirically supported treatments were developed for specific diagnostic groups. Resources for behavioral clinicians interested in providing such treatments to primary care patients are described next.

Effective Consultation/Liaison for Anxiety in Primary Care Settings

Empirically supported psychosocial treatments for the anxiety disorders are cognitive-behavioral in nature. These treatment protocols typically begin with some form of psychoeducation component. Clinicians explain the adaptive nature of anxiety and fear and associated physiology as well as how such processes have developed into the problematic symptoms of an anxiety disorder. Rationale for future treatment components is provided. Patients are encouraged to begin regular daily monitoring of anxiety levels and cues. Next, the clinician teaches skills patients can use as coping responses to internal and external anxiety triggers. Deep-breathing techniques, progressive muscle relaxation, and imagery relaxation procedures are all examples. Third, clinicians introduce cognitive therapy as a way to identify and to examine automatic anxious thoughts and underlying beliefs. Finally, some form of exposure to feared bodily sensations, images, environmental stimuli, and/or situations is conducted.

Some experts are developing new unified CBT treatment protocols that target fundamental processes underlying all the anxiety disorders (Barlow, Allen, & Choate, 2004). However, current empirically supported interventions are tailored to each anxiety disorder. Fortunately, many of these manualized protocols have become accessible to primary care behavioral providers. Concise and straightforward therapist treatment guides and patient workbooks containing pre-printed therapy forms are available increasingly. These materials are listed below, each of which outline a treatment protocol with empirical research support. Many of these resources are available through Oxford University Press (www.oup.com) in their "Treatments That Work" series. One final clinician resource was designed specifically for the managed care context: *Treatment plans and interventions for depression and anxiety disorders* (Leahy & Holland, 2000). This book provides brief treatment plan protocols and client handouts for all of the anxiety disorders.

Panic disorder (with or without agoraphobia). Panic Control Treatment (PCT) developed by Barlow, Craske, and their colleagues targets the fear of bodily sensations, or "fear of fear," that characterizes this particular anxiety disorder. This CBT protocol is summarized and demonstrated with a case example in Craske and Barlow (2001). A step-by-step Therapist Guide and accompanying Workbook for patients known as the *Mastery of your anxiety and panic,* 4th ed. or MAP-4 program (Craske & Barlow, 2006a; Barlow & Craske, 2006) is commercially available from Oxford University Press. An additional Client Workbook for Agoraphobia was available with the previous version of these materials (Craske & Barlow, 2000). A new MAP Workbook for Primary Care Settings has recently become available as well (Craske & Barlow, 2007).

Generalized anxiety disorder. Two cognitive-behavioral protocols for GAD are presented in accessible therapist materials. These protocols treat chronic somatic anxiety symptoms and muscle tension with muscle relaxation techniques. In addition, cognitive therapy and imagery exposure techniques target excessive worry and increased perceptions of threat. The *Mastery of your anxiety and worry,* 2nd ed. program (MAW-2) also consists of a Therapist Guide (Zinbarg, Craske, & Barlow, 2006) and Workbook for patients (Craske & Barlow, 2006b). These materials as well are commercially available through Oxford University Press. A therapist manual entitled *Treating generalized anxiety disorder* describes a similar protocol developed by Rygh and Sanderson (2004). This Guilford Press clinician resource contains several client handouts and therapy transcript examples.

Other practical suggestions for clinicians implementing CBT for GAD can be found in book chapters by Newman (2000), by Brown, O'Leary, and Barlow (2007), and by Leahy (2004). A final resource describes a particularly promising CBT protocol: *Cognitive-behavioral treatment for generalized anxiety disorder* (Dugas & Robichaud, 2007). This book is more comprehensive than the resources described above, and it contains several clinical procedures that may hold additional value in the treatment of GAD. For example, clinical procedures targeting intolerance of uncertainty, meta-cognitive worry beliefs, and poor problem orientation are described.

Social phobia/social anxiety disorder. The Cognitive-Behavioral Group Therapy (CBGT) developed by Heimberg and colleagues is considered the state-of-the-art cognitive behavioral treatment for social phobia. This treatment is illustrated in a book chapter by Turk, Heimberg, and Hope (2001) and is described for clinicians in a detailed treatment manual entitled *Cognitive-behavioral group therapy for social phobia* (Heimberg & Becker, 2002). This treatment is presented in a streamlined fashion for clinicians in a therapist guide and accompanying client workbook entitled *Managing social anxiety: A cognitive-behavioral therapy approach* (Hope, Heimberg, & Turk, 2006; Hope, Heimberg, Juster, & Turk, 2004), both available from Oxford University Press. An additional resource for clinicians treating adolescents entitled *Cognitive-behavioral therapy for social phobia in adolescents: Stand up, speak out* (Albano & DiBartolo, 2007) is now available as well.

Specific phobia. This anxiety disorder can be treated effectively with exposure techniques within a brief period of time. Both a therapist guide and workbook are available from Oxford University Press entitled *Mastering Your Fears and Phobias* (2nd ed.) (Craske, Antony, & Barlow, 2006; Antony, Craske, & Barlow, 2006).

Post-traumatic stress disorder. Cognitive-behavioral treatment of this complicated anxiety disorder typically involves some form of imagery exposure and cognitive therapy components. In cognitive processing therapy, exposure is conducted through writing assignments and subsequent therapy discussions of the traumatic event. This treatment is described with a case example in a book chapter by Resick and Calhoun (2001). An alternative form of exposure therapy for PTSD involves prolonged exposure. Both a Therapist Guide entitled *Prolonged exposure therapy for PTSD: Emotional processing of traumatic experiences* (Foa, Hembree & Rothbaum, 2007) and a Workbook entitled *Reclaiming your life from a traumatic experience: A prolonged exposure treatment program* (Rothbaum, Foa, & Hembree, 2007) are available from Oxford University Press. An alternative Client Workbook, *Reclaiming your life after rape: Cognitive-behavioral therapy for posttraumatic stress disorder* (Rothbaum & Foa, 2004), also is available. A Workbook for teenagers entitled *Reclaiming your life from PTSD: Teen Workbook* (Chrestman, Gilboa-Schechtman, & Foa, in press) is scheduled to be released in the spring of 2008. An additional Therapist Guide and Workbook were specifically tailored to individuals suffering from the effects of a serious motor vehicle accident: *Overcoming the trauma of your motor vehicle accident: A cognitive-behavioral treatment program* (Hickling & Blanchard, 2006a; 2006b).

Obsessive-compulsive disorder. Exposure and ritual (response) prevention is considered the leading psychosocial treatment for OCD. These therapy procedures are clearly demonstrated for clinicians in a book chapter by Foa and Franklin (2001). This treatment is presented in the *Mastery of obsessive-compulsive disorder: A cognitive-behavioral approach* Therapist Guide and Client Kit (Foa & Kozak, 2004a; 2004b) available from Oxford University Press.

Detailed therapy procedures and suggestions also can be found in the practitioner manual by Steketee (1993). A more concise and accessible Therapist Protocol entitled *Overcoming obsessive-compulsive disorder* (Steketee, 1999a) and an accompanying Client Manual (Steketee, 1999b) are available from New Harbinger Publications. In addition, a Therapist Guide and Workbook for the hoarding subtype of OCD are available from Oxford University Press: *Compulsive hoarding and acquiring* (Steketee & Frost, 2006a; 2006b).

Other Considerations to Support the PCP

The anxiety symptoms seen in some primary care patients may be the result of underlying medical conditions such as thyroid problems or hypoglycemia. Behavioral care providers might support the PCP by working with patients to increase compliance with necessary medical testing and treatment for these conditions. Along similar lines, many patients with anxiety disorders have comorbid medical diagnoses including asthma, chronic obstructive pulmonary disease (COPD), and irritable bowel syndrome (IBS). Behavioral providers can assist with the medical management of these conditions as well. In addition, the behavioral care provider might serve as a liaison between the patient and the PCP by clarifying which symptoms or sensations require medical intervention versus which symptoms and sensations simply reflect anxiety and are harmless. Furthermore, the behavioral provider might educate the PCP about the primary aims of cognitive-behavioral treatment as well as the behavioral advantages of an SSRI or other anti-depressant medication approach over benzodiazepine medications.

Self-Help Resources

Numerous self-help books are available to patients struggling with anxiety. Fortunately, an increasing number of these resources are based on empirically supported CBT methods. Reliable information about anxiety disorders also has become available to the public. For example, the website of the Anxiety Disorders Association of America (www.adaa.org) provides straightforward information on background statistics, diagnosis, and treatment options for individuals suffering from any of the anxiety disorders. Patients can download a brochure and take a self-test online to determine whether they might be diagnosed with an anxiety disorder. An online "Guide to Treatment" explains various types of psychotherapy and medication treatments with suggestions for choosing a therapist. Finally, a "Find a Therapist" online referral source is available on the ADAA website as well. Patients who prefer a book or who do not have Internet access may benefit from reading *Anxiety disorders: Everything you need to know* (Caldwell, 2005). The short paperback book provides basic psychoeducation information for each of the anxiety disorders as well as brief descriptions of treatment options. Both of these resources provide useful information to patients in accessible lay language.

For patients seeking self-help methods of treatment, the list below provides specific resources for each type of anxiety condition:

Panic and Phobias

Antony, M., & McCabe, R. (2004). *10 simple solutions to panic: How to overcome panic attacks, calm physical symptoms, and reclaim your life*. Oakland, CA: New Harbinger.
Bourne, E. (2000). *The anxiety and phobia workbook*. Oakland, CA: New Harbinger.

Brown, D. (1996). *Flying without fear.* Oakland, CA: New Harbinger.
Pollard, C. A., & Zuercher-White, E. (2003). *The agoraphobia workbook: A comprehensive program to end your fear of symptom attacks.* Oakland, CA: New Harbinger.
Zuercher-White, E. (1998). *An end to panic: Breakthrough techniques for overcoming panic disorder.* Oakland, CA: New Harbinger.

Generalized Anxiety and Worry

Hazlett-Stevens, H. (2005). *Women who worry too much: How to stop worry and anxiety from ruining relationships, work, and fun.* Oakland, CA: New Harbinger.
Leahy, R. L. (2005). *The worry cure: Seven steps to stop worry from stopping you.* New York: Harmony Books.

Shyness and Social Anxiety

Antony, M. (2004). *10 simple solutions to shyness.* Oakland, CA: New Harbinger.
Antony, M., & Swinson, R. (2000). *The shyness and social anxiety workbook: Proven techniques for overcoming your fears.* Oakland, CA: New Harbinger.
Markway, B., Carmin, C., Pollard, C. A., & Flynn, T. (1992). *Dying of embarrassment: Help for social anxiety and social phobia.* Oakland, CA: New Harbinger.
Rapee, R. M. (1998). *Overcoming Shyness and Social Phobia: A Step-by-Step Guide.* Lanham, MD: Jason Aronson.
Stein, M., & Walker, J. (2002.) *Triumph over shyness: Conquering shyness and social anxiety.* New York: McGraw-Hill.

Trauma Recovery

Follette, V. M., & Pistorello, J. (2007). *Finding life beyond trauma.* Oakland, CA: New Harbinger.
McCraig, M., & Kubany, E. S. (2003). *Healing the trauma of domestic violence.* Oakland, CA: New Harbinger.

Obsessions and Compulsions

Foa, E. B., & Wilson, R. (2001). *Stop obsessing! How to overcome your obsessions and compulsions.* New York: Bantam.
Grayson, J. (2003). *Freedom from obsessive-compulsive disorder: A personalized recovery program for living with uncertainty.* New York: Tarcher.
Purdon, C., & Clark, D. A. (2005). *Overcoming obsessive thoughts: How to gain control of your OCD.* Oakland, CA: New Harbinger.

Referral and Stepped Care

Once the primary care provider has detected a likely anxiety disorder, the patient can be referred to some form of behavioral treatment. In some primary care settings, behavioral health services might not be readily available. In such cases, patients might be referred to the ADAA website and given a list of self-help resources immediately. If patients have not experienced relief from symptoms by the time behavioral treatment begins, the behavioral provider might follow session procedures as outlined in the published therapist guides described above. Patients exhibiting severe or complicated clinical presentations who do not benefit from such brief protocols would then be referred to specialized mental health services for further treatment.

Key Readings

Barlow, D. H. (2007). *Clinical handbook of psychological disorders: A step-by-step treatment manual* (4th ed.). New York: Guilford.
Leahy, R. L., and Holland, S. J. (2000). *Treatment plans and interventions for depression and anxiety disorders.* New York: Guilford.

References

Albano, A. M., & DiBartolo, P. M. (2007). *Cognitive-behavioral therapy for social phobia in adolescents: Stand up, speak out: Therapist guide.* New York: Oxford University Press.
Antony, M. M., Craske, M. G., & Barlow, D. H. (2006). *Mastering your fears and phobias: Workbook* (2nd ed.). New York: Oxford University Press.
Barlow, D. H., Allen, L. B., & Choate, M. I. (2004). Toward a unified treatment for emotional disorders. *Behavior Therapy, 35*, 205–230.
Barlow, D. H., & Craske, M. G. (2006). *Mastery of your anxiety and panic: Client workbook* (4th ed.). New York: Oxford University Press.
Brown, T. A., O'Leary, T. A., & Barlow, D. H. (2001). Generalized anxiety disorder. In D. H. Barlow (Ed.), *Clinical handbook of psychological disorders: A step-by-step treatment manual* (3rd ed.) (pp. 154–208). New York: Guilford.
Bufka, L. F., Crawford, J. I., & Levitt, J. T. (2002). Brief screening assessments for managed care and primary care. In M. M. Antony, & D. H. Barlow (Eds.), *Handbook of assessment and treatment planning for psychological disorders* (pp. 38–63). New York: Guilford.
Caldwell, J. P. (2005). *Anxiety disorders: Everything you need to know.* Buffalo, NY: Firefly Books Inc.
Chrestman, K. R., Gilboa-Schechtman, E., & Foa, E. B. (in press). *Reclaiming your life from PTSD: Teen Workbook.* New York: Oxford University Press.
Craske, M. G., Antony, M. M., & Barlow, D. H. (2006). *Mastering your fears and phobias: Therapist guide* (2nd ed.). New York: Oxford University Press.
Craske, M. G., & Barlow, D. H. (2000). *Mastery of your anxiety and panic: Client workbook for agoraphobia* (3rd ed.). New York: Oxford University.
Craske, M. G., & Barlow, D. H. (2001). Panic disorder and agoraphobia. In D. H. Barlow (Ed.), *Clinical handbook of psychological disorders: A step-by-step treatment manual* (3rd ed.) (pp. 1–59). New York: Guilford.
Craske, M. G., & Barlow, D. H. (2006a). *Mastery of your anxiety and panic: Therapist guide* (4th ed.). New York: Oxford University Press.
Craske, M. G., & Barlow, D. H. (2006b). *Mastery of your anxiety and worry: Client workbook* (2nd ed.). New York: Oxford University Press.
Craske, M. G., & Barlow, D. H. (2007). *Mastery of your anxiety and panic: Workbook for Primary Care Settings.* New York: Oxford University Press.

Dugas, M. J., & Robichaud, M. (2007). *Cognitive-behavioral treatment for generalized anxiety disorder: From science to practice.* New York: Routledge/Taylor & Francis.

Edlund, M. J., & Swann, A. C. (1987). The economics and social costs of panic disorder. *Hospital and Community Psychiatry, 38,* 1277–1279, 1288.

Foa, E. B., & Franklin, M. E. (2001). Obsessive-compulsive disorder. In D. H. Barlow (Ed.), *Clinical handbook of psychological disorders: A step-by-step treatment manual* (3rd ed.) (pp. 209–263). New York: Guilford.

Foa, E. B., Hembree, E. A., & Rothbaum, B. O. (2007). *Prolonged exposure therapy for PTSD: Emotional processing of traumatic experiences: Therapist guide.* New York: Oxford University Press.

Foa, E. B., & Kozak, M. J. (2004a). *Mastery of obsessive-compulsive disorder: A cognitive-behavioral approach: Therapist Guide.* New York: Oxford University Press.

Foa, E. B., & Kozak, M. J. (2004b). *Mastery of obsessive-compulsive disorder: A cognitive-behavioral approach: Client kit.* New York: Oxford University Press.

Goisman, R. M., Warshaw, M. G., & Keller, M. B. (1999). Psychosocial treatment prescriptions for generalized anxiety disorder, panic disorder, and social phobia, 1991–1996. *American Journal of Psychiatry, 156,* 1819–1821.

Harvey, A. G. (2002). Trouble in bed: The role of pre-sleep worry and intrusions in the maintenance of insomnia. *Journal of Cognitive Psychotherapy: An International Quarterly, 16,* 161–177.

Heimberg, R. G., & Becker, R. E. (2002). *Cognitive-behavioral group therapy for social phobia: Basic mechanisms and clinical strategies.* New York: Guilford.

Hickling, E. J., & Blanchard, E. B. (2006a). *Overcoming the trauma of your motor vehicle accident: A cognitive-behavioral treatment program: Therapist guide.* New York: Oxford University Press.

Hickling, E. J., & Blanchard, E. B. (2006b). *Overcoming the trauma of your motor vehicle accident: A cognitive-behavioral treatment program: Workbook.* New York: Oxford University Press.

Hope, D. A., Heimberg, R. G., Juster, H. A., & Turk, C. L. (2004). *Managing social anxiety: A cognitive-behavioral therapy approach: Client Workbook.* New York: Oxford University Press.

Hope, D. A., Heimberg, R. G., & Turk, C. L. (2006). *Managing social anxiety: A cognitive-behavioral therapy approach: Therapist guide.* New York: Oxford University Press.

Kennedy, B. L., & Schwab, J. J. (1997). Utilization of medical specialists by anxiety disorder patients. *Psychosomatics, 38,* 109–112.

Kessler, R. C., Berglund, P., Demler, O., Jin, R., Merikangas, K. R., & Walters, E. E. (2005). Lifetime prevalence of age-of-onset distributions of DSM-IV disorders in the National Comorbidity Survey Replication. *Archives of General Psychiatry, 62,* 593–602.

Kessler, R. C., Chiu, W. T., Demler, O., & Walters, E. E. (2005). Prevalence, severity, and comorbidity of 12-month DSM-IV disorders in the National Comorbidity Survey Replication. *Archives of General Psychiatry, 62,* 617–627.

Kobak, K. A., Taylor, L. H., Dottl, S. L., Greist, J. H., Jefferson, J. W., Burroughs, D., et al. (1997). A computer-administered telephone interview to identify mental disorders. *Journal of the American Medial Association, 278,* 905–910.

Leahy, R. L. (2004). Cognitive-behavioral therapy. In R. G. Heimberg, C. L. Turk, & D. S. Mennin (Eds.), *Generalized anxiety disorder: Advances in research and practice* (pp. 265–292). New York: Guilford Press.

Leahy, R. L., & Holland, S. J. (2000). *Treatment plans and interventions for depression and anxiety disorders.* New York: Guilford.

Markowitz, J. S., Weissman, M. M., Ouellette, R., Lish, J. D., & Klerman, G. L. (1989). Quality of life in panic disorder. *Archives of General Psychiatry, 46,* 984–992.

Newman, M. G. (2000). Generalized anxiety disorder. In M. Hersen, & M. Biaggio (Eds.), *Effective brief therapies: A clinician's guide* (pp. 157–178). San Diego, CA: Academic Press.

Newman, M. G., Holmes, M., Zuellig, A. R., Kachin, K. E., & Behar, E. (2006). The reliability and validity of the Panic Disorder Self-Report: A new diagnostic screening measure of panic disorder. *Psychological Assessment, 18*, 49–61.

Newman, M. G., Kachin, K. E., Zuellig, A. R., Constantino, M. J., & Cashman-McGrath, L. (2003). The Social Phobia Diagnostic Questionnaire: Preliminary validation of a new self-report diagnostic measure of social phobia. *Psychological Medicine, 33*, 623–635.

Newman, M. G., Zuellig, A. R., Kachin, K. E., Constantino, M. J., Przeworski, A., Erickson, T., et al. (2002). Preliminary reliability and validity of the Generalized Anxiety Disorder Questionnaire-IV: A revised self-report diagnostic measure of generalized anxiety disorder. *Behavior Therapy, 33*, 215–233.

Resick, P. A., & Calhoun, K. S. (2001). Posttraumatic stress disorder. In D. H. Barlow (Ed.), *Clinical handbook of psychological disorders: A step-by-step treatment manual* (3rd ed.) (pp. 60–113). New York: Guilford.

Rothbaum, B. O., & Foa, E. B. (2004). *Reclaiming your life after rape: cognitive-behavioral therapy for posttraumatic stress disorder: Client workbook*. New York: Oxford University Press.

Rothbaum, B. O., Foa, E. B., & Hembree, E. A. (2007). *Reclaiming your life from a traumatic experience: A prolonged exposure treatment program: Workbook*. New York: Oxford University Press.

Roy-Byrne, P. P., & Wagner, A., (2004). Primary care perspectives on generalized anxiety disorder. *Journal of Clinical Psychiatry, 65*(Suppl. 13), 20–26.

Rygh, J. R., & Sanderson, W. C. (2004). *Treating generalized anxiety disorder: Evidence-based strategies, tools, and techniques*. New York: Guilford Press.

Sareen, J., Cox, B. J., Clara, I., & Asmundson, G. J. G. (2005). The relationship between anxiety disorders and physical disorders in the U.S. National Comorbidity Survey. *Depression and Anxiety, 21*, 193–202.

Sheehan, D. V., & Lecrubier, Y. (2002). *MINI International Neuropsychiatric Interview for DSM-IV* (English Version 5.0.0). Tampa: University of South Florida.

Sheehan, D. V., Lecrubier, Y., Harnett-Sheehan, K., Amorim, P., Janavs, J., Weiller, E., et al. (1998). The Mini-International Neuropsychiatric Interview (M.I.N.I.): The development and validation of a structured diagnostic psychiatric interview for DSM-IV and ICD-10. *Journal of Clinical Psychiatry, 59*(Suppl. 20), 22–33.

Siegel, L., Jones, W. C., & Wilson, J. O. (1990). Economic and life consequences experienced by a group of individuals with panic disorder. *Journal of Anxiety Disorders, 4*, 201–211.

Spitzer, R. L., Kroenke, K., & Williams, J. B. (1999). Validation and utility of a self-report version of PRIME-MD: The PHQ primary care study. Primary Care Evaluation of Mental Disorders. Patient Health Questionnaire. *Journal of the American Medical Association, 282*, 1737–1774.

Spitzer, R. L., Williams, J. B. W., Kroenke, K., Linzer, M., deGruy, F. V., Hahn, S. R., et al. (1994). Utility of a new procedure for diagnosing mental disorders in primary care: The PRIME-MD 1000 study. *Journal of the American Medical Association, 272*, 1749–1756.

Stein, M. B., & Heimberg, R. G. (2004). Well-being and life satisfaction in generalized anxiety disorder: Comparison to major depressive disorder in a community sample. *Journal of Affective Disorders, 79*, 161–166.

Steketee, G. S. (1993). *Treatment of obsessive compulsive disorder*. New York: Guilford.

Steketee, G. S. (1999a). *Overcoming obsessive-compulsive disorder: Therapist protocol*. Oakland, CA: New Harbinger.

Steketee, G. S. (1999b). *Overcoming obsessive-compulsive disorder: Client manual*. Oakland, CA: New Harbinger.

Steketee, G. S., & Frost, R. O. (2006a). *Compulsive hoarding and acquiring: Therapist guide*. New York: Oxford University Press.

Steketee, G. S., & Frost, R. O. (2006b). *Compulsive hoarding and acquiring: Workbook*. New York: Oxford University Press.

Swinson, R. P., Cox, B. J., & Woszcyna, C. B. (1992). Use of medical services and treatment for panic disorder with agoraphobia and for social phobia. *Canadian Medical Association, 147*, 878–883.

Tollefson, G. D., Tollefson, S. L., Pederson, M., Luxenberg, M., & Dunsmore, G. (1991). Comorbid irritable bowel syndrome in patients with generalized anxiety and major depression. *Annals of Clinical Psychiatry, 3*, 215–222.

Turk, C. L., Heimberg, R. G., & Hope, D. A. (2001). Social anxiety disorder. In D. H. Barlow (Ed.), *Clinical handbook of psychological disorders: A step-by-step treatment manual* (3rd ed.) (pp. 114–153). New York: Guilford.

Wang, P. S., Lane, M., Olfson, M., Pincus, H. A., Wells, K. B., & Kessler, R. C. (2005). Twelve-month use of mental health services in the United States. *Archives of General Psychiatry, 62*, 629–640.

Yonkers, K. A., Bruce, S. E., Dyck, I. R., & Keller, M. B. (2003). Chronicity, relapse, and illness – Course of panic disorder, social phobia, and generalized anxiety disorder: Findings in men and women from 8 years of follow-up. *Depression and Anxiety, 17*, 173–179.

Zimmerman, M., & Mattia, J. I. (1999). The reliability and validity of a screening questionnaire for 13 DSM-IV Axis I disorders (the Psychiatric Diagnostic Screening Questionnaire) in psychiatric outpatients. *Journal of Clinical Psychiatry, 60*, 677–683.

Zimmerman, M., & Mattia, J. I. (2001a). The Psychiatric Diagnostic Screening Questionnaire: Development, reliability, and validity. *Comprehensive Psychiatry, 42*, 175–189.

Zimmerman, M., & Mattia, J. I. (2001b). A self-report scale to help make psychiatric diagnoses: The Psychiatric Diagnostic Screening Questionnaire (PDSQ). *Archives of General Psychiatry, 58*, 787–794.

Zinbarg, R. E., Craske, M. G., & Barlow, D. H. (2006). *Mastery of your anxiety and worry: Therapist guide* (2nd ed.). New York: Oxford University Press.

Assessing and Managing Chronic Pain in the Primary Care Setting

Melanie P. Duckworth, Tony Iezzi, and M. Todd Sewell

Chronic Pain in the Primary Care Setting

Pain is experienced by almost everyone at some point in time. For most persons, the experience of pain is brief and uncomplicated, with pain remitting fully in the absence of medical intervention. For a small but significant proportion of the population, the experience of pain, due to its duration, intensity, and functional impacts, will precipitate contact with a health care provider. It has been observed that two of every five visits to a primary care provider (PCP) are made due to pain (Mantyselka, Turunen, Ahonen, & Kumpusalo, 2001). Pain conditions are common among patients attending primary care, with an estimated 20% of these patients diagnosed with persistent or chronic pain conditions (Gureje, Von Korff, Simon, & Gater, 1998).

Despite the significant number of persons presenting to health care providers for evaluation and management of pain, pain is an experience that patients find difficult to communicate and that care providers find difficult to quantify. According to the International Association for the Study of Pain (IASP), pain is defined as "an unpleasant sensory and emotional experience associated with actual or potential tissue damage, or described in terms of such damage" (Merskey & Bogduk, 1994, p. 210). The most widely accepted classification of pain reflects a pain-injury association. *Acute pain* is commonly defined as pain that does not last longer than six months and that remits when the underlying cause of pain has healed. Pain that persists for longer than six months is referred to as *chronic pain* (IASP, 1986). Although the IASP definitions of acute pain and chronic pain are widely recognized and accepted, the acute pain and chronic pain are frequently used to describe pain that persists up to three months and longer than three months, respectively.

Another category of pain that is garnering increased research attention is widespread pain. Widespread pain is defined as pain present at two contralateral quadrants of the body and in the axial skeleton, and persisting for at least two months

M.P. Duckworth (✉)
Department of Psychology/MS298, University of Nevada, Reno, Reno, NV 89557, USA
e-mail: melanied@unr.edu

L.C. James, W.T. O'Donohue (eds.), *The Primary Care Toolkit*,
DOI 10.1007/978-0-387-78971-2_13, © Springer Science+Business Media, LLC 2009

(Wolfe et al., 1990). All of these categories of pain (acute, chronic, and widespread) are important because they have implications for the recovery of physical function and quality of life.

Screening and Assessment of Chronic Pain in the Primary Care Setting

Pain is one of the most common clinical presentations that PCPs are called upon to evaluate and manage (Gureje et al., 1998). Pain symptoms may be experienced consequent to an injury, in conjunction with various disease conditions, or in the absence of an identifiable cause. When evaluating a patient's report of pain, the PCP is tasked with establishing the duration, intensity, and quality of the patient's pain symptoms and determining the relation of that pain to disease conditions, physical injuries, and/or health behaviors present in the patient's medical history.

Information regarding the parameters of pain is usually obtained through verbal reporting and physical examination of the patient. The PCP works to establish the location, duration, intensity, and quality of pain (e.g., burning, dull, radiating, stabbing) and to determine those factors that seem to be associated with changes in pain intensity or quality (i.e., time of day, activity level, level of fatigue, medication, emotional distress). In managing a patient's experience of acute pain, the PCP must be cognizant of the most effective strategies for both reducing pain *and* restoring normal function. The PCP may employ a variety of interventions to managing acute pain, including education, exercise, chiropractic manipulation and mobilization, massage therapy, physiotherapy, and pharmacotherapy. It is generally agreed that the key components of pain management include early and gradual resumption of normal activities and avoidance of bed rest (Deyo, Diehl, & Rosenthal, 1986; Malmivaara et al., 1995; Waddell, 1987). In the context of acute pain management, a behavioral health specialist can assist the PCP in tailoring the information and providing advice to address patient concerns and behaviors (e.g., fear of re-injury, catastrophizing, pain avoidance) that are thought to significantly interfere with recovery. Based on their 2002 review of the literature on whiplash-associated disorders, McClune, Burton, and Waddell indicated the following messages as having the potential to reduce the risk of chronicity:

- Serious physical injury is rare.
- Reassurance about good prognosis is important.
- Over-medicalization is detrimental.
- Recovery is improved by early return to normal (pre-collision) activities, self exercise, and manual therapy.
- Positive attitudes and beliefs are helpful in regaining activity levels.
- Collars, rest, and negative attitudes and beliefs delay recovery and contribute to chronicity.

The strength of these messages lies in the fact that they are evidence-based. *Reassurance about good prognosis is important.* It is generally assumed that physician-delivered messages and instructions regarding patient health and health practices are of particular import to patients and are more likely to be heeded than messages and instructions received from others with less medical knowledge and authority. The strength of physician-delivered health instructions has been empirically tested in the contexts of smoking and alcohol use. In both contexts, physician-delivered health instructions have served to significantly reduce patient engagement in risky health behaviors (Fleming, Barry, Manwell, Johnson, & London, 1997; Ockene, Adams, Hurley, Wheeler, & Herbert, 1999; Ockene et al., 1991). In the face of persisting reports on pain and suffering, a PCP should avoid unqualified statements that indicate that "nothing is physically wrong" with the injured person. In the absence of positive diagnostic findings that would suggest physical compromise, the PCP might speak of the limitation in current diagnostic technology and reassure the patient that monitoring of symptoms will be continued.

Over-medicalization is detrimental. In responding to pain, patients employ a number of different pain relief strategies. Using a postal survey, Turunen, Mantyselka, Kumpusalo, and Ahonen (2004) identified respondents from the general population who reported the experience of pain during the past seven days, and evaluated respondents' use of pain relief strategies employed to manage their pain during the previous six months. Respondents indicated the use of a variety of pain relief strategies, including over-the-counter medications, exercise, prescription medicines, and visiting a physician. Supporting the warning against over-medicalization is the fact that pain persistence was predicted by respondents' use of multiple pain treatments. Using data from interviews conducted with 17,543 randomly sampled residents of New South Wales, Australia, Blyth, March, Brnabic, and Cousins (2004) determined that chronic pain and chronic pain with activity interference predict health care utilization, with high levels of pain-related disability being most predictive of health care utilization.

Recovery is improved by early return to normal activities. Malmivaara et al. (1995) compared the levels of recovery achieved by patients with acute low back pain who were assigned to one of three treatment conditions: two days of bed rest, back-mobilizing exercises, or the continuation of ordinary activities as tolerated. Patients who were prescribed to continue normal activities as tolerable differed significantly from those who were assigned the other two treatment conditions across a host of pain and functional status variables. Patients who continued their normal activities as tolerable despite pain experienced briefer pain duration, lower pain intensity, increased lumbar flexion, and improved work function as measured by patient report, including the number of days absent from work. The authors described patients who had been prescribed rest as experiencing the slowest recovery.

In the face of the most judicious application of pain intervention strategies and the most articulate communication of recovery information and advice, some patients reported prolonged pain and impairment even weeks after the initial PCP visit. This persistence of pain and impairment may point to the need for individually tailored pain treatment plans in which specific functional limitations (e.g., difficulties in standing, sitting, bending, lifting, etc.) and support needs (e.g., limited number of telephonic contacts or visits to a behavioral health specialist aimed at reinforcing recovery behaviors and managing barriers to such behaviors) are identified and managed. The behavioral health specialist is perfectly positioned to perform a more detailed analysis of pain-related functional limitations and support needs and to put into action a pain treatment plan that will result in more optimal outcomes for such patients.

Ahles et al. (2006) have proposed that the provision of information that specifically addresses the concerns of a patient (INFO), feedback to the PCP regarding the patient's specific problems and concerns (FEED), and minimal telephonic contact with a nurse-educator (NE) can be more effective than usual care in the management of pain experienced by primary care patients with and without psychosocial problems. The benefits of a combined INFO + FEED + NE intervention include significant improvements on the bodily pain, role physical, and role emotional scales of the Medical Outcomes Study 36-item Short Form (Ware, Snow, Kosinski, & Gandek, 1993) as well as improvement on the Functional Interference Estimate scale (Toomey, Mann, Hernandez, & Abashian, 1993). The benefits of the combined intervention were maintained at 12-month assessment, with the authors noting that, on average, only three telephone contacts were required to achieve and maintain these improvements. This, of course, confirms the cost-effectiveness of such minimal contact approaches (Blount et al., 2007).

It is also possible that a patient's report of continuing pain and impairment reflects the interaction of an entire array of physical, psychological, and social influences. These influences are usually first made clear to the PCP through the patient's report of increasing pain, suffering, disability, *and* emotional distress. Chronic pain is frequently accompanied by distress reactions, including symptoms of anxiety and depression. Here again, the behavioral health specialist is perfectly positioned to assist the PCP in determining the clinical significance of such distress reactions and to facilitate an appropriate referral should psychological symptoms warrant more intensive management. There are certain symptoms and behaviors that would indicate to the PCP that consultation and/or referral is in order. In making a determination regarding the clinical import of emotional distress reactions and the need to enlist the assistance of behavioral/mental health specialists, the following symptoms and behaviors should be considered significant:

- severe physical injury
- significant pain or illness behaviors
- increasing *widespread* pain
- lack of acceptance of the chronicity of pain
- kinesiophobia or fear of re-injury
- excessive resistance or lack of compliance in returning to the workplace
- simultaneous use of multiple, uncoordinated treatments
- high levels of somatization (i.e., preoccupation with physical symptoms)
- excessive medication-seeking behavior and *repeated* misuse of prescribed medications

- passive coping and pain catastrophizing (i.e., evidencing an exaggerated response to pain)
- increased alcohol and/or illicit substance use/abuse
- prominent marital discord
- repeated episodes of property destruction and/or physical assault
- prominent and multiple systems issues
- little or no social support
- increasing severity of depression in the face of treatment with anti-depressants
- increasing suicidal ideations and setting a plan for suicide

These symptoms and behaviors are associated with a cascade of pain-related lifestyle disruptions that move from lost work days, to increased financial burden, to increased interpersonal and intrapersonal distress. Research suggests that these pain-related lifestyle disruptions are predictive of the long-term recovery and well-being of patients with chronic pain (Blincoe et al., 2002; DePalma, Fedorka, & Simko, 2003; Duckworth, Iezzi, & Lewandowski, 2008; Mayou, & Bryant, 2003). For a PCP who attempts to manage a patient's pain symptoms and functional limitations in the face of such disruptions, it is essential that an integrated and coordinated treatment plan be undertaken. Consultation liaison services become particularly relevant to the management of such patients in the primary care setting.

Consultation Liaison for Chronic Pain Management in Primary Care Setting

In the primary care setting, consultation liaison has been a traditional avenue in which representatives of different disciplines are brought together to address a chronic pain condition that has multiple determinants (e.g., biological, psychological, and social). Traditionally, the PCP's use of consultation liaison services would have occurred after all medical interventions for pain management had been exhausted, and would have involved a redefinition of the patient's pain conditions as due to psychological factors and requiring psychiatric rather than medical management. Today, PCP's and other health specialists who work in the area of pain management embrace a biopsychosocial model of pain and, out of that model, work collaboratively across all phases of the patient's pain conditions to manage pain, reduce functional limitations, and maximize outcomes (Brown & Folen, 2005; Simon & Folen, 2001; Tovian, 2006). These services, if delivered in this manner, have been found to be cost-effective (Blount et al., 2007).

The importance of early and coordinated evaluation and management of pain rests in the strength of early pain reports in predicting pain persistence and future pain-associated disability. Gureje, Simon, and Von Korff (2001) examined the persistence of pain syndromes among primary care patients. Using data from the World Health Organization's international study of psychological problems in general health care, the authors tested the contribution of baseline reports of pain, other somatic symptoms, and anxiety and depression to the persistent experience of these symptoms at 12-month follow-up. Persistent pain at baseline was predicted by the presence of a psychological disorder, poor self-rated health, and occupational role disability and was equally predictive of the onset of a psychological disorder. Nearly 50% of those primary care patients with persistent pain at baseline had not recovered at 12-month follow-up, with non-recovery of function best predicted by the number of pain sites reported at baseline. Symptoms of anxiety and depression did not predict the continuation of persistent pain at 12-month follow-up. Through their coordinated efforts, the PCPs ensure effective address of pain occurring across multiple body sites, and the behavioral health specialists evaluate and address the psychological difficulties and role disabilities that contributed to initial reports of persistent pain.

Guiding Chronic Pain Patients toward Pain Acceptance

No matter how effective the strategies employed by the PCP to manage acute pain, some injured persons will experience the persistence of pain and the associated physical limitations and lifestyle disruptions. It is in the face of chronic pain that the PCP will be required to shift from treatment that is consistent with a *pain relief* model to treatment that is consistent with a *pain coping* model. A pain coping model emphasizes pain acceptance. McCracken (1998) defines acceptance of pain as involving responses to pain-related experiences that do not include attempts at pain control or pain avoidance as well as engagement in valued actions and pursuit of personal goals regardless of these experiences. Of course, for the PCP, the ultimate goals of pain acceptance are (1) avoidance of medical procedures that are either inappropriate for the management of persisting pain or that have been proven less effective for the management of pain that persists long after the expected recovery from a physical injury has been achieved; and (2) increased patient acceptance of the adjustments to physical and lifestyle functions that are required to ensure the most optimal post-injury quality of life that is possible.

The importance of pain acceptance and valued actions and goals to functional outcomes among pain patients has been tested empirically. In a recent study on the adjustment to chronic pain experienced by 117 chronic pain patients, Esteve, Ramirez-Maestre, and Lopez-Martinez (2007) found that acceptance of pain determines one's functional status and functional impairment as measured by the Impairment and Function Inventory (IFI; Ramirez-Maestre, & Valdivia, 2003 as cited in Esteve et al., 2007). The importance of pursuing valued actions in the presence of pain is further supported by Smith and Zautra (2004). These researchers tested the role of a sense of purpose in life in predicting recovery from knee replacement surgery. They determined a sense of purpose in life to be related to less anxiety, less depression, and less functional disability following surgery.

Pain acceptance is not something that patients arrive at independently or embrace easily. In moving a pain patient away from pain relief and towards pain acceptance, the behavioral health specialist encourages the patient to reflect on the less-than-satisfactory outcomes of the past pain relief attempts, to assess the loss in quality of life that has been experienced as a function of pain avoidance and the pursuit of pain relief, to entertain the possibility of a life that is lived in the presence of pain, to identify valued actions and roles that define one's life, and to identify those functional and lifestyle adjustments that would be required to live as normal and satisfying a life as possible in the presence of pain. This shift in focus from pain relief to the pursuit of valued actions and goals is critical to the patient's willingness to engage effectively in a comprehensive pain management plan. Once the shift has occurred, the behavioral health specialist is in a position to recommend and assist the patient in implementing a variety of interventions, including exercise and goal-setting aimed at reclaiming normal functioning across vocational and avocational domains (i.e., household, recreational, social, familial, and interpersonal).

Managing Pain-Related Psychological Conditions

The importance of the relationship between pain and psychological variables was made most salient in an impressive literature review conducted by Linton (2000). He identified 37 prospective studies out of a larger group of 913 studies that examined psychological risk factors in back and neck pain. The study findings were evaluated using a grading system that ranged from Level A (support from two or more good-quality prospective studies) to Level D (no studies meeting the criteria were available); based on his evaluation of the studies, Linton concluded the following (p. 1153):

1. Psychosocial variables are clearly linked to the transition from acute to chronic pain disability (Level A evidence).
2. Psychological factors are associated with reported onset of back and neck pain (Level A evidence).
3. Psychosocial variables generally have more impact than biomedical or biomechanical factors on back pain disability (Level A evidence).
4. No evidence exists to support the idea of a 'pain prone' personality link (Level D evidence).
5. Results are mixed with regard to whether personality and traits are risk factors (Level C evidence).
6. Cognitive factors (attitudes, cognitive style, fear-avoidance beliefs) are related to the development of pain and disability (Level A evidence).

   a. Passive coping is related to pain and disability (Level A evidence).
   b. Pain cognitions (e.g., catastrophizing) are related to pain and disability (Level A evidence).
   c. Fear-avoidance beliefs are related to pain and disability (Level A evidence).

7. Depression, anxiety, distress, and related emotions are related to pain and disability (Level A evidence).

8. Sexual and/or physical abuse may be related to chronic pain and disability (Level D evidence).
9. Self-perceived poor health is related to chronic pain and disability (Level A evidence).
10. Psychosocial factors may be used as predictors of the risk for developing long-term pain and disability (Level A evidence).

A number of psychological treatments have been developed for the management of chronic pain and the associated psychosocial consequences of chronic pain. Meta-analyses and systematic reviews have supported the effectiveness of psychological treatments for chronic pain (Hoffamn, Papas, Chatkoff, & Kerns, 2007; Thorn, Cross, & Walker, 2007). Behavioral health specialists are ideally suited to manage the more intractable features of chronic pain, including marked psychological distress, maladaptive cognitions, maladaptive coping styles, functional limitations, and disruptions across lifestyle domains.

Although a number of different interventions have been established as effective for the management of chronic pain and the associated psychological difficulties and lifestyle impairments, many of these interventions share an emphasis on goal-setting across work, household, recreational, and social domains; behavioral activation; pain confrontation versus pain avoidance; and emotion regulation and reduction of interpersonal discord. These interventions also focus on reducing pain behaviors (e.g., reducing reliance on pain medication, decreasing over-reliance on others, decreasing time spent resting or in bed).

Supporting the Primary Care Physician's Efforts to Managing Chronic Pain

Behavioral health specialist may be considered essential to efforts aimed at reducing the number and complexity of treatment targets faced by the PCP who is attempting to manage a patient with chronic pain. Chronic pain is often associated with functional limitations that contribute to a range of lifestyle impairments. Chronic pain patients who experience pain-related functional limitations often experience clinically significant symptoms of psychological distress, including depression and anxiety (Simon & Folen, 2001). The behavioral health specialist not only addresses the psychological management of chronic pain but also plays a primary role in recommending pharmacotherapy for mood disorders and assisting with the monitoring of opioid medication use (Brown & Folen, 2005).

The behavioral health specialist is expert in evaluating the various impacts of chronic pain. A comprehensive pain assessment conducted by a behavioral health specialist usually relies on a semi-structured interview and extensive psychological testing. Psychological tests document changes in psychological functioning, quality of life, and coping. Measures of general psychological functioning include the Minnesota Multiphasic Personality Inventory-II (Butcher, Dahlstrom, Graham, Tellegen, & Kaemmer, 1989), Millon Clinical Multiaxial Inventory-III (Millon et al., 1994), and the Symptom Checklist-90-Revised (Derogatis, 1983). Specific measures of depression and anxiety can include the Beck Depression Inventory-II (Beck, Steer, & Brown, 1996) and Beck Anxiety Inventory (Beck & Steer, 1990). The Sickness Impact Profile (Bergner, Bobbitt, Carter, & Gilson, 1981) and the Medical Outcomes Study Short-Form (Ware, Snow, Kosinski, & Gandek, 1993) are good measures of quality of life, while the Coping Strategies Questionnaire (Keefe, Crisson, Urban, & Williams, 1990) and Pain Catastrophizing Scale (Sullivan, Bishop, & Pivak, 1995) provide a good index of coping style. The Multidimensional Pain Inventory (Kerns, Turk, & Rudy, 1985) is one of the best measures of pain severity, quality of life, and affective distress.

The aim of interviewing and testing is to provide both ideographic (i.e., within the individual) and nomothetic (i e., the individual compared to other patients) perspectives on the chronic pain patient. The information provided by the behavioral health specialist allows the PCP to more fully appreciate and develop better management strategies that are tailored to the needs of respective chronic pain patient.

The behavioral health specialist also brings to the primary care setting a sophisticated knowledge of the various demographic, psychological, and social factors to have been found to best predict the persistence of pain and disability. In consort with the PCPs efforts, behavioral health specialists can assist in forecasting the probable course of the chronic pain patient. A number of studies suggest that neck pain (Sterling, Jull, & Kenardy, 2006) and widespread pain (Wynne-Jones, Jones, Silman, & MacFarlane, 2006) can best be predicted by a prediction model that includes sociodemographic, physical, and psychological variables. The PCP and the behavioral health specialist work together to identify and manage the immediate and future care needs of chronic pain patients.

A Stepped Care Approach to Chronic Pain Management

Interventions that are used to managing pain may be placed on a continuum from least intensive/restrictive to most intensive/restrictive based on a variety of factors, including patient effort required, level of PCP contact required, and the cost of intervention. A stepped care model of healthcare delivery is one in which patients are first provided with less intensive/restrictive interventions. The patient's response to treatment is then evaluated. More intensive/restrictive interventions are employed only in the absence of an adequate treatment response to the least intensive/restrictive interventions. Different models of stepped care for management of chronic illness have been proposed (Davison, 2000; Otis, MacDonald, & Dobscha, 2006; Von Korff & Moore, 2001; Von Korff & Tiemens, 2000), with a number of these models being specific to pain management. The most effective stepped care approaches to pain management share an emphasis on sequenced interventions that: (1) address patients' pain-related worries and concerns, restore normal functioning, and discourage activity avoidance; (2) provide structured support for physical exercise and activity engagement efforts; and (3) provide more intensive psychological interventions aimed at addressing clinically significant emotional distress and lifestyle impairment. For patients who experience more intractable pain, a comprehensive chronic pain program may be required (Gatchel & Okifuji, 2006).

Otis et al. (2006) have recommended a three-step approach to pain management. In step 1, intervention strategies are aimed at "identifying and addressing specific patient concerns about pain and enhancing patient readiness for self-care" (p. 1335). These authors describe some of the most common patient concerns including the fear that pain is suggestive of some underlying physical pathology as well as the fear that getting involved in an activity may contribute to re-injury. Again, intervention at this step is aimed at alleviating such patient concerns and ensuring that patients feel supported in the efforts to resume normal functioning. Chronic pain patients who benefit most from step 1 interventions are those who tend to experience less intense pain, rely less on medication, be more active across a variety of lifestyle domains, and experience less intense emotional distress. In the general chronic pain literature, such patients would be described as adaptive copers (Kerns et al., 1985). In step 2, a more active approach to pain management is undertaken, with emphasis placed on the identification of patient-specific functional difficulties and the development and implementation of a treatment plan that would address those patient-specific functional difficulties. It is at this step that the behavioral health specialist would re-evaluate the treatment needs of the patient and determine which additional intervention strategies might serve best in maximizing the treatment outcomes. A variety of interventions are considered, including patient participation in a professional- or peer-led psychoeducational group and/or brief individual therapy. Step 3 involves the use of more intensive psychological interventions aimed at managing psychological distress and addressing lifestyle impairments across occupational, interpersonal, and social domains of function. Otis and colleagues suggest that this step of treatment is appropriate for patients who have not responded optimally to interventions provided in the early treatment steps and who continue to report significant levels of pain, pain-related disability, and clinically significant emotional distress.

A maximally effective stepped care approach to the management of chronic pain is one that appreciates that patients who report chronic pain vary with respect to the number of functional limitations and lifestyle impairments that accompany the chronic pain conditions and require different levels of interventions to achieve the desired functional outcomes (Turk, 2005).

Chronic Pain Self-Help Resources

There are numerous self-help resources available to patients with chronic pain who may be interested in self-initiated efforts toward pain management. These resources are largely in the form of pain management books and Internet sites targeted directly at lay persons. Although the effectiveness of any individual resource is generally not available to the patient with chronic pain, he or she may rely on the credentials of the authors (e.g., authors who emphasize empirical research) or the Internet site hosts (e.g., Internet sites that are hosted by universities or other research institutions) to guide their selection of self-help materials.

Self-Help Books

- Caudill-Slosberg, M. A., & Caudill, M. A. (2001). *Managing pain before it manages you, revised edition*. New York, NY: Guilford Press.
- Dahl, J., & Lundgren, T. (2006). *Living beyond your pain: using acceptance & commitment therapy to ease chronic pain*. Oakland, CA: New Harbinger Publications.
- Gatchel, R. (2004). *Clinical essentials of pain management*. Washington, DC: American Psychological Association.
- Melzack, R., & Wall, P. (2004). *The challenge of pain*. New York, NY: Penguin Global.
- Sternbach, R. A. (1987). *Mastering pain: A twelve-step program for coping with chronic pain*. New York, NY: Ballantine Publishing.
- Thorn, B. E. (2004). *Cognitive therapy for chronic pain: A step-by-step guide*. New York, NY: Guilford Press.
- Turk, D. C., & Winter, F. (2005). *The pain survival guide: How to reclaim your life (APA lifetools)*. Washington. DC: American Psychological Association.
- Waddell, G. (2004). *The back pain revolution*. Oxford, UK: Churchill Livingstone.

Self-Help Websites

- http://www.ahrq.gov/
- http://www.ampainsoc.org/
- http://www.chronicpain.org/
- http://www.headaches.org/
- http://www.fmaware.org/
- http://www.iasp-pain.org/
- http://www.mayoclinic.com/health/chronic-pain/
- http://www.nationalpainfoundation.org/
- http://www.pain.com/
- http://www.theacpa.org/

Key Readings on the Assessment and Management of Chronic Pain

The key readings listed below were selected to provide the behavioral health specialist with readings that address issues important to the comprehensive assessment and cost-effective management of chronic pain conditions and delineate the role of the behavioral health specialist in identifying and generating a treatment plan to manage those psychosocial factors that are considered to contribute to the chronicity of pain and pain-related disability.

- Brown, K. S., & Folen, R. A. (2005). Psychologists as leaders of multidisciplinary chronic pain management teams: A model for health care delivery. *Professional Psychology: Research and Practice, 36*, 587–594.
- Fordyce, W. E. (1988). Pain and suffering: A reappraisal. *American Psychologist, 43*, 276–283.
- Gatchel, R., Peng, Y. B., Peters, M. L., Fuchs, P. N., & Turk, D. C. (2007). The biopsychosocial approach to chronic pain: Scientific advances and future directions. *Psychological Bulletin, 133*, 581–624.
- Linton, S. J. (2000). A review of psychological risk factors in back and neck pain. *Spine, 25*, 1148–1156
- Melzack, R. (1999). From the gate to the neuromatrix. *Pain,* (Suppl. 6), S121–S126.
- Otis, J. D. (2007). *Managing chronic pain: A cognitive-behavioral therapy approach therapist guide (Treatments that work)*. New York, NY: Oxford University Press.
- Simon, E. P., & Folen, R. A. (2001). The role of the psychologist on the multidisciplinary pain management team. *Professional Psychology: Research and Practice, 32*, 125–134.
- Sternbach, R. A. (1987). *Mastering pain: A twelve-step program for coping with chronic pain*. New York, NY: Ballantine Publishing.
- Tait, R. C., & Chibnall, J. T. (2005). Racial and ethnic disparities in the evaluation and treatment of pain: Psychological perspectives. *Professional Psychology: Research and Practice, 36*, 595–601.
- Turk, D. C. (2005). The potential of treatment matching for subgroups of patients with chronic pain: Lumping versus splitting. *Clinical Journal of Pain, 21*,, 44–55.
- Turk, D. C., & Burwinkle, (2005). Clinical outcomes, cost-effectiveness, and the role of psychology in treatments for chronic pain sufferers. *Professional Psychology: Research and Practice, 36*, 602–610.
- Turk, D. C., & Gatchel, R. J. (Eds). (2002). *Psychological approaches to pain management, second edition: A practitioner's handbook*. New York, NY: Guilford Press.
- Turk, D. C., & Melzack, R. (Eds). (2001). *Handbook of pain assessment (2nd ed.)*. New York, NY: Guilford Press.
- Turk, D. C., & Okifuji, A. (2002). Psychological factors in chronic pain: evolution and revolution. *Journal of Consulting and Clinical Psychology, 70*, 678–690.

Conclusions

An integrated care effort between the PCP and the behavioral health specialist is absolutely essential to the process of ensuring the optimal management of patients with chronic pain. In trying to reduce the likelihood that injured persons will develop chronic conditions (e.g., chronic pain), the PCP presents an optimistic picture of recovery, encourages the pursuit of normal activities, discourages rest and activity avoidance, and normalizes the injured person's fears regarding re-injury and continuing functional compromise. The behavioral health specialist is critical in identifying emotional reactions that patients with chronic pain experience. The PCP and the behavioral health specialist work in consort to determine the overall impact of pain on the range of quality of life domains (e.g., work, family, recreation) and to assist the patient in maximizing recovery.

References

Ahles, T. A., Wasson, J. H., Seville, J. L., Johnson, D. J., Cole, B. F., Hanscom, B. et al. (2006). A controlled trial of methods for managing pain in primary care patients with or without co-occurring psychosocial problems. *Annals of Family Medicine, 4*, 341–350.

Beck, A. T., Steer, R. A., & Brown, G. K. (1996). *The beck depression inventory-II*. San Antonio, TX: Psychological Corporation.

Beck, A. T., & Steer, R. A. (1990). *Beck anxiety inventory manual*. San Antonio, TX: Psychological Corporation.

Bergner, M., Bobbitt, R. A., Carter, W. B., & Gilson, B. S. (1981). The Sickness Impact Profile: Development and final revision of a health measure. *Medical Care, 8*, 787–805.

Blincoe, L., Seay, A., Zaloshnja, E., Miller, T., Romano, E., Luchter, S., et al. (2002). *The Economic Impact of Motor Vehicle Crashes 2000*. Washington, DC: National Highway Traffic Safety Administration.

Blount, A., Schoenbaum, M., Kathol, R., Rollman, B. L., Thomas, M., O'Donohue, W. T., et al. (2007). The economics of behavioral health services in medical settings: A summary of the evidence. *Professional Psychology: Research and Practice, 38*, 290–297.

Blyth, F. M., March, L. M., Brnabic, A. J. M., & Cousins, M. J. (2004). Chronic pain and frequent use of health care. *Pain, 111*, 51–58.

Brown, K. S., & Folen, R. A. (2005). Psychologists as leaders of multidisciplinary chronic pain management teams: A model for health care delivery. *Professional Psychology: Research and Practice, 36*, 587–594.

Butcher, J. N., Dahlstrom, W. G., Graham, J. R., Tellegen, A. M., & Kaemmer, B. (1989). *MMPI-2: Minnesota Multiphasic Personality Inventory-2. Manual for administration and scoring.* Minneapolis, MN: University of Minnesota Press.

Davison, G. C. (2000). Stepped care: Doing more with less? *Journal of Consulting and Clinical Psychology, 68*, 580–585.

DePalma, J. A., Fedorka, P., & Simko, L. C. (2003). Quality of life experienced by severely injured trauma survivors. *AACN Clinical Issues: Advanced Practice in Acute & Critical Care Psychosocial Issues, 14*, 54–63.

Derogatis, L. R. (1983). *SCL-90-R administration, scoring, and procedures manual-II*. Towson, MD: Clinical Psychometric Research.

Deyo, R. A., Diehl, A. K., & Rosenthal, M. (1986). How many days of bed rest for acute low back pain? A randomized clinical study. *New England Journal of Medicine, 315*, 1064–1070.

Duckworth, M. P., Iezzi, T., & Lewandowski, M. (2008). Managing MVC-related sequelae in the primary care setting: Normalizing experiences of emotional distress. In M. P. Duckworth, T. Iezzi, & W. T. O'Donohue (Eds.), *Motor vehicle collisions: Medical, psychosocial, and legal consequences.* New York, NY: Academic Press/Elsevier.

Esteve, R., Ramirez-Maestre, C., & Lopez-Martinez, A. E. (2007). Adjustment to chronic pain: The role of pain acceptance, coping strategies, and pain-related cognitions. *Annals of Behavioral Medicine, 33*, 179–188.

Fleming, M. F., Barry, K. L., Manwell, L. B., Johnson, K., & London, R. (1997). Brief physician advice for problem alcohol drinkers: A randomized controlled trial in community-based primary care practices. *Journal of the American Medical Association, 277*, 1039–1045.

Gatchel, R. J., & Okifuji, A. (2006). Evidence-based scientific data documenting the treatment and the cost-effectiveness of comprehensive pain programs for chronic nonmalignant pain. *Journal of Pain, 7*, 779–793.

Gureje, O., Simon, G. E., & Von Korff, M. (2001). A cross-national study of the course of persistent pain in primary care. *Pain, 92*, 195–200.

Gureje, O., Von Korff, M. Simon, G. E., & Gater, R. (1998). Persistent pain and well-being: A World Health Organization study in primary care. *Journal of the American Medical Association, 280*, 147–151.

Hoffamn, B. M., Papas, R. K., Chatkoff, D. K., & Kerns, R. K. (2007). Meta-analysis of psychological interventions for chronic low back pain. *Health Psychology, 26*, 1–9.

International Association for the Study of Pain. (1986). Classification of Chronic Pain. *Pain, 3*(Suppl. 3), 1–226.

Keefe, F. J., Crisson, J., Urban, B. J., & Williams, D. (1990). Analyzing chronic low back pain: the relative contribution of pain coping strategies. *Pain, 40*, 293–301.

Kerns, R. D., Turk, D. C., & Rudy, T. E. (1985). The West Haven-Yale Multidimensional Pain Inventory. *Pain, 23*, 345–356.

Linton, S. J. (2000). A review of psychological risk factors in back and neck pain. *Spine, 25*, 1148–1156.

Malmivaara, A., Kakkinen, U., Aro, T., Heinrichs, M. L., Koskenniemi, L., & Kuosma, E., et al. (1995). The treatment of acute low back pain – Bed rest, exercises, or ordinary activity? *New England Journal of Medicine, 332*, 351–355.

Mantyselka, P. T., Turunen, J. H. O., Ahonen, R. S., & Kumpusalo, E. O. (2001). Chronic pain and poor self-rated health. *Journal of the American Medical Association, 290*, 2435–2442.

Mayou, R., & Bryant, B. (2003). Consequences of road traffic accidents for different types of road users. *Injury, International Journal of the Care of the Injured, 34*, 197–202.

McClune, T., Burton, A. K., & Waddell, G. (2002). Whiplash associated disorders: a review of the literature to guide patient information and advice. *Emergency Medicine Journal, 19*, 499–506.

McCracken, L. M. (1998). Learning to live with pain: Acceptance of pain predicts adjustment in persons with chronic pain. *Pain, 74*, 21–27.

Merskey, H., & Bogduk, N. (1994). *Classification of chronic pain: Descriptions of chronic pain syndromes and definitions of pain terms.* Seattle, WA: IASP Press.

Millon, T., Millon, C., & Davis, R. (1994). *Millon clinical inventory-III manual.* Minneapolis, MN: National Computer Systems.

Ockene, J. K., Adams, A., Hurley, T. G., Wheeler, E. V., & Herbert, J. R. (1999). Brief physician- and nurse practitioner-delivered counseling for high-risk drinkers. *Archives of Internal Medicine, 159*, 2198–2205.

Ockene, J. K., Kristeller, J., Goldberg, R., Amick, T. L., Pekow, P. S., Hosmer, D. et al. (1991). Increasing the efficacy of physician-delivered smoking interventions. *Journal of General Internal Medicine, 6*, 1–8.

Otis, J. D., MacDonald, A., & Dobscha, S. K. (2006). Integration and coordination of pain management in primary care. *Journal of Clinical Psychology: In Session, 62*, 1333–1343.

Simon, E. P., & Folen, R. A. (2001). The role of the psychologist on the multidisciplinary pain management team. *Professional Psychology: Research and Practice, 32*, 125–134.

Smith, B. W., & Zautra, A. J. (2004). The role of purpose in life in recovery from knee surgery. *International Journal of Behavioral Medicine, 11*, 197–202.

Sterling, M., Jull, G., & Kenardy, J. (2006). Physical and psychological factors maintaining long-term predictive capacity post-whiplash injury. *Pain, 122*, 102–108.

Sullivan, M. J. L., Bishop, S., & Pivik, J. (1995). The Pain Catastrophizing Scale: Development and validation. *Psychological Assessment, 7*, 524–532.

Thorn, B. E., Cross, T. H., & Walker, B. B. (2007). Meta-analyses and systematic reviews of psychological treatments for chronic pain: Relevance to an evidence-based practice. *Health Psychology, 26*, 12–12.

Toomey, T., Mann, D., Hernandez, J., & Abashian, S. (1993). Psychometric characteristics of a brief measure of pain-related functional impairment. *Archives of Physical Medicine and Rehabilitation, 74,* 1305–1308.

Tovian, S. M. (2006). Interdisciplinary collaboration in outpatient practice. *Professional Psychology: Research and Practice, 37,* 268–272.

Turk, D. C. (2005). The potential of treatment matching for subgroups of patients with chronic pain: Lumping versus splitting. *Clinical Journal of Pain, 21,* 44–55.

Turunen, J. H. O., Mantyselka, P. T., Kumpusalo, E. O., & Ahonen, R. S. (2004). How do people ease their pain? A population-based study. *Journal of Pain, 5,* 498–504.

Von Korff, M., & Moore, J. C. (2001) Stepped care for back pain: Activating approaches for primary care. *Annals of Internal Medicine, 134,* 911–917.

Von Korff, M., & Tiemens, B. (2000). Individualized stepped care of chronic illness. *Western Journal of Medicine, 172,* 133–137.

Waddell, G. (1987). A new clinical model for the treatment of low back pain. *Spine, 12,* 632–644.

Ware, J. E., Snow, K. K., Kosinski, M., & Gandek, B. (1993). *SF-36 Health Survey: Manual and interpretation guide.* Boston, MA: The Health Institute, New England Medical Center.

Wolfe, F., Smythe, H. A., Yunus, M. B., Bennett, R. M., Bombardier, C., Goldenberg, D. L. et al. (1990). The American College of Rheumatology 1990 criteria for the classification of fibromyalgia: Report of the multicenter criteria committee. *Arthritis and Rheumatism, 33,* 160–72.

Wynne-Jones, G., Jones, G. T., Wiles, N. J., Silman, A. J., & MacFarlane, G. J. (2006). *The Journal of Rheumatology, 33,* 968–974.

Promoting Treatment Adherence Using Motivational Interviewing: Guidelines and Tools

Lisa Hagen Glynn and Eric R. Levensky

What Is Treatment Adherence?

Treatment adherence describes the "extent to which patients follow the instructions they are given for prescribed treatments" (Haynes et al., 2005, p. 2). Conversely, treatment non-adherence refers to the degree to which patients do not follow treatment recommendations. Examples of non-adherence behaviors include missing or being late to appointments, not beginning a recommended treatment, not completing homework, not taking medication as prescribed, and terminating treatment early (Levensky & O'Donohue, 2006).

Treatment non-adherence is a complex and multifaceted problem that is often difficult to remedy. The identified causes of patient non-adherence are numerous, but can be grouped into general categories of factors related to the patient (e.g., insufficient knowledge, resources, or motivation; depression; substance abuse; and problematic health-related beliefs), the specific illness (e.g., lack of immediate consequences to health and functioning, symptoms that exacerbate non-adherence), the treatment (e.g., complex medication regimens, high cost), and the patient–provider relationship (e.g., distrust, discomfort, and miscommunication) (Konkle-Parker, 2001; Levensky & O'Donohue, 2006).

On average, approximately 25% (and as high as 92%; Meichenbaum & Turk, 1987) of medical patients are non-adherent to recommended treatment regimens (DiMatteo, 2004). This high prevalence represents great monetary costs (Atreja, Bellam, & Levy, 2005), not to mention wasted time and frustration for providers and patients. Even more importantly, treatments cannot work if they are not implemented, and non-adherence to treatment can lead to dangerous or lethal

L.H. Glynn (✉)
Dept. of Psychology, University of New Mexico, MSC03 2220, Albuquerque, NM 87131–1161, USA
e-mail: lglynn@unm.edu

E. Levensky (✉)
Clinical Psychologist, Department of Behavioral Medicine Program, New Mexico VA Health Care System, Behavioral Health Care Line (116), 1501 San Pedro SE, Albuquerque, NM 87108, USA
e-mail: levensky@unm.edu

L.C. James, W.T. O'Donohue (eds.), *The Primary Care Toolkit*,
DOI 10.1007/978-0-387-78971-2_14, © Springer Science+Business Media, LLC 2009

consequences. Patients who do not follow treatment recommendations have higher rates of treatment failure, potential of increased side effects, unexplained or unexpected secondary medical problems, and greater rates of mortality (e.g., Carroll, 1997; Ho et al., 2006; Miller, Hill, Kottke, & Ockene, 1997; Simpson et al., 2006).

Promising work has been done in the development and evaluation of methods to promote patient adherence to treatment recommendations; for an overview of this literature, see O'Donohue and Levensky (2006). In particular, motivational interviewing (MI), introduced in 1983 by William Miller, has shown promise as a counseling method to promote change. MI is a patient-centered approach to facilitating behavior that was initially developed for the treatment of addictions, and has been widely adapted to facilitate change across a range of patient health behaviors, including those related to the management and prevention of chronic diseases. MI is well suited for use in many healthcare settings, as it can be adapted to very brief (10- to 15-minute) patient encounters.

This chapter will present an overview of the empirical support, principles, and techniques of MI and will provide guidelines and tools for the application of this approach to brief interactions within a primary care setting.

What Is Motivational Interviewing?

Motivational interviewing is a "client-centered, directive method for enhancing intrinsic motivation to change by exploring and resolving ambivalence" (Miller & Rollnick, 2002, p. 25) that has its roots in the substance-treatment field. Motivational interviewing stands in contrast to approaches in which ambivalence is viewed as a sign of patient resistance that must be vigorously broken down for the patient to succeed in changing; rather, MI conceptualizes ambivalence as a normal process along the path to change. By weighing pros and cons of both change and the status quo, the patient finds a way to resolve these opposing forces. The provider serves as patient-centric moderator and thoughtful questioner, gently guiding the discussion toward a target behavior and its role within a patient's life.

Why Adopt a Patient-Centered Approach to Treatment Adherence?

Adopting a patient-centered approach can improve adherence to medication and regimens and lead to better health behavior outcomes (Williams, Frankel, Campbell, & Deci, 2000). Because patients often know themselves better than their providers do, their ideas about how and why they adhere (or do *not* adhere) to a treatment plan can be extremely useful. Moreover, a less-than-perfect adherence plan created and adhered to by a patient can be more valuable than a perfect plan prescribed by a provider but not adhered to. Assuming that the providers have all of the solutions to treatment non-adherence can be misguided and counter-productive, whereas relinquishing ownership of the patient–provider interaction might actually encourage the patient to invest in – and benefit more from – the treatment and its outcome.

Efficacy of Motivational Interviewing

Over 60 trials (Miller, 2004) have supported the use of MI for a number of target behaviors, including alcohol use, smoking, diet, exercise, medication adherence, and dental cavity prevention (e.g., Dunn, Deroo, & Rivara, 2001; Golin et al., 2006; Hettema, Steele, & Miller, 2006; Soria, Legido, Escolano, Lopez Yeste, & Montoya, 2006; Vasilaki, Hosier, & Cox, 2006; Weinstein, Harrison, & Benton, 2006; Welch, Rose, & Ernst, 2006).

Motivational Interviewing and Primary Care

Motivational interviewing can be a useful approach to improving treatment adherence in primary care settings for a number of reasons. First, MI is directive, which is important to providers who need to accomplish specific tasks during a visit and are bound to provide certain services and information. Second, MI is non-confrontational, and thus lends itself well to interactions with 'difficult' or frustrating patients. Third, MI focuses on resolving ambivalence about the costs and benefits of adhering to specific prescribed treatments (e.g., medications) or other health behaviors (e.g., quitting smoking). Finally, MI is versatile and can be used in brief interactions, which is ideal for the constraints of most primary healthcare settings

How Does Motivational Interviewing Work?

Motivational interviewing is believed to work through a combination of strong patient–provider relationship and specific techniques that encourage the patient to discuss the possibility of behavior change.

Patient–Provider Relationship

The interaction style of the provider appears to be of particular importance in creating an environment for collaboration and change, predicting long-lasting effects upon patients and treatment outcomes (e.g. Miller, Benefield, & Tonigan, 1993; Moyers, Miller, & Hendrickson, 2005; Patterson & Forgatch, 1985). Provider behaviors consistent with MI (e.g., showing empathy and support, promoting autonomy, and rolling with patient resistance) have been shown to hasten patient behavior change, whereas MI-inconsistent behaviors (advising, warning, confronting, and attempting to convince; discussed in detail later in this chapter) can lead to patient resistance that prevents change for months or years later (Moyers & Martin, 2006). Consequently, maintaining an MI-consistent style of collaboration, evocation, and autonomy (known as 'MI spirit'; Miller & Rollnick, 2002) throughout the interaction is advisable, leading patients toward self-exploration and eventual behavior change.

Eliciting and Reinforcing Change Talk

A primary goal of MI is for providers to elicit patient discussion of making health behavior changes (e.g., take prescribed medications; increase healthy eating and physical activity) and then reinforce or promote patient statements in favor of change (Miller & Moyers, 2007). Called "change talk" or "self-motivational statements" (Miller & Rollnick, 2002), patient discussion of change is believed to influence actual future behavior change (Amrhein, Miller, Yahne, Palmer, & Fulcher, 2003; Moyers et al., 2007). Change talk tends to follow MI-consistent statements from providers, whereas patient resistance usually follows providers' MI-inconsistent statements (Moyers & Martin, 2006). When change talk occurs, providers have the task of reinforcing it through specific techniques (e.g., reflective listening and supportive statements), which increase the probability of both eventual change and also more change talk, further increasing the likelihood of change. Importantly, patient statements *against* change ('counter-change talk', or 'sustain talk') are believed to decrease the likelihood of future change, and so it is important not to encourage patients to speak at length about reasons not to change. Skills for eliciting change talk are discussed later in the chapter.

What Is Not Motivational Interviewing?

As discussed in Miller and Rollnick (2002), several characteristics distinguish MI from many other provider techniques. First, MI is not confronting, belittling, or judging. However, this method should not be confused with non-directive reflective listening, a series of provider questions, or just 'being nice' to patients. Second, the use of specific techniques to elicit change talk is often valuable and is a part of what distinguishes MI from other approaches. Nonetheless, reducing MI to just a 'cookbook' of specific techniques contradicts the spirit of MI and can be ineffective. Indeed, a recent review of MI research (Hettema et al., 2006) found that the use of manualized MI treatments actually *decreased* the efficacy of MI-based interventions. More important than following the procedures step-by-step is adopting the MI 'way of being': creating an environment of collaboration and acceptance that normalizes ambivalence and allows patients to change *if*, *when*, and *how* they choose to do so. With this caveat in mind, the sections that follow outline how providers can apply the principles and techniques of MI to improve treatment adherence.

What Are the Principles of Motivational Interviewing?

Motivational interviewing is guided by four principles: developing discrepancy, expressing empathy, rolling with resistance, and supporting self-efficacy (Miller & Rollnick, 2002). When implementing MI, the provider attempts to interact with the patient in a manner that instantiates these principles (see Provider Reference 2 for an outline).

Developing Discrepancy

By developing discrepancy we mean helping patients recognize differences between their current behaviors and the behaviors that would be consistent with their long-term goals and values. This technique can be used when patients are pre-contemplative about making a change (i.e., importance is low). You can help patients notice reasons that change might be necessary or desirable by inquiring about personal values and how the behavior 'fits in,' querying about pros and cons of change and the status quo, and correcting misconceptions and filling gaps in information (after obtaining their permission).

Example
Patient: I'm worried that smoking in the car might not be good for my kids, but I also really like how it makes me relaxed when I drop them off for school.
Provider: You want to be a good parent, and you don't see smoking fitting in with that ideal.

Example
Patient: It hadn't really occurred to me to get more exercise. I eat well, so my health hasn't ever been a problem.
Provider: It's never been a concern for you before. I'm wondering if I could share some findings with you about getting your body moving and its benefits in preventing heart disease.

Expressing Empathy

Expressing empathy involves conveying understanding of your patients as they are, but not necessarily agreeing with their point of view. You can use this technique often throughout the interaction to enhance rapport and show patients that you are listening, particularly when approaching difficult and emotional topics or when encountering resistance. You might try using many more reflections than questions (a three-to-one ratio) and many more open questions than closed questions (Miller & Rollnick, 2002).

Example
Patient: Giving up drinking has been awful! I can't go out anymore because all of my friends drink, and when I stay home I get bored.
Provider: This might be the hardest thing you've ever had to do, and yet you've managed to not drink for a whole month.

Example
Patient: Ever since my wife died, I haven't been able to get off the couch to do anything.
Provider: That has been so devastating for you, and it's been really tough getting back into your exercise routine.

Rolling with Resistance

Rolling with resistance means avoiding confronting or arguing for change, and instead reflecting your patients' words and feelings. You can use this technique when encountering resistance or intense negative emotions.

Example
Provider: I see from your chart that you've used drugs in the past. Tell me about your current drug use.
Patient: I've had doctors talk to me about getting treatment plenty of times before and I have a lot of stuff to do today. Can we just skip to the part where you tell me I have a drug problem so we can get to what I really need?
Provider: Wow! It sounds like you have some really good reasons for not wanting to talk about this right now, and I respect your right to decide how we use our time. Tell me how I can help you today.

Example
Patient: So you're going to tell me that I need to take better care of my feet. Damned nurses always do when I come to this clinic.
Provider: You're sick and tired of everyone else telling you what to do.

Supporting Self-Efficacy

Supporting self-efficacy means instilling confidence in your patients that they have the ability to change if they choose to do so. During a visit, this entails assuring your patients that only they can decide whether to change, complimenting their strengths or efforts to change, relating the current change opportunity to their past successes in changing, and refusing to take the 'expert role.' You can use this principle throughout the visit, especially when patients ask for direct advice or imply that someone else should take responsibility for their decisions.

Example
Patient: I'm just so confused about whether to have this operation. What do you think is best?
Provider: I'll be glad to share some of my ideas about the surgery, but first I'd like to hear your thoughts about it.

Example
Patient: It's so difficult to wake up at 5:00 a.m. to catch the hospital shuttle, but it's the only way I can get to my appointments.
Provider: Even though it's inconvenient, you still choose to make that effort for your health.

How Do I Put the Principles of Motivational Interviewing into Practice?

To put the four principles of MI into practice, MI providers use four common counseling skills known as "OARS": *O*pen-ended questions, *A*ffirmations, *R*eflective listening, and *S*ummaries. (See Provider Reference 2 for an outline of these skills.)

Open Questions

Open questions are those that encourage patients to elaborate, make them feel respected, and elicit change talk; these are in contrast to closed questions that require only a brief 'yes/no' answer, which discourage patients from providing more information than requested. In MI, statements such as "tell me about. . ." are considered open questions because they invite elaboration, although technically they are not questions.

> *Examples*
> Provider: What would help you to be more successful at taking your pills?
> Provider: How could your family support you in making this change happen?
> Provider: Tell me how your life would be different if you quit smoking.

Affirmations

Affirmations are statements that reinforce positive choices, highlight patient strengths, and support self-efficacy. Using affirmations can also help you to build rapport.

> *Examples*
> Provider: It takes a real commitment to remember your medication four times every day. I can see how important it is to you to feel better.
> Provider: Despite everything that has happened this week, you still managed to keep your appointments. I really appreciate that you're here today.

Reflective Listening

Reflective listening is 'following along' with your patients by restating what they have said, clarifying, adding meaning, and highlighting emotions as appropriate. Reflective listening allows you to influence the interaction by selectively reinforcing patient statements in favor of change, while conveying respect and allowing your patients to play the 'expert' on the issue.

There are two primary types of reflections: simple and complex. Simple reflections simply restate what patients have said, whereas complex reflections add meaning to what the patient has said. One type of complex reflection is double-sided reflection, which presents both sides of your patient's ambivalence using an 'on one hand...and on the other hand' format.

Example: *Simple reflection*
Patient: Even with the meds I've been really down lately.
Provider: The medications don't seem to be helping with your depression.

Example: *Complex reflection*
Patient: My knee has been much better after I started going to physical therapy twice a week.
Provider: It's really making a difference for you.

Example: *Double-sided reflection*
Patient: I don't want to catch something, but condoms really ruin it for me.
Provider: On one hand you want sex to be spontaneous, and on the other you're worried that not using protection could be risky.

Summaries

Summaries refer to periodically summing up your patients' stories, adding insight and reinforcing statements in favor of change. Doing so permits your patients to synthesize information, recognize discrepancies, and re-evaluate beliefs. Summaries should reflect the ambivalence that they have expressed, and double-sided reflections can help achieve this. Summarization also builds rapport and supports self-efficacy by allowing your patients to correct any misunderstandings.

Examples
Provider: We've talked about several things today, so let me make sure that I understood everything: You had your first heart attack five years ago. You changed your diet and joined the gym in your neighborhood, but found it really difficult to continue because it didn't fit in with the lifestyle of the rest of your family. On one hand you like eating the foods that you like and you want to be able to eat with your family, and on the other hand you want live to see milestones in your children's lives and you're concerned about what might happen with your health if you don't make some changes.

Provider: I'd like to sum up what you've told me so far, and please jump in if I missed anything: The dental hygienist noted that your gums were swollen and bleeding during your exam and suggested that you might need surgery if you don't start taking better care of your mouth. You think that flossing is a real pain and don't see how such a minor thing could make a difference, and at the same time you want to avoid surgery at all costs. What do you make of this?

Special Issues in Applying Motivational Interviewing to Primary Care

This section describes several applications of MI to primary care, including agenda setting, using Importance and Confidence Rulers, weighing pros and cons, providing information in an MI-consistent manner, and avoiding traps. Many of these concepts are central to MI, but were first described by Rollnick, Mason, and Butler (1999). Please refer to the eight handouts (Patient Worksheets 1–6 and Provider References 1–2) available at the end of this chapter.

Setting an Agenda

By necessity, encounters with primary care patients are typically brief, and providers often wish to focus upon behaviors that are central to overall health but not necessarily of immediate or primary concern to patients (e.g., medication compliance, tobacco smoking, and diet or exercise modification). That is, patients usually arrive with their own agenda, which might or might not coincide with that of the provider, and what can be discussed is limited by time. Therefore, choosing a focus is an important first task. MI is directive in that a target health behavior must be chosen early in the interview. This should be a discussion initiated by the provider but led by the patient. Ways of engaging the patient in a discussion include asking permission to discuss a particular behavior (e.g., smoking tobacco) and asking the patient to name an area of concern with the help of a 'menu of options' (see Patient Worksheet 1), in which the provider lists several health behavior topics but leaves space for the patient to fill in a topic of concern. Offering a choice to patients about what to discuss (and when) supports autonomy and encourages them to play an active role in the treatment.

Using the Menu of Options

1. Prior to using the menu with your patient, fill in a few topics that you encounter most frequently in your practice (e.g., smoking, diet, exercise, testing blood sugars, taking medication, drinking alcohol, and stress). Depending upon the scope of your practice, the range of topics can be broad or narrow.
2. Describe the menu, explaining its purpose and highlighting the topics that you bring up with your other patients with similar medical conditions (e.g., type II diabetes).
3. Point out the blank squares and ask the patient which other items he/she might like to include.
4. Together, decide which topics are most important and set an agenda for the visit. If the patient circles several topics, ask him/her to rank them in the order of relative importance.

Using Rulers

The two most useful tools for assessing and enhancing patient readiness for health behavior changes are the Importance and Confidence Rulers (Patient Worksheet 2). These 'rulers' represent the continua of importance and confidence using an 11-point scale. A '0' represents the least importance or confidence ('not at all'), and '10' the most ('extremely'). Asking your patients to rank their importance and confidence could helps you to know how to proceed. (For a flowchart of these guidelines, please see Provider Reference 1.)

Ruler Steps:

1. Ask permission to talk about the target behavior.
2. Introduce the scale, remembering to define the anchors (high and low points).
3. Be sure to include the target behavior in your question.
4. Example questions:

   - Importance: "On a scale from 0 to 10, with 0 being 'not at all important' and 10 being 'extremely important,' how important is it to you to exercise more?"
   - Confidence: "On a scale from 0 to 10, with 0 being 'not at all confident' and 10 being 'extremely confident,' how confident are you that you could make these changes to your diet?"

5. Reflect the patient's answer (e.g., "You're at a '6.' So right now you're feeling more confident than not.").
6. Ask follow-up questions to elicit change talk.

   - When patients give a numerical rating, ask why a *lower* number was not chosen (e.g., "Why are you at a '4' and not a '0'?"). Alternatively, you can ask what would have to happen for the rating to be higher (e.g., "What would it take for you to move up to an '8'? "). These questions should prompt patients to provide reasons to change, or 'change talk.'
   - Asking why the patient did not choose a higher number (e.g., "Why are you a '2' and not a '5') is *not* recommended. Doing so can encourage patients to talk about reasons *not* to change (i.e., offer 'counter-change talk'), and thus talk themselves into not changing.

Decisional Balance

The Decisional Balance Exercise allows patients to list the pros and cons of changing or of not changing health-related behaviors, and then to assign subjective weights (of importance) to each. This exercise can be an efficient way to elicit change talk.

To have your patient complete the Decisional Balance Exercise (see Patient Worksheet 3), first ask the patient to list the benefits of not changing, and then ask about the downsides of not changing. (Alternately, or in addition, you can ask about the downsides and then the benefits of changing.) Try ending by asking patients about reasons *to* change, which often elicits change talk and provides an easy transition into a change plan discussion. After the patient has listed the pros and cons, explain that different reasons are important to different people, and ask the patient to assign a weight (or importance) to each reason. Have the patient visualize an old-fashioned scale, and ask which side (pros or cons) stacks up heavier and why. Then, using a brief but well-constructed double-sided reflection, summarize the patient's ambivalence and simultaneously increase importance. Finally, ask the patient to reflect upon his/her conclusions.

Example

Provider: You've listed taking a break with friends, managing stress, and controlling your weight as things that you enjoy about smoking; and breathing more easily on the stairs, setting a good example for your nieces, and not smelling like smoke as things that would be good about quitting. How do these balance for you? Which side weighs more heavily?

Patient: Reducing stress is pretty important, and so are being able to breathe and making sure that my nieces don't start. Time with friends, my weight, and the smell aren't really a big deal to me. The scale is tipping a little toward quitting.

Provider: On one hand, you really enjoy smoking and it does some positive things for you, and on the other hand you're concerned about your own health and the future health of your nieces. What do think you might do?

Ask-Provide-Ask

As a medical provider, you often will need to convey information to your patients about to their illness or treatment. In MI, giving information is viewed as a neutral behavior, not detrimental to rapport or outcomes, but it must be done with care. In general, refraining from giving information is the rule, unless patients ask you for specific information or unless you first ask permission to do so. Giving information in a way that respects patients' autonomy and contributions to the visit is essential to adopting an MI-consistent style.

The 'ask-provide-ask' model of giving information allows you to provide any information needed to complete the visit while still welcoming patient contribution and surrendering the expert role: first begin by *asking* patients what they already know about their condition or regimen, then *provide* additional information or gently correct patient misconceptions (using care to ask permission first), and then *ask* patients about their perceptions of the information you have provided. This process allows patients to share their perspectives and ask important questions that might influence adherence, and enables providers to check patients' understanding and drive away confusion.

Examples: Ask

Provider: What do you already know about managing your diabetes?

Provider: You've received a lot of information today. So I can make sure that we're on the same page, please tell me your understanding of your condition.

Provider: What are your thoughts about changing to this new medication?

Provider: What are your reactions to this diagnosis?

Examples: Provide

Provider: Would it be OK if I offered a few suggestions about weight control that have worked well for some of my patients?

Provider: If you'd like, I can tell you about some ways to make rehabilitating your shoulder a little easier.

Provider: These are all good ideas about how to get to the gym more often. May I offer some others that might also be worth considering?

Examples: Ask

Provider: What do you think about the ideas that we've talked about today?

Provider: We've discussed a number of ways to decrease your risk of HIV and other STIs. What would you like to try?

Provider: Which of these strategies appeal to you most?

Traps

Miller and Rollnick (2002) describe several 'traps' that can entangle providers and thwart successful visits. Among these, the 'expert' and 'question-answer' traps are perhaps most relevant to primary care practice. The expert trap refers to the provider serving as an expert on how the patient can best go about making health behavior changes, rather than allowing the patient to generate these solutions. The question–answer trap describes how providers ask a series of close-ended questions as in a general health assessment, which serves only to gather information and not to help understand or validate patients. In both cases, a trap can relegate patients to a passive role and discourage them from leading, or even participating in, their own care. The result of non-involvement can be non-adherence, because patients feel less of a personal investment in their participation.

Example: Falling into the expert trap

Patient: I know that I need to do something about my blood pressure, but I just don't know where to start.

Provider: You could try eating less fat and getting more exercise.

Patient: Do you think that would help?

Provider: Definitely. The key to keeping your blood pressure in control is getting rid of excess fat, which you may do through diet or exercise, but a combination is usually better. Also, reducing your sodium is a good idea, and you should try to control stress.

Patient: That seems like a lot I should remember to do. Isn't there a medication I can try instead?

Provider: For people with slightly elevated blood pressure, lifestyle change is what's recommended – your condition isn't severe enough for a drug. Here's a pamphlet about how to manage your blood pressure before it gets worse.

Patient: Are people really able to stick with this?

Example: *Avoiding the expert trap*

Patient: I know that I need to do something about my blood pressure, but I just don't know where to start.

Provider: I'll be glad to offer a few suggestions, but I'm curious about what you've thought of already.

Patient: I've been seeing those blood-pressure drug ads on TV, but I'm worried about things that can go wrong.

Provider: You've thought about possibly taking medication, and at the same time you're worried about the risks.

Patient: Yeah, I'd rather not risk it, but I don't want to have a heart attack either.

Provider: That's understandable. Would you mind if I shared a little information with you about some alternatives to medication?

Patient: Oh, sure. I didn't know there were any.

Provider: You're right; there can be some side effects in medication, although many people do benefit from it. But, for people with slightly elevated blood pressure, lifestyle change is actually what's recommended – most people don't take medication at this point, although it's something that we can talk about more later if you're interested. 'Lifestyle change' is another way to saying 'change your diet and exercise,' and it doesn't involve medication.

Patient: Oh, so I can do this without taking a drug? That sounds better. But how do I know what to change?

Provider: I'd like to hear some ideas from you, and if you're interested I can offer you a pamphlet about managing your blood pressure.

Patient: This sounds pretty do-able.

The dialogs in Table 1 portray two brief primary care encounters about adherence to an antibiotic regimen. The left side depicts a non-MI encounter and the right side an encounter using MI skills.

Making the Transition

After you have identified and discussed the target behavior, it is time to assess patient readiness to change. Although a few patients are able to make sudden, drastic change ("quantum change;" Miller & C'de Baca, 2001, p. 4), most patients are thought to approach potential change through a process of weighing benefits against drawbacks of health behavior changes (and of their alternatives). Broaching change with patients before they are ready – that is, jumping ahead of their current

Table 1. Sample Patient-Provider Dialogue: Brief Encounter Without and With MI

Non-MI Dialogue	Provider Techniques	MI Dialogue	Provider Techniques
Provider: I didn't expect to see you back so soon. So you're having some trouble with the antibiotic I prescribed?	Closed question	**Provider**: I didn't expect to see you back so soon. Tell me about your experience with the antibiotics I prescribed.	Open question
Patient: Yes! I've felt awful for three days. I kept feeling like I was going to puke, and my sinuses are still killing me. I'm missing work again right now and I can't afford to miss any more, so I need to get better.		**Patient**: I've felt awful for three days. I kept feeling like I was going to puke, and my sinuses are still killing me. I'm missing work again right now and I can't afford to miss any more, so I need to get better.	
Provider: Did you remember to take food with it?	Closed question	**Provider**: You've put in a lot of effort to be here today. It sounds like you've been feeling just miserable. Let's see if we can work together to figure out how you can feel better. What have you tried so far?	Rolling with resistance (using reflection); Support; Collaboration ; Open Question; Ask
Patient: Well, I tried eating something with the pills, but I was always still so nauseous from my last dose that I couldn't keep it down. I finally quit taking it yesterday.		**Patient:** Well, I tried eating something with the pills, but I was always still so nauseous from my last dose that I couldn't keep it down. I finally quit taking it yesterday.	
Provider: You should never stop taking any medicine without talking to me first, especially antibiotics. If you don't finish your course of antibiotics it will lead to resistant bacteria and then the drug won't work for you or anyone else.	Confronting; Warning; Taking expert role	**Provider**: So the food didn't really help much. What else have you tried?	Reflection; Open question

Table 1. (continued)

Non-MI Dialogue	Provider Techniques	MI Dialogue	Provider Techniques
Patient: But I can't really keep taking it if it makes me sicker.		**Patient**: Actually, that was about it. But the stomach problems went away when I quit taking it, so at least only my head hurts now.	
Provider: But if you don't keep taking it you can't get well. I need you to work with me if you want your infection to go away.	Warning	**Provider**: So you were feeling pretty sick to your stomach, but then you felt better right away after you quit taking the pills. Nausea is a common side effect of this medication, so that makes sense. I do have a couple of concerns about you stopping your medication that I'd like to share with you, if that's OK.	Reflection; Supporting self-efficacy (patient's interpretation of symptoms); Asking permission to give information
Patient: Actually, I did a lot of reading before I made this appointment, and one website said there's a liquid version I could take and it might be easier on my stomach. Can you give me that instead?		**Patient**: Oh, sure.	
Provider: The Internet can be a great source of misinformation. The liquid is usually for kids. So that doesn't seem like a good option for you.	Confronting	**Provider**: Although your stomach might feel better, your sinuses are probably still infected, which might be why your headache is getting worse again. Another thing we worry about when patients stop taking antibiotics early is that bacteria can become resistant to the medication, which means that antibiotics might not work for you or others in the future. What are your thoughts about that?	Provide; Ask: Giving information; Open question
Patient: OK. Then tell me what you want me to do.		**Patient**: Hmmm…I didn't realize that could happen with these pills, and I get sinus infections a lot. So that doesn't seem very good. I guess I should keep taking the same thing. Actually, I did a lot of reading before I made this appointment, and one website said there's a liquid version I could take and it might be easier on my stomach. Can you give me that instead?	

Table 1. (continued)

Non-MI Dialogue	Provider Techniques	MI Dialogue	Provider Techniques
Provider: The first thing you should do is start taking your pills again. I'll have to extend your prescription, but it might not be too late to get a little benefit from taking them. I think that if you eat a little more with the pill, maybe some crackers, then...	Advising; Taking expert role	**Provider:** It's great that you've done some of your own research already. If you don't mind, I'll try to add to what you already know. The liquid is usually for kids, but like you said it can also be good for adults who have trouble tolerating the pills. We can try that, and if it doesn't work we can try something different.	Supporting; Asking permission to give information
Patient: (*Jaw tightening*) Like I said, it didn't work. I need something else.		**Patient:** I'm willing to give it a try!	
Provider: OK, I'll give you the liquid, but I'm going to need you to take all of it as prescribed this time.	Warning	**Provider:** Thanks for not giving up after the side effects; I know it can be hard to stick with something that's making you feel worse. Here's your prescription. What questions do you have?	Supporting; Open question; Ask
Patient: Fine. I just need to get out of here so I can get back to work.		**Patient:** Actually, I think I understand fine. I'm just taking the liquid when I would've taken the pills.	
Provider: Here's your prescription. It should last you another ten days, and then you should probably come back for a check-up. Be sure to make that appointment with the receptionist before you leave today because we fill up quickly here.	Giving information; Advising; Warning	**Provider:** Right. Just to summarize, the plan is for you to take the liquid every eight hours – that's three times a day – for ten more days. But feel free to call me if any questions come up or if the medication still isn't working for you in a few days. If necessary, I can call in a different prescription to the pharmacy, so you don't have to miss any more work.	Collaborating
Patient: Thanks. My boss will love that (*sarcastic*).		**Patient:** Thanks! My boss will love that (*relieved*).	

stage of change – can be detrimental to the rapport and can lead to poorer treatment outcomes (Miller & Rollnick, 2002).

Assessing readiness early in the visit is crucial because it tells the provider how to proceed. You might already have a feel for readiness based upon what the patient has told you, or you might need to ask some more specific questions first before deciding how to proceed with your patient.

Is My Patient 'Ready, Willing, and Able'?

Being prepared to make a change has two main components: importance and confidence (Miller & Rollnick, 2002). Importance refers to patients' beliefs about the degree to which change is worthwhile or necessary. Confidence describes the patients' beliefs in their ability to change. Importance and confidence each fall on a continuum. Thus, patients may be high in both, low in both, or high in one component but low in another. Overarching importance and confidence is readiness, or priority that a particular change takes place in a patient's life. Most patients need to rate themselves high on both importance and confidence in order to be 'ready' to change a target behavior, so a provider should help patients increase any rating that is low.

Patients can believe that change is important and wish to change (importance), and simultaneously feel that they lack the ability or skills to *enact* change (confidence). When importance is low, ask permission of the patient to offer information about why change is important. Conversely, patients can be confident that they *could* change if necessary (confidence), but might not believe that change is necessary (importance). When confidence is low, ask about barriers to success. When both importance and confidence are low, first work to increase importance and then confidence. Conversely, when both importance and confidence are high, patients are likely ready to change. When a patient is ready to change, your role is to provide enthusiastic encouragement and help with creating a change plan. (See Using Rulers above for instructions; see Provider Reference 1 for a flowchart of these steps.)

Creating a Change Plan

When your patient ranks high in both importance and confidence, it is time to create a change plan together. A change plan is a strategy to help the patient to enact change. A change plan include a listing of the patient's goals and ratings, as well as his/her plans for achieving those goals. (See Patient Worksheets 4 and 6 for adherence tips and change plan.)

To create a change plan with your patient, begin by asking an open question, such as "What would you like to do next?" Work with the patient to 'brainstorm' specific strategies for adherence, offering your own suggestions only after your patient has offered his or hers (and after asking permission to do so). Praise the patient genuinely for taking charge of his/her treatment. If you have major concerns about the plan (e.g., due to safety issues), ask permission to express those with a statement like "You mentioned that you plan to [*restate the plan of concern*]. I'm wondering if I can share some concerns that I have about that." However, remember that an imperfect change strategy generated by the patient will be more likely to promote adherence than a flawless one suggested by the provider. The goal is to drive toward behavior change, and the patient should be in the driver's seat, even if it means that it will take a little longer to arrive at your destination.

Skill Building

Sometimes patients are ready to change but lack the essential skills, knowledge, and resources to do so. Skill building refers here to methods of providing information and behavioral repertoires that may facilitate patients overcoming common barriers to treatment adherence. Although skill-building techniques may be unnecessary for some patients (particularly those who have a successful record of adhering to past treatments and rank themselves high in importance and confidence), most can benefit from their use.

Examples of skill-building methods include memory aids, self-monitoring tools, and rehearsal. Memory aids include pillboxes or blister packages, written reminders (e.g., notes to self, calendars), electronic reminder systems (e.g., timer, alarm clock, pager, and electronic medication lids), and utilizing a support network (e.g., inviting a friend or pet to exercise, asking a family member to remind about medication, joining a support group). Self-monitoring skills refer to methods that help patients recognize adherence and non-adherence behaviors and environmental contingencies that precede them. Self-monitoring involves patients keeping a diary identifying when they adhered to treatment (or not) and which events, behaviors, thoughts, and emotions occurred immediately prior and afterward. This can help them become more aware of the chain of stimuli and reactions that can hinder or improve their adherence. (See Patient Worksheet 5 for a self-monitoring form and sample treatment diary.) Rehearsal includes techniques such as problem-solving (e.g., anticipating problems with adherence) and practicing skills (e.g., drink refusal, seeking social support), which help patients think ahead and plan around barriers to adherence (Fig. 1).

Example: Rehearsal
Provider: Would it be OK to talk about situations that might be difficult for you and what you might do to keep on track?
Patient: Sure. I'm a little worried about weekends because that's when I usually go out to eat. Also, my son's birthday party is coming up and I'm afraid that I might pig out on cake and ice cream.
Provider: How do you think you might make those situations easier for yourself?

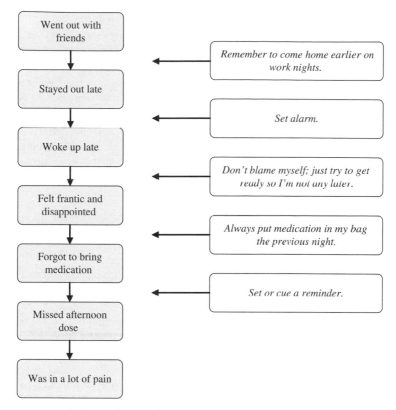

Fig. 1 Example: Behavior chain and solutions

Patient: I think that I'd eat a snack before we go out so I'm not so hungry, and skipping the cocktail might help me order something more healthful. At the party, I'll try to stick to one small piece of cake, and I guess I could put away the leftovers as soon as the kids have been served.

Combining Motivational Interviewing and Skill Building

Although MI and skill-building approaches are different in method, they share the goal of promoting change, and often they can be successfully reconciled and used in complement. Both approaches are directive, meaning that they advocate for change in a target behavior. They differ in that MI views the patient as expert (patient-centered) and the skills-building approach view the provider as expert (provider-centered).

Once you establish that your patient is ready to change (see Section *Is My Patient 'Ready, Willing, and Able'?*), combining the two approaches can be relatively simple. For example, working collaboratively with the patient can set the tone for a skill-building session. Begin by asking patients an open question about their impression of their medical condition and how it ought to be treated. Next, ask the patient to offer problem-solving solutions first. Then, ask permission to advise, share your opinion, or give information. If patients are unwilling to hear your recommendations, it is likely that they are unready to change, and your energy would be better spent in ways other than arguing for change; if they are willing to discuss the issue further, you have built valuable rapport, conveyed respect, and supported autonomy. Then, you may proceed with the skill-building information as usual, stopping intermittently to summarize and reflect. In short, MI prepares the ground, and skill-building plants the seeds for growth.

Summary

- Treatment non-adherence is a pervasive and costly health care problem.
- Patients might hold the solutions to their own problems. Providers can facilitate exploration of these.
- Motivational interviewing-based approaches might improve adherence by increasing motivation toward change.
- Skill-building techniques might increase instrumental skills necessary to adhere to treatment.
- Motivational interviewing and skill-building can be used in conjunction to achieve better treatment outcomes.

Resources

- http://www.motivationalinterview.org
  Website maintained by the Motivational Interviewing Network of Trainers; includes current information from the MI community and a bibliography of MI-related research.
- Meichenbaum, D., & Turk, D. C. (1987). *Facilitating treatment adherence: A practitioner's guidebook*. New York: Plenum.
  An overview of adherence promotion in health care; includes lists of treatment adherence examples and suggestions.
- Miller, W. R., & Rollnick, S. (2002). *Motivational interviewing: Preparing people for change* (2nd ed.) New York: Guilford Press.
  The landmark MI book; includes a chapter about MI and treatment adherence.
- O'Donohue, W.T., & Levensky, E.R., Ed. (2006). *Promoting Treatment Adherence: A practical handbook for health care providers*. Thousand Oaks, CA: Sage.
  Explores many aspects of treatment adherence.
- Rollnick, S., Mason, P., & Butler, C. (1999). *Health behavior change: A guide for practitioners*. New York: Churchill Livingstone.
  Techniques for applying MI principles to healthcare settings.

Table 2. Sample Dialogue Integrating MI and Skill-Building

Diet and Exercise Dialogue	Techniques/Handouts Used
Building Motivation	
Provider: Thanks for taking the time to come in today. So, from the nurse's notes, it looks like you're here because you're hoping to quit smoking.	Affirming (praises patient for coming and invites discussion)
Patient: Yeah. Well, kinda. Actually, my partner made the appointment for me. I don't really care one way or the other about quitting, but I'm just sick of hearing about cigarettes every night when I get home.	Ambivalence
Provider: You're not here because *you* want to quit smoking; you're here because your partner wants you to be.	Reflection
Patient: Pretty much.	
Provider: Then it must have been difficult for you to keep this appointment, but you came here anyway. So tell me what you might like to discuss with me today.	Reflection; open question
Patient: OK. Does it have to be about smoking?	
Provider: I'm here to talk about whatever your concerns are, and whether smoking is included in that is up to you. Here's a chart of common issues that I talk about with my patients. (*Provider shows a menu of options.*) These are just some ideas, and the blank squares are for you to add any topics that are important to you but aren't on the list.	Setting agenda; collaboration
Patient: Oh, OK. Thanks. I mean, quitting smoking might be a good idea (*nervous laugh*), but I can always get a patch or something if I can't stand the nagging anymore. I'm more worried about my weight.	
Provider: So *your* real concern today is how you can lose weight, and smoking isn't even on your radar right now.	Reflection
Patient: I'm a little embarrassed to admit, but yeah, that's about right.	
Patient: I'm hearing that you really don't want to talk about your smoking today, and I won't ask you more about it. But, because it's an important topic, would it be OK if we came back to it another day?	Reflection; asking permission
Patient: I think that would be OK. Thanks.	
Provider: Thank you for being open to that later. So on the topic of losing weight...I'd like to ask about how important it is to you. Using this zero-to-ten scale, where zero means 'not at all important' and ten means 'extremely important,' how important is it to you to lose weight?	Directly assessing importance
Patient: I would say that I'm about '9.'	
Provider: So this is something that you really need to do.	Reflection
Patient: Definitely. I tried on my old swimsuit the other day and my family laughed at me! I know that they were just teasing, but I was so embarrassed that I just tossed the suit in the garbage. I also hate losing my breath on the stairs at work, and I wish that I could play softball with my church league again, but I'm so out of shape.	Ambivalence

Table 2. (continued)

Diet and Exercise Dialogue	Techniques/Handouts Used
Provider: You see a lot of reasons that you should make some changes.	Reflection
Patient: Yes, I do. But I just don't know how I'd do it. My family wants to spend evenings together, and I can't bring everyone to a gym with me. Plus, we're pretty short on money these days with our oldest away at college.	Ambivalence
Provider: So on one hand you're seeing a lot of obstacles to losing weight, and on the other hand it's really important to you, and you owe it to yourself to slim down so you can be the person you're used to being. What a challenge.	Double-sided reflection
Patient: That's right! I want to do it, but when it gets down to actually trying something, it's just too complicated.	Ambivalence
Provider: You're not sure you'd even know where to start.	Reflection
Patient: Right. (*Sigh.*) I wish that you could just tell me how to do it, because I really don't want to fail again.	Counter-change talk
Provider: It sounds like your confidence is down right now. I'm glad to share some ideas that I have, but first I'd like to ask what you have thought of so far.	Indirectly assessing confidence; avoiding expert trap
Patient: I've thought about trying to get up early to go walking, but I have to get the family ready for work.	Ambivalence
Provider: Everyone else seems to have needs that come before yours.	Reflection
Patient: I hadn't really thought about it that way, but you're right. I need to make some time for myself if this is going to work. I just don't know when.	Change talk; ambivalence
Provider: I'm wondering whether I could share some suggestions that some of my other patients have found useful for them.	Asking permission
Patient: Oh, that would be great. Thanks.	
Building Skills	
Provider: One thing that seems to work really well for some people is to involve a support system – like getting your whole family involved in preparing meals from scratch. What do you think of this idea?	Normalizing; soliciting patient feedback
Patient: Well, I do most of the cooking, but I could teach them to chop vegetables or look for healthful recipes online. But I think that I need to start exercising, too, and I don't know how to make time.	Change talk; ambivalence
Provider: You see, how could you make changes in diet, but exercise still seems impossible?	Reflection
Patient: I don't think I'd say 'impossible,' but it will be a challenge. Maybe I could start walking around the block and bring the kids with me. It's not much, but...	Change talk; ambivalence
Provider: It's a start!	Reflection
Patient: You read my mind.	
Provider: What else might help you to exercise more?	Open question
Patient: Hmmm...I had an exercise bike but it's been broken for a few years now and just tossed in the garage. Maybe I could fix that up and ride while I watch TV.	Change Talk
Provider: That's a really good idea.	Supporting

Table 2. (continued)

Diet and Exercise Dialogue	Techniques/Handouts Used
Patient: It's not a perfect solution, but it would be nice during the winter when it's too cold to walk outside.	Ambivalence
Provider: You're right. Something else that might be helpful, if you'd like, is to keep a diary of all of your food and exercise for two weeks, as well as the thoughts or emotions that you're having. It might not be for you, but some people find it helpful to track these because it can point out patterns that keep you from your goal. If you decide to try this, here's a worksheet that you can use.	Supporting Self-efficacy; self-monitoring worksheet (with sample diary)
Patient: It would probably help with my forgetfulness! I'm not sure it will work, but I'd be willing to at least give it a try.	Change talk
Provider: If you're worried about remembering, I have a couple of other worksheets that you might find useful, but again, what you try is up to you. The first one is a general list of ways to remind yourself to follow the plan that we're creating—like setting a timer or asking a friend to exercise with you. The second is an outline of what we've discussed today. If you're interested, we can write down goals that you have, any suggestions that I have that you think might be important, and a reminder about when to schedule your next appointment.	Tips for Adherence Worksheet; Change Plan Worksheet
Patient: Those look helpful, too. If I get started on this tonight, I'll have a better shot at staying motivated, but I do want to talk this over with my partner first. Maybe I could sneak in a walk, though.	Change talk
Wrapping Up	
Provider: Great! I can see that you've really been struggling with whether this is something you want to do, and yet you're willing to give it a try. That's really admirable, and I appreciate your willingness to discuss it with me. We'll have to wrap up in a moment, so I'd like to summarize what we discussed today so I can be sure that I understand your plan. If I heard you correctly, you're going to start by talking this over with your partner to make sure that it's something that you want to do and to see how it might fit into your family's routine. If you decide to go ahead with this, you're going to start by walking around the block with your kids and asking them to help with food preparation. You might also think about fixing up your bike for the winter, and you'll consider using a diary to track your eating and exercise. It sounds like you have a pretty good idea of what you want to do. Did I miss anything?	Supporting and Affirming; Summarizing; Reinforcing Change Talk; Change Plan
Patient: No, I think you got the gist, and yes, I guess I do. I'd love to come back here next time after making some progress.	Change talk
Provider: Whether you do or not, I'm here to help you, and if this first plan needs some revision, we can certainly do that together. Feel free to call me in the meantime if any questions come up.	Supporting
Patient: I will. Thanks for all your help.	Change talk
Provider: Thanks for coming in today. Good luck with your plan!	Affirming

References

Atreja, A., Bellam, N., & Levy, S. R. (2005). Strategies to enhance patient adherence: making it simple. *Medscape General Medicine, 7*(1), 4.

Amrhein, P. C., Miller, W. R., Yahne, C. E., Palmer, M., & Fulcher, L. (2003). Client commitment language during motivational interviewing predicts drug use outcomes. *Journal of Consulting and Clinical Psychology, 71*(5), 862–878.

DiMatteo, M. R. (2004). Variations in patients' adherence to medical recommendations: a quantitative review of 50 years of research. *Medical Care, 42*(3), 200–209.

Carroll, K. M. (1997). Manual-guided psychosocial treatment. A new virtual requirement for pharmacotherapy trials? *Archives General Psychiatry, 54*(10), 923–928.

Dunn, C., Deroo, L., & Rivara, F. P. (2001). The use of brief interventions adapted from motivational interviewing across behavioral domains: A systematic review. *Addiction, 96*(12), 1725–1742.

Golin, C. E., Earp, J., Tien, H.-C., Stewart, P., Porter, C., & Howie, L. (2006). A 2-arm, randomized, controlled trial of a Motivational Interviewing-based intervention to improve adherence to Antiretroviral Therapy (ART) among patients failing or initiating ART. *Journal of Acquired Immune Deficiency Syndromes, 42*(1), 42–51.

Haynes, R. B., Yao, X., Degani, A., Kripalani, S., Garg, A., & McDonald, H. P. (2005). Interventions for enhancing medication adherence. *Cochrane Database of Systematic Reviews, 4* (CD000011).

Hettema, J., Steele, J., & Miller, W. R. (2006). Motivational Interviewing. *Annual Review of Clinical Psychology, 1*, 91–111.

Ho, P. M., Rumsfeld, J. S., Masoudi, F. A., McClure, D. L., Plomondon, M. E., Steiner, J. F., et al. (2006). Effect of medication nonadherence on hospitalization and mortality among patients with diabetes mellitus. *Archives of Internal Medicine, 166*(17), 1836–1841.

Konkle-Parker, D. J. (2001). A motivational intervention to improve adherence to treatment of chronic disease. *Journal of the American Academy of Nurse Practitioners, 13*(2), 61–68.

Levensky, E. R., & O'Donohue, W. T. (2006). Patient adherence and nonadherence to treatments: An overview for health care providers. In *Promoting Treatment Adherence*. Thousand Oaks, CA: Sage.

Meichenbaum, D., & Turk, D. C. (1987). *Facilitating treatment adherence: A practitioner's guidebook.* New York: Plenum.

Miller, N. H., Hill, M., Kottke, T., & Ockene, I. S. (1997). The multilevel compliance challenge: recommendations for a call to action. A statement for healthcare professionals [Electronic Version]. *Circulation, 95*, 1085–1090. Retrieved Feb 18 from http://circ.ahajournals.org/cgi/content/full/95/4/1085.

Miller, W. R., & C'de Baca, J. (2001). *Quantum change: When epiphanies and sudden insights transform ordinary lives.* New York: Guilford Press.

Miller, W. R. (2004). Motivational interviewing in the service of health promotion. *Art of Health Promotion in American Journal of Health Promotion, 18*(3), 1–10.

Miller, W.R., Benefield. R.G. & Tonigan, J.S. (1993). Enhancing motivation for change in problem drinking. A controlled comparison of two therapist styles. *Journal of Consulting and Clinical Psychology, 61*, 455–461.

Miller, W. R., & Moyers, T. B. (2007). Eight stages in learning motivational interviewing. *Journal of Teaching in the Addictions, 5*(1), 3–17.

Miller, W. R., & Rollnick, S. (2002). *Motivational interviewing: Preparing people for change* (2nd ed.) New York: Guilford Press.

Moyers, T. B., & Martin, T. (2006). Therapist influence on client language during motivational interviewing sessions. *Journal of Substance Abuse Treatment, 30*(3), 245–251.

Moyers, T. B., Miller, W. R., & Hendrickson, S. M. L. (2005). How does motivational interviewing work? Therapist interpersonal skill predicts client involvement within motivational interviewing sessions. *Journal of Consulting and Clinical Psychology, 73*(4), 590–598.

Moyers, T. B., Martin, T., Christopher, P. J., Houck, J. M., Tonigan, J. S., & Amrhein, P. C. (2007). Client language as a mediator of Motivational Interviewing efficacy: Where is the evidence? *Alcoholism: Clinical and Experimental Research, 31*(S3), 40S-47S.

O'Donohue, W.T., & Levensky, E.R., Ed. (2006). *Promoting treatment adherence: A practical handbook for health care providers.* Thousand Oaks, CA: Sage.

Patterson, G. R., & Forgatch, M. S. (1985). Therapist behavior as a determinant for client noncompliance: a paradox for the behavior modifier. *Journal of Consulting and Clinical Psychology, 53*(6), 846–851.

Rollnick, S., Mason, P., & Butler, C. (1999). *Health behavior change: A guide for practitioners.* New York: Churchill Livingstone.

Simpson, S. H., Eurich, D. T., Majumdar, S. R., Padwal, R. S., Tsuyuki, R. T., Varney, J., et al. (2006). A meta-analysis of the association between adherence to drug therapy and mortality. *British Medical Journal, 333*(7557), 15.

Soria, R., Legido, A., Escolano, C., Lopez Yeste, A., & Montoya, J. (2006). A randomised controlled trial of motivational interviewing for smoking cessation. *The British Journal of General Practice, 56*(531), 768–774.

Vasilaki, E. I., Hosier, S. G., & Cox, W. M. (2006). The efficacy of motivational interviewing as a brief intervention for excessive drinking: a meta-analytic review. *Alcohol and Alcoholism, 41*(3), 328–335.

Weinstein, P., Harrison, R., & Benton, T. (2006). Motivating mothers to prevent caries: confirming the beneficial effect of counseling. *Journal of the American Dental Association, 137*(6), 789–793.

Welch, G., Rose, G., & Ernst, D. (2006). Lifestyle and behavior. Motivational Interviewing and diabetes: what is it, how is it used, and does it work? *Diabetes Spectrum, 19*(1), 5–11.

Williams, G. C., Frankel, R. M., Campbell, T. L., & Deci, E. L. (2000). Research on relationship-centered care and healthcare outcomes from the Rochester biopsychosocial program: A self-determination theory integration. *Families, Systems, & Health, 18*(1), 79–90.

Patient Worksheet 1: Menu of Options

Directions: Below are several boxes containing topics that many patients want to talk about. Please circle the topics that are most important to you today. If a topic that you want to talk about is not listed you can write it in an empty box.

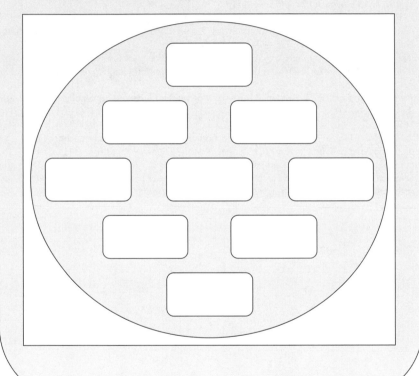

Patient Worksheet 2: Rulers

Behavior change being considered: _____

Directions:

Below are two 'rulers' to measure how you feel right now about changing your behavior. Each scale goes from 0 to 10, where 0 is 'not at all' and 10 is 'extremely'. Using the Importance Ruler, circle the number indicating how important it is for you to make the change. Using the Confidence Ruler, circle the number indicating how confident are you that you could make the change if you wanted to.

Importance Ruler

0	1	2	3	4	5	6	7	8	9	10
Not at All Important					Neither Important nor Unimportant					Extremely Important

Confidence Ruler

0	1	2	3	4	5	6	7	8	9	10
Not at All Confident					Neither Confident nor Unconfident					Extremely Confident

Patient Worksheet 3: Decisional Balance (Pros and Cons) Exercise

Behavior change being considered: _____

Directions: Below are spaces for reasons that you might want to change or not change a behavior. Please list some of these reasons and then we can discuss them together.

Cons of Changing	Pros of Changing
1.	1.
2.	2.
3.	3.
4.	4.
5.	5.
6.	6.
7.	7.
Pros of Not Changing	Cons of Not Changing
1.	1.
2.	2.
3.	3.
4.	4.
5.	5.
6.	6.
7.	7.

How do these factors balance for you? _____

_____

Patient Worksheet 4: Hints for Sticking with Treatment Recommendations

Appointments:

- Post a reminder message somewhere noticeable (like on the refrigerator or near the telephone)
- Request that your health care provider to give you a reminder phone call the day before
- Ask a trusted other to remind you when it is time to leave
- Plan ahead for transportation, time off work, and babysitters
- Leave early to allow enough time for traffic, weather, or other unexpected delays

Medications:

- Carry a notebook to your appointment and write down instructions from your provider, and ask questions if you do not understand completely
- Bring all your medications with you to your appointment
- Use pill boxes, tear-off calendars, or electronic medication cap reminders
- Set alarms
- Think of cues for taking your medications (like brushing teeth, your lunch, or watching a favorite TV show)
- Pack your medication dose and bring it with you in case you cannot make it home in time
- Write reminders to yourself on sticky notes and place them where you will be at medication time (like on the mirror, steering wheel, or coffee maker)

Social Support:

- Invite a friend or family member to start a new activity with you (like walking, flossing, or cooking healthful foods)
- Join (or start!) a support group on the internet or at your local hospital or religious institution
- Take a class at your local community center, gym, or college

Self Support:

- Set goals and revise them occasionally
- Keep a diary of your progress and note any reasons for not following your plan
- Reward yourself regularly when you follow your treatment plan (like taking an outing, asking your partner to make your favorite dish, making time for your hobby, or adding money to a piggy bank for a special cause)
- Write a list of reasons why you need to stick with your treatment and tape it somewhere you can see often (like in your bedroom or office)
- Plan out your daily routine the night before and practice anything that might make adherence difficult
- Substitute a more desirable behavior for a less desirable one (like going out for fresh air instead of a cigarette, or eating an omelet instead of a pastry)

Patient Worksheet 5: Self-Monitoring Exercise (with Sample Treatment Diary)

Sample Treatment Diary				
Date and Time	Event	What Happened Before	What I Did	What Happened After
9/15, 7:00 AM	Craved a cigarette	Woke up	Chewed nicotine gum	Felt better, but restless
9/15, 10:15 AM	Smoked one cigarette	Coworker offered one during break	Smoked	Felt calm, but guilty
9/15, 6:30 PM	Almost smoked	Went out for drinks with friends	Refused cigarette	Difficult because I was drinking, but proud of myself

_____'s Treatment Diary				
Date and Time	Event	What Happened Before	What I Did	What Happened After

Patient Worksheet 6: Appointment Summary and Change Plan

_____'s Appointment Summary   Date _____

My Medications

Medication Name	Times Per Day	Dose	Special Instructions

My Instructions

My next appointment is: _____

Provider instructions: _____

If I may have questions, whom to contact: _____

My Change Plan

My Goals	Importance	Confidence	My Plans for Achieving these Goals
1.			1.
2.			2.
3.			3.

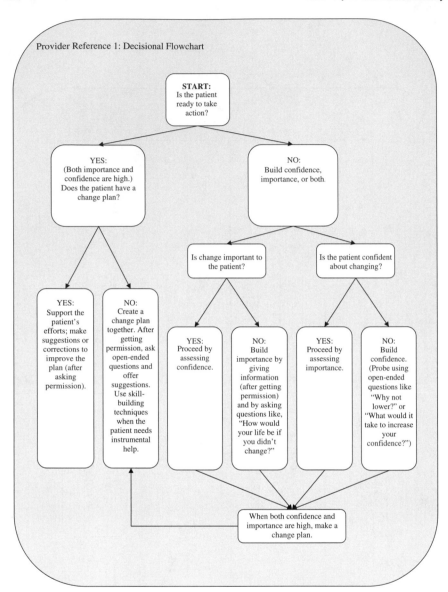

Provider Reference 1: Decisional Flowchart

Provider Reference 2: Principles and Skills of Motivational Interviewing

Four Principles of Motivational Interviewing

Develop Discrepancy
- Help patients recognize differences between current and ideal behavior or self

Express Empathy
- Convey understanding of patients as they are, but do not necessarily agree with their point of view

Roll with Resistance
- Avoid confrontation or arguing for change; instead reflect the patient's words and feelings

Support Self-Efficacy
- Assure patients that only they can decide whether to change; compliment patient strengths or efforts to change; refuse to take an 'expert role'

Four Skills of Motivational Interviewing (OARS)

Open Questions
- Queries that encourage the patient to elaborate
- Convey respect and elicit change talk
- Contrast with close-ended questions

Affirmations
- Statements reinforcing choices toward change
- Highlight patient strengths
- Support self-efficacy
- Build rapport

Reflective Listening
- 'Following along' with patients by restating what they have said
- Clarifying, adding meaning, and highlighting emotions
- Reinforcing change talk
- Convey respect and allow patients to play the 'expert'

Summaries
- Periodically summing up patients' stories, adding insight and reinforcing change talk
- Permit patients to synthesize information, recognize discrepancies, and re-evaluate beliefs
- Build rapport, support self-efficacy, and allow correction of misunderstandings

Diabetes – Guidelines and Handouts

Lauren Woodward Tolle

What Is Diabetes?

Diabetes is a chronic illness in which an individual stops producing or properly using insulin. Insulin is a hormone that assists in converting sugars, starches, and other foods into usable energy (American Diabetes Association, ADA, 2007). Diabetes can lead to long-term health complications, including stroke, heart disease, neuropathy, retinopathy, and kidney disease among others; however, with proper management of diabetes, individuals can lower the risk of these complications. There are several methods for diagnosing diabetes, including (1) a fasting plasma glucose test, (2) an oral glucose tolerance test, and (3) a random plasma glucose test. The fasting plasma glucose test (FPG) is often the preferred method and involves testing blood glucose after an individual has not eaten for at least 8 hours. Table 1 reflects how diabetes can be diagnosed using the FPG (NIDDK, 2005).

The American Diabetes Association estimates that approximately 20.8 million, or 7% of the United States' population, including both children and adults, have diabetes (2007); however, it is estimated that only 14.6 million people have been diagnosed and the remaining 6.2 million remain undiagnosed (National Institute of Diabetes and Digestive and Kidney Diseases, NIDDK, 2005). The cause of diabetes is still largely unknown; however, genetics and lifestyle factors (overweight and inactivity) appear to be agents for the onset of the disease. There are several different types of diabetes – the major types being type 1, type 2, and gestational diabetes (ADA, 2007). Type 1 diabetes, formerly referred to as insulin-dependent or juvenile-onset diabetes, is frequently diagnosed in childhood, as early as infancy through adolescence. As obesity rates in the United States continue to increase, the incidence of type 2 diabetes, never reported in children earlier, is now on the rise in young people (NIDDK, 2005). Among racial/ethnic groups, in the United States, in 2005, the age-adjusted prevalence of diabetes was 17.9 % among American Indian and

L.W. Tolle (✉)
Department of Psychology/296, University of Nevada, Reno, Reno, NV, 89557-0296, USA
e-mail: ltolle@unr.nevada.edu

L.C. James, W.T. O'Donohue (eds.), *The Primary Care Toolkit*,
DOI 10.1007/978-0-387-78971-2_15, © Springer Science+Business Media, LLC 2009

Table 1 Fasting plasma glucose test

Plasma Glucose Result (mg/dL)	Diagnosis
99 and below	Normal
100 to 125	Pre-diabetes (impaired fasting glucose)
126 and above	Diabetes*

*Confirmed by repeating the test on a different day.

Alaskan Natives, 14.8% among non-Hispanic African Americans, 13.7% among Hispanic/Latino Americans, and 8% among non-Hispanic Caucasian Americans (NIDDK, 2005).

Type 1 Diabetes

Approximately 1 in 400–600 children in the United States have type 1 diabetes (NIDDK, 2005; Wysocki, Greco, & Buckloh, 2003). The peak age of onset is middle childhood; however, diagnosis can occur in early childhood through late adolescence. Type 1 diabetes involves an autoimmune destruction of pancreatic cells that produce insulin; thus, glucose remains in the bloodstream, blood glucose increases, and glucose is eventually passed through the urine (Hanas, 2005). Effective management of type 1 diabetes involves strict glucose monitoring with synthetic insulin administration through shots, pens, or an insulin pump following a dietary and exercise regimen, which includes counting grams of carbohydrates consumed at each meal.

Type 2 Diabetes

Type 2 diabetes, also formerly referred to as adult-onset diabetes, involves not a destruction of insulin producing cells as is seen with type 1 diabetes but a growing resistance to insulin. Individuals with type 2 diabetes are prescribed pills that increase the body's sensitivity to insulin and also increases the release of insulin from the pancreas. Some individuals may also be prescribed insulin. A combination of overweight or obesity as well as a lack of physical activity have been found to be risk factors for developing type 2 diabetes. Effective management of type 2 diabetes, similar to type 1 diabetes, involves taking medication, making wise food choices, getting adequate physical activity, and managing one's blood pressure and cholesterol (NIDDK, 2005).

Gestational Diabetes

Some women, often in the late stages of their pregnancy, can develop gestational diabetes or high blood glucose levels. Gestational diabetes occurs in approximately 2–4% of pregnancies, or 135,000 cases per year (ADA, 2007; Rubin, 2004), and frequently disappears after childbirth, although they may be at risk of developing type 2 diabetes later on (NIDDK, 2005). Gestational diabetes occurs as the growing fetus and placenta produce hormones, some of which can contribute to the resistance of insulin.

For more information about these types of diabetes, including their diagnosis, treatment, complications, and risk factors, visit the National Institute of Diabetes and Digestive and Kidney Diseases fact sheet at: http://diabetes.niddk.nih.gov/dm/pubs/diagnosis/diagnosis.pdf

Screening and Assessment in Primary Care

Many individuals know of their diagnosis of type 1 diabetes after being admitted into a hospital. However, given the number of cases that go undiagnosed, we give below some common symptoms of diabetes (ADA, 2007):

- Frequent urination
- Excessive thirst
- Extreme hunger
- Unexplained weight loss
- Increased fatigue
- Irritability
- Blurry vision

In addition, it is important to distinguish symptoms of very low blood glucose (hypoglycemia) and very high blood glucose (hyperglycemia and ketoacidosis):

Hypoglycemia:
- Shakiness
- Dizziness
- Headache
- Sweating
- Sudden moodiness
- Confusion or difficulty in concentrating
- Seizure

Hyperglycemia:
-High blood glucose
-High levels of glucose in the urine

-Frequent urination
-Increased thirst

What Is Effective Consultation/Liaison for This Problem?

Talking to an individuals' diabetes treatment team, specifically, their endocrinologist, endocrine nurse, nutritionist, or others including their primary care physician, will be helpful in understanding unique considerations in creating a targeted treatment plan for each individual (i.e., how recently they have been diagnosed, if they have recently switched to insulin pump, etc.). If the individual were to be a child or an adolescent, consulting with their parents/caregivers concerning the management of child's diabetes and identifying what potential barriers to better treatment exist

Table 2 Interpretation of Glycosylated Hemoglobin (HbAlc) Results

	HbA1c (%)	Mean Blood Glucose	
		mg/dL	mmol/L
Action suggested	14.0	380	21.1
	13.0	350	19.3
	12.0	315	17.4
	11.0	280	15.6
	10.0	250	13.7
	9.0	215	11.9
Good	8.0	180	10.0
	7.0	150	8.2
Excellent	6.0	115	6.3
	5.0	80	4.7

might help. If the individuals have access to the result of their previous glycated hemoglobin test (HbA1c%), this may be helpful in knowing the current stability of their blood glucose levels or metabolic control, and what step should be taken for keeping it lower and more stable. The hemoglobin A1c% reveals an individual's metabolic control or average blood glucose level for the past three months. Table 2 can assist clinicians in explaining patients where their HbA1c% falls and caution when any action may be taken.

As is apparent in Table 2, an HbA1c above 9% is considered high and reflects that steps should be immediately taken to tighten one's metabolic control. It is important to take into consideration other factors outside of the individual's control that might be driving an individual's blood glucose. For example, physiological changes in puberty, including the human growth hormone, can increase blood glucose. Physical illness can also increase blood glucose levels.

Practice Guidelines

There are a variety of appropriate interventions for individuals and families with diabetes depending on the individual's treatment needs. Frequently, and understandably due in part to its difficulty, individuals with diabetes show poor adherence to their diabetes treatment regimen. Studies have found that up to 80% of patients administer insulin incorrectly, 58% of individuals with diabetes do not administer the correct dosage of insulin, as many as 77% test their blood glucose incorrectly, and up to 75% were not adhering to their prescribed dietary or exercise regimen properly (Watkins, Williams, Martin, Hogan & Anderson, 1967; Wing, Epstein, Nowalk, & Lamparski, 1986). In addition, research indicates that most individuals with diabetes do not interpret the results of their blood glucose tests correctly, and many may also not begin adhering to the treatment regimen until they feel the physical symptoms (i.e., of going low or being high) (Sarafino, 2000; Taylor, 1999). Finally, individuals who may initially follow a strict regimen, often drop off over time, and have been found to make crude estimations of required units of insulin/grams of carbohydrates consumed (Wysocki et al., 2003). Part of the problem with adherence in this population that unlike asthma medication, or birth control pills, although being hyperglycemic can feel unpleasant, the effects of nonadherence are not immediate and thus the punishing consequences of not adhering appropriately have less impact on individuals in the moment (Taylor, 1999). Though other factors may be more salient with a given individual, as adherence rates are so high and often contribute and are interrelated with other problems, interventions presented across populations will largely involve improving adherence and the related psychosocial variables. The following interventions have found empirical support with the given presenting problems.

Children with Diabetes

Several factors have been found to be associated with better treatment adherence in children. One, in particular, that finds a consistent positive relationship is that of better parental knowledge on diabetes (Chisholm et al., 2007; La Greca, Follansbee, & Skyler, 1990; Wysocki et al., 2003). Primary management of a child's diabetes regimen is often conducted by the parent/caregiver, whose knowledge on diabetes and its effective management is crucial for the child. In addition, adherence behaviors in childhood can set an individual for better management later on, when they are managing their care by themselves. A positive relationship with the child's physician, adequate health care coverage, supportive peer relationships, psychologically healthy parents, and low conflict, supportive families have all been found to be predictors of better adherence in children (Anderson, Svoren & Laffel, 2007, Marteau, Johnston, Baum & Bloch, 1987). In addition, parents who have more effective parenting skills in general has been associated with better adherence in children with diabetes. Greening, Stoppelbein, Konishi, Jordan, and Moll (2007) found that instilling structured, daily routines mediated the relationship between child behavior problems and poor treatment adherence. A number of educational resources are available for parents to not only improve diabetes knowledge but also to improve parenting skills. Given below is a list of recommended resources:

- Hanas, R. (2005). *Type 1 Diabetes: A guide for children, adolescents, young adults – and their caregivers.* New York: Marlowe & Company.
- Rubin, A. L. (2004). *Diabetes for dummies.* Hoboken, NJ: Wiley.
- Loy, V. N. (2001). *Real life parenting of kids with diabetes.* New York: American Diabetes Association.
- Phelan, T. W. (2004). *1-2-3 Magic: Effective discipline for children 2–12* (3rd ed.). New York: Parentmagic, Inc.
- American Diabetes Association: www.diabetes.org
- WebMD: diabetes.webmd.com

Primary caregivers of children with diabetes, which has been found in the literature to predominantly be the child's mother, are at an increased risk of depression for up to 1 year post-diagnosis (Wysocki et al., 2003). Children and adolescents with diabetes are also at an increased risk of psychological problems, including depression, anxiety, and eating disorders (Wysocki et al.). Children may also be hesitant to disclose their diagnosis to peers, and combined with frequent absences from school due to medical appointments, etc., children with diabetes may be at an increased risk of self-stigmatizing their diabetes. Children can place social acceptance in front of diabetes care in social contexts for fear of looking strange or standing out. Normalization of this as well as encouragement to disclose to peers can assist in improving treatment adherence in children in the social contexts.

Adolescents with Diabetes

Adolescents have been found to have more problems with diabetes management than children or adults for a variety of reasons (Anderson, Auslander, Jung, Miller & Santiago, 1990; Hanna, DiMeglio & Fortenberry, 2005). Research indicates that the mean age at which individuals with diabetes are hospitalized due to poor adherence, ketoacidosis, or hypoglycemia is between 14 and 15 years of age (Glasgow et al., 1991). One factor that complicates adherence in adolescence is that this is frequently a time period in which adolescents are attempting to demonstrate their autonomy in taking responsibility for their diabetes management. Unfortunately, this has not been found to be associated with improved adherence, rather it is associated with poorer adherence (Ingersoll et al., 1990; Palmer et al., 2004; Pendley et al., 2002). Other factors that have been found to be associated with poorer adherence in adolescence include physiological changes taking place in them during this developmental period, social pressures/stigma about adhering in peer situations, lack of understanding about diabetes management, poor body image, and most notably family conflict (Anderson, Svoren & Laffel, 2007; Wysocki, 1993; Wysocki et al., 2003).

Adolescents with type 1 diabetes, especially females, may be at increased risk of eating disorders (Grylli Wagner, Hafferl-Gattermeyer, Schober, & Karwautz, 2005; Rodin et al., 2002). This risk may be associated in part to the weight gain from administering insulin, as well as the constant focus diabetes requires with regard to food choices and the nutritional content of food (Antisdel & Chrisler, 2000). In addition, the ease in which weight loss can be accomplished simply by omitting insulin shots and maintaining a consistent state of hyperglycemia – leading to higher HbA1c – may tempt individuals with high body dissatisfaction. It has been estimated that as many as 31% of female adolescents and adults with diabetes purposefully omit their insulin, causing the term 'diabulimia' to arise (Polonksy et al., 1994). In cases where underweight adolescents are reporting high HbA1c levels, it is important to assess for insulin omission or other disordered eating patterns to determine if an eating disorder is present.

Several interventions have been conducted in attempting to improve treatment adherence in adolescents with diabetes. Specifically, coping skills training has been helpful in improving metabolic control and lowering HbA1c; adolescents

Table 3 A sample contract

Using this form, fill out a contract with your teen agreeing on all aspects of their diabetes management. Remember to be comprehensive when you complete this contract, and keep in mind that in order for it to work, it is necessary to come together and compromise on your decisions so that both you and your teen are satisfied.

Contract time frame:_____

Monitoring blood glucose (including keeping track of the monitoring form, remembering to test before meal and bedtime, ensuring that diabetes testing supplies and kit are available at necessary times, preparing for times when feeling low, etc.):
My role:_____
My teen's role:_____
What I'm going to do to ensure I stick with my role:_____
_____
_____

What my teen is going to do to ensure they stick with their role:_____
_____
_____

What I'm willing to agree to if I don't stick with my role:_____
_____
_____

What my teen's willing to agree to if they don't stick with their role:_____
_____
_____

What we will do to celebrate sticking to our roles:_____
_____
_____

Insulin administration (including correctly administering appropriate units of insulin, knowing how to correctly use shots, insulin pens, or the pump – whichever your teen is using, having appropriate supplies with them in public, etc.)
My role:_____
My teen's role:_____
What I'm going to do to ensure that I stick with my role:_____
_____
_____

What my teen's going to do to ensure that they stick with their role:_____
_____
_____

What I'm willing to agree to if I don't stick with my role:_____
_____
_____

Table 3 (continued)

What my teen is willing to agree to if they don't stick with their role:_____

_____
_____
_____

What we will do to celebrate sticking with our roles: _____

_____
_____

Date we will review and possibly renegotiate our contract:_____

Parent(s)/Caregiver(s)
signature(s):_____

Teen signature:_____

who received coping skills training reported a higher quality of life than those who did not receive such training (Davidson, Boland & Grey, 1997). Behavioral family systems therapy has gained efficacy in improving adolescent adherence to diabetes regimen as well as improving family communication and conflict resolution (Wysocki et al., 2000, 1999; Wysocki, Greco, Harris, Bubb, & White, 2001). Multisystemic family therapy has gained effectiveness in improving blood glucose monitoring, reducing poor adherence-related hospitalizations, and significantly improving metabolic control in adolescents with type 1 diabetes (Ellis et al., 2004). Finally, other interventions that have been found to improve adherence include behavioral contracting and motivational interviewing (Channon, Smith, & Gregory, 2003; Wysocki, Green, & Huxtable, 1989). The transition from parent responsibility to adolescent responsibility in adherence behaviors can be difficult, and contracting around this may be effective in reducing family conflict as well as maintaining stable metabolic control. Table 3 reflects a sample family contract that families can use to negotiate responsibility around diabetes adherence, establishing clear consequences to not following through as well as implicit rewards for maintaining responsibility.

Adults with Diabetes

Numerous interventions have been found to be helpful in improving diabetes management in adults. Cognitive behavioral strategies including motivational interviewing (Clark & Hampson, 2001), coping skills training (Grey et al., 1998; Rabin, Amir, Nardi, & Ovadia, 1986), self-monitoring (Bielamowicz, Miller, Elkins, & Ladewig, 1995; Hendricks & Hendricks, 2000), stimulus control (Cabrera-Pivaral et al., 2000), relaxation (Zetter, Duran, Waadt, Herschbach & Strian, 1995), social support-seeking (Brown, Kouzekanani, Garcia, & Craig , 2002), and stress management (Surwit et al., 2002) are all evidence-based strategies that have been effective in improving diabetes management in adults.

Self-monitoring of one's blood glucose (SMBG) has been found to be associated with better diabetes control in adults (Peyrot & Rubin, 1988). SMBG provides individuals with immediate feedback on their glucose control, and can be used to assess individuals' treatment efficacy and the effects of diet and exercise on their blood glucose (Banjeri, 2007). In addition, individuals can examine patterns in their blood glucose levels, which may require an adjustment in their treatment (Wysocki, Hough, Ward, Allen, & Murgai, 1992). Researchers conclude that simply monitoring one's blood glucose numbers is not enough to lead to behavior change, but that individuals must use these data to alter their insulin doses or injection-meal intervals for SMBG to be useful (Delameter et al., 1988). Table 4 includes a sample of a blood glucose monitoring form for patients to use.

Assessment Measures

There are numerous diabetes-related measures that may be helpful to a primary care practitioner in tailoring an intervention to a given individual. The following is not intended to be a comprehensive list; however, it gives the practitioner an idea of the available options.

- The *Measurement of Diabetes Knowledge Scales* (DKN) (Beeney, Dunn & Welch, 1994) was developed for use with type 1 and type 2 diabetes patients to quickly assess their knowledge on diabetes. The DKN scales include three parallel scales that are similar in content and item type and show very similar mean and standard deviations as well as intercorrelations (Beeney, Dunn & Welch, 2006). Reliability coefficients for the three scales have ranged from 0.77 to 0.97 (Beeney et al., 2006). The DKN scales are intended for use with adult diabetes patients.
- The *Barriers to Diabetes Self-Care Scale* (Glasgow, McCaul, & Schafer, 1986) is a 31-item self-report instrument that assesses the frequency with which an individual encounters various barriers to diabetes self-care. The scale is designed for individuals with either type 1 or type 2 diabetes of age 12 and above. This scale has been found to have adequate validity and reliability with Cronbach's alphas for the total score ranging from 0.84 to 0.86.
- The *Diabetes Family Behavior Checklist* (DFBC) (Schafer, McCaul, & Glasgow, 1986) is a measure of family interactions between individuals with type 1 diabetes and their family members, assessing their support in various areas of diabetes management (insulin administration, glucose monitoring, dietary regimen, and exercise). The measure was designed to be used by individuals of age 12 and older.
- The *Self Care Inventory* (SCI) (La Greca, Follansbee, & Skyler, 1990) is a 14-item Likert scale that assesses how well individuals have followed their prescribed diabetes regimen for the previous month. The scale was designed for use by adolescents and adults.

Table 4 Sample Blood Glucose Self-Monitoring Form

Day of the Week	Breakfast (grams of carbohydrates) (time, BG, units of insulin given)	Lunch (grams of carbohydrates) (time, BG, units of insulin given)	Dinner (grams of carbohydrates) (time, BG, units of insulin given)	Bedtime (time, BG, units of insulin given)	Exercise Y N	Sick Y N	Overall Mood for the Day from 0–10 (0 = terrible; 10 = best ever)
Monday Date:							
Tuesday Date:							
Wednesday Date:							
Thursday Date:							
Friday Date:							
Saturday Date:							
Sunday Date:							

Self-Help Resources

There are promising self-help options available for individuals with diabetes seeking self-help resources. Boren et al. (2006) examined the utility of a diabetes education call center intervention in which individuals could call and listen to one of 24 four-minute messages on topics of diabetes management (e.g., prevention, management and coping, diet and activity) and found that it significantly impacted glucose monitoring behavior and improved both general diabetes and insulin-specific knowledge.

With the advent of web-based interventions and increased opportunities to seek support, social support and informational online forums have sprouted and attracted thousands of members. Online social support forums for individuals with diabetes have also been found to be a positive source of support, and may be a step toward examining the long-term effects of being a part of an online support group (Barrera, Glasgow, McKay, Bowles, & Feil, 2002). Support groups have also been found to improve self-efficacy and self-care behaviors and decrease glycosylated hemoglobin (A1c) in older patients (DeCoster & George, 2005). Several online forums, message boards, and chat rooms are available to adolescents, parents, and adults with diabetes. The following are some that are available:

- www.diabeteschat.net
- www.childrenwithdiabetes.net
- www.diabetes123.com
- www.community.diabetes.org
- www.mydiabetes.com

In addition to online support groups, computer interventions appear to have gained efficacy in improving diabetes management. Williams, Lynch, and Glasgow (2007) developed a patient-centered, computer-assisted intervention program to increase perceived autonomy support and perceived competence and outcome on diabetes management. The computer-assisted intervention was tested on 866 individuals with type 2 diabetes and found that perceived autonomy increased, which led to increased perceived competence and finally improved diabetes self-care outcomes. In addition, www.fitandhealthykids.com is an empirically validated website dealing with overweight and obesity in children (Moore, 2006).

Researchers aiming to reach younger generations through technology have developed video games attempting to improve diabetes knowledge and health outcomes in children and adolescents. The Health Hero video games series included two messages about diabetes self-management (Lieberman, 1997), and children with diabetes were found to maintain engagement with these games, and their disclosure of diabetes to friends was found to increase the longer they played. Most recently, GlucoBoy, a blood sugar monitoring game, allows individuals to plug their glucometer device into GameBoy before pricking their finger and putting the strip on their glucometer. The players are awarded points for monitoring their blood glucose, using which they are able to unlock games or purchase things online. In addition, the more frequently their blood glucose levels stay in the desired ranges, the more points they will get. To the present author's knowledge, this device has not been empirically tested.

In addition to websites and games, various books and workbooks are available to individuals with diabetes to assist in their self-management:

- Roybal & Funnell (2004). *Managing diabetes your way workbook: Living with type 2 diabetes.* NY: Ulysses Press.
- Betschart (2001). *It's time to learn about diabetes: A workbook on diabetes for children.* NY: John Wiley & Sons.
- Tolle & O'Donohue (submitted). *Adolescents with type 1 diabetes: Help with the hard stuff/Parents of adolescents with type 1 diabetes: Help with the hard stuff.*
- Labbat & Maggi (1997). *Weight management for type 2 diabetes: An action plan.* NY: Wiley.

Referral and Stepped Care

For families or individuals in which self-management of diabetes is of primary concern, and are otherwise functioning at a high level, it is important to consider what stepped care options from those listed above might be more appropriate than more intensive approaches. For families or individuals with more serious comorbid psychological problems, such as an eating disorder, severe depression, or other serious mental health problems (e.g., schizophrenia), more intensive psychotherapeutic options should be considered. Consultation with the individual's physician or multidisciplinary team should take place to ensure that the optimal treatment plan is selected or when any recommendation is made that could impact medical treatment of the individual's diabetes.

Conclusion

Individuals with diabetes are confronted with a myriad of barriers in their disease management. A lack of diabetes knowledge, family conflict, social pressures, high body dissatisfaction, burnout, and lack of time/motivation are just a few that have been discussed. Individuals with diabetes are at an increased risk to experience depression and poor coping. Cognitive behavioral strategies have been found to be efficacious in improving diabetes management, especially type 1 and type 2, across all age ranges. Multiple sources of social support, information, and interventions are available via the internet, video games as well as self-help books designed to improve management of diabetes. Continued research is needed to establish the effectiveness of these stepped care approaches as adjuncts to medical care.

References

American Diabetes Association. (2007). *All about diabetes*. Accessed at http://www.diabetes.org/about-diabetes.jsp December 12, 2007.

Anderson, B. J., Auslander, W. F., Jung, K. C., Miller, J. P. & Santiago, J. V. (1990). Assessing family sharing of diabetes responsibilities.*Journal of Pediatric Psychology, 15*(4), 477–492.

Anderson, B. J., Svoren, B. & Laffel, L. (2007). Initiatives to promote effective self-care skills in children and adolescents with diabetes mellitus. *Disability Management Health Outcomes, 15*(2), 101–108.

Antisdel, J. E. & Chrisler, J. C. (2000). Comparison of eating attitudes and behaviors among adolescent and young women with type 1 diabetes and phenylketonuria. *Developmental and Behavioral Pediatrics, 21,* 81–86.

Banjeri, M. A. (2007). The foundation of diabetes self-management. *The Diabetes Educator, 33*(4), 87–90.

Barrera, M., Glasgow, R. E., McKay, H. G., Bowles, S. M., & Feil, E. G. (2002). Do internet-based support interventions change perceptions in social support? An experimental trial of approaches for supporting diabetes self-management. *American Journal of Community Psychology, 30*(5), 637–654.

Beeney, L. J., Dunn, S. M. & Welch, G. (1994). Measurement of diabetes knowledge – the development of the diabetes knowledge scales. In C. Blare (Ed.), *Handbook of psychology and diabetes: A guide to psychological measurement in diabetes research and practice*. Langhorne, PA England: Harwood Academic Publishers.

Beeney, L. J., Dunn, S. M. & Welch, G. (2006). Measurement of diabetes knowledge – the development of the diabetes knowledge scales. In C. Blare (Ed.) *Handbook of psychology and diabetes*. New York: Psychology Press.

Bielamowicz, M. K., Miller, W. C., Elkins, E. & Ladewig, H. (1995). Monitoring behavioral changes in diabetes care with the diabetes self-management record. *Diabetes Educator, 21,* 426–431.

Boren, S. A., De Leo, G., Chanetsa, F. F., Donaldson, J., Krishna, S., & Balas, E. A. (2006). Evaluation of a diabetes education call center intervention. Telemedicine & e-health 12(4), 457–465.

Brown, S. A., Kouzekanani, K., Garcia, A. A., & Craig, L. H. (2002). Culturally competent diabetes self management education for Mexican Americans. *Diabetes Care, 25,* 259–268.

Cabrera-Pivaral, C. E., Gonzalez-Perez, G., Vega-Lopez, G., Gonzalez-Hita, M., Centeno-Lopez, M., Gonzalez-Ortiz, M., Martinez-Abundis, E., & Ojeda, A. G. (2000). Effects of behaviorally modifying education in the metabolic profile of the Type 2 diabetes mellitus patient. *Journal of Diabetes and its Complications, 14,* 322–326.

Channon, S., Smith, V. J. & Gregory, J. W. (2003). A pilot study of motivational interviewing in adolescents. *Archives of Disease in Childhood, 88,* 680–683.

Chisholm, V., Atkinson, L., Donaldson, C., Noyes, K., Payne, A., & Kelnar, C. (2007). Predictors of treatment adherence in young children with type 1 diabetes. *Journal of Advanced Nursing, 57*(5), 482–493.

Clark, M., & Hampson, S. E. (2001). Implementing a psychosocial intervention to improve lifestyle self-management in patients. *Patient Education and Counseling, 42,* 247–256.

Davidson, M., Boland, E. A., & Grey, M. (1997). Teaching teens to cope: Coping skills training for adolescents with insulin-dependent diabetes mellitus. *Journal of the Society of Pediatric Nurses, 2*(2), 65–72.

DeCoster, V. A. & George, L. (2005). An empowerment approach for elders living with diabetes: A pilot study of a community-based self help group – the diabetes club. *Educational Gerontology, 31*(9), 699–713.

Delameter, A. M., Davis, S., Bubb, J., Smith, J., White, N. H., & Santiago, J. V. (1988). Self-monitoring of blood glucose by adolescents with diabetes: Technical skills and utilization of data. *Diabetes Educator, 15,* 56–61.

Ellis, D. A., Naar-King, S., Frey, M., Templin, T., Rowland, M. & Greger, N. (2004). Use of multisystemic therapy to improve regimen adherence among adolescents with type 1 diabetes in poor metabolic control: A pilot investigation*Journal of Clinical Psychology in Medical Settings, 11*(4), 315–324.

Glasgow, R. E., McCaul, K. D., & Schafer, L. C. (1986). Barriers to regimen adherence among persons with insulin-dependent diabetes. *Journal of Behavioral Medicine, 9*(1), 65–77.

Glasgow, A. M., Weissberg-Benchell, J., Tynan, W. D., Epstein, S. F., Driscoll, C., Turek, J., et al. (1991). Readmissions of children with diabetes mellitus to a children's hospital. *Pediatrics, 88*, 98–104.

Greening, L., Stoppelbein, L., Konishi, C., Jordan, S. S. & Moll, G. (2007). Child routines and youths' adherence to treatment for type 1 diabetes. *Journal of Pediatric Psychology, 32*(4), 437–447.

Grey, M.,Yu, C , Boland, E. A., Sullivan-Bolyai, S. Davidson, M., & Tamborlane, W. V. (1998). Short term effects of coping skills training as adjunct to intensive therapy in adolescents. *Diabetes Care, 21*, 902–908.

Grylli, V., Wagner, G., Hafferl-Gattermeyer, A., Schober, E., & Karwautz, A. (2005). Disturbed eating attitudes, coping styles, and subjective quality of life in adolescents with type 1 diabetes. *Journal of Psychosomatic Research, 59*(2), 65–72.

Hanas, R. (2005). *Type 1 diabetes: A guide for children, adolescents, young adults – and their caregivers* (3rd ed.). New York: Marlowe & Company.

Hanna, K. M., DiMeglio, L. A. & Fortenberry, J. D. (2005). Parent and adolescent versions of the diabetes-specific parental support for adolescents' autonomy scale. *Journal of Pediatric Psychology, 30*, 257–271.

Hendricks, L. E., & Hendricks, R. T. (2000). The effect of diabetes self-management education with frequent follow-up on the health outcomes of African American men. *Diabetes Educator, 26*, 995–100.

Ingersoll, G. M., Hibbard, R. A., Kronz, K. K., Fineberg, N. S., Marrero, D. G., & Golden, M. P. (1990). Pediatrics residents' attitudes about insulin-dependent diabetes mellitus and children with diabetes. *Academic Medicine, 65(10)*, 643–645.

La Greca, A. M., Follansbee, D., & Skyler, J. S. (1990). Developmental and behavioral aspects of diabetes management in youngsters. *Children's Health Care, 19*, 132–139.

Lieberman, D. A. (1997). Interactive video games for health promotion: Effects on knowledge, self-efficacy, social support and health. In R. L. Jr. Street, W. R. Gold, & T. Manning (Eds.). *Health promotion and interactive technologies: Theoretical applications and new directions* (pp. 103–120). Mahwah, NJ: Lawrence Erlbaum Associates, Inc.

Marteau, T. M., Johnston, M., Baum, J. D. & Bloch, S. (1987). Goals of treatment in diabetes: A comparison of doctors and parents of children with diabetes. *Journal of Behavioral Medicine, 10*(1), 33–48.

Moore, B. A. (2006). *Fit and healthy kids*. Unpublished dissertation. University of Nevada, Reno.

National Institute of Diabetes and Digestive and Kidney Diseases – NIDDK (2005). *Diagnosis of Diabetes*. Bethesda MA: National Institute of Health.

Palmer, D. L., Berg, C. A., Wiebe, D. J., Beveridge, R. M., Korbel, C. D., Upchurch, R., et al. (2004). The role of autonomy and pubertal status in understanding age differences in maternal involvement in diabetes responsibility across adolescence. *Journal of Pediatric Psychology, 29*, 35–46.

Pendley, J. S., Kasmen, L., Miller, D., Donze, J., Swenson, C., & Reeves, G. (2002). Peer and family support in children and adolescents with type 1 diabetes. *Journal of Pediatric Psychology, 27*, 429–438.

Peyrot, M., & Rubin, R. R. (1988). Insulin self-regulation predicts better glycemic control. *Diabetes, 37*, 53A.

Polonksy, W. H., Anderson, B. J., Lohrer, P. A., Aponte, J. E., Jacobson, A. M. & Cole, C. F. (1994). Insulin omission in women with IDDM. *Diabetes Care, 17*(10), 1178–1185.

Rabin, C , Amir, S., Nardi, R.. & Ovadia, B. (1986). Compliance and control: Issues in group training for diabetes. *Health & Social Work, 11*, 141–151.

Rodin G, Olmsted MP, Rydall AC, Maharaj SI, Colton PA, Jones JM,et al. (2002). Eating disorders in young women with type 1 diabetes. *Journal of Psychosomatic Research, 53*, 943 949.

Rubin, A. L. (2004). *Diabetes for dummies*. Hoboken, NJ: Wiley.

Sarafino, E. P. (2000). *Health psychology: Biopsychosocial interactions*. 4th Ed. New York: Wiley.

Schafer, L. C., McCaul, K. D. & Glasgow, R. E. (1986). Supportive and nonsupportive family behaviors: Relationships to adherence and metabolic control in persons with type 1 diabetes. *Diabetes Care, 9*, 179–185.

Surwit, R. S., Feinglos, M. N., van Tilburg, M. A. L., Edwards, C. L., Zucker, N., Williams. P, et al. (2002). Stress management improves long-term glycemic control in type 2 diabetes. *Diabetes Care, 25*, 30–34.

Taylor, S. E. (1999). *Health Psychology*. Boston, MA: McGraw Hill.

Watkins, J. D., Williams, T. F., Martin, D. A., Hogan, M. D. & Anderson, E. (1967). A study of diabetic patients at home. *American Journal of Public Health, 57*, 452–459.

Williams, G. C., Lynch, M. F., & Glasgow, R. E. (2007). Computer-assisted intervention improves patient-centered diabetes care by increasing autonomy support. *Health Psychology, 26*, 728–734.

Wing, R. R., Epstein, L. H., Nowalk, M. P. & Lamparski, D. M. (1986). Behavioral self-regulation in the treatment of patients with diabetes mellitus. *Psychological Bulletin, 99*, 78–89.

Wysocki, T. (1993). Associations among teen-parent relationships, metabolic control,and adjustment to diabetes in adolescents. *Journal of Pediatric Psychology, 18*(4), 441–452.

Wysocki, T. Greco, P. & Buckloh, L. M. (2003). Childhood diabetes in a psychological context. In M C. Roberts (Ed.) *Handbook of pediatric psychology* (3rd ed., pp.304–320). New York: Guilford Press.

Wysocki, T., Greco, P., Harris, M. A., Bubb, J., & White, N. H. (2001). Behavior therapy for families of adolescents with diabetes: Maintenance of treatment effects. *Diabetes Care, 24*(3), 441–446.

Wysocki, T., Green, L. B., & Huxtable, K. (1989). Blood glucose monitoring by diabetic adolescents. Compliance and metabolic control. *Health Psychology, 8*, 267–284.

Wysocki, T., Harris, M. A., Greco, P., Bubb, J., Danda, C. E., Harvey, L. M., et al. (2000). Randomized, controlled trial of behavior therapy for families of adolescents with insulin-dependent diabetes mellitus. *Journal of Pediatric Psychology, 25*(1), 23–33.

Wysocki, T., Hough, B. S., Ward, K. M., Allen, A. A., & Murgai, N. (1992). Use of blood glucose data by families of children and adolescents with DM1. *Diabetes Care, 15*, 1041–1044.

Wysocki, T., Miller, K. M., Greco, P., Harris, M. A., Harvey, L. M., Elder-Danda, C. L., et al. (1999). Behavior therapy for families of adolescents with diabetes: Effects on directly observed family interactions. *Behavior Therapy, 30*, 496–515.

Zetter, A , Duran, G., Waadt, S., Herschbach, P.,& Strian, F. (1995). Coping with fear of long-term complications in diabetes mellitus: A model clinical program. *Psychotherapy Psychosomatic, 64*, 178–184.

Attention-Deficit Hyperactivity Disorder in Primary Care

Brie A. Moore

Current DSM-IV Diagnostic Criteria

According to the *Diagnostic and Statistical Manual of Mental Disorders, Fourth Edition (DSM-IV)*, criteria for this disorder require one of two patterns of symptoms: inattention or hyperactivity/impulsivity, as delineated below. Currently, three subtypes of attention-deficit hyperactivity disorder (ADHD) are recognized: (1) primarily inattentive, (2) primarily hyperactive/impulsive, and (3) combined type. The inattentive subtype consists of individuals who exhibit inattentive behaviors but not hyperactive or impulsive behaviors. The hyperactive/impulsive subtype consists of the presence of hyperactive and impulsive features, without inattentive behaviors. The combined subtype presents with inattention and hyperactivity/impulsivity.

According to *DSM-IV*, the individual must exhibit six or more of the following symptoms of inattention. These symptoms must have persisted for at least 6 months, and must be causing significant impairment in the child's functioning:

Inattention

- Often fails to give close attention to details or makes careless mistakes in school-work, work, or other activities
- Often has difficulty sustaining attention in tasks or play activities
- Often does not seem to listen when spoken to directly
- Often does not follow through on instructions and fails to finish schoolwork, chores, or duties in the workplace (not due to oppositional behavior or failure to understand instructions)
- Often has difficulty organizing tasks and activities
- Often avoids, dislikes, or is reluctant to engage in tasks that require sustained mental effort (such as schoolwork or homework)

B.A. Moore (✉)
CareIntegra, Inc., University of Nevada, Reno, NV, USA
e-mail: brieamoore@yahoo.com

L.C. James, W.T. O'Donohue (eds.), *The Primary Care Toolkit*,
DOI 10.1007/978-0-387-78971-2_16, © Springer Science+Business Media, LLC 2009

- Often loses things necessary for tasks or activities (toys, school assignments, pencils, books, tools, etc.)
- Is often easily distracted by irrelevant stimuli
- Is often forgetful in daily activities

On the other hand, the individual must exhibit six or more of the following symptoms of hyperactivity/impulsivity. These symptoms must have persisted for at least 6 months, and must be causing significant impairment in the child's functioning:

Hyperactivity

- Often fidgets with hands or feet or squirms in seat
- Often leaves seat in classroom or in other situations in which remaining seated is expected
- Often runs about or climbs excessively in situations in which it is inappropriate (in adolescents or adults, it may be limited to subjective feelings of restlessness)
- Often has difficulty playing or engaging in leisure activities quietly
- Is often 'on the go' or acts as if 'driven by a motor'
- Often talks excessively

Impulsivity

- Often blurts out answers before questions have been completed
- Often has difficulty awaiting a turn
- Often interrupts or intrudes on others' conversations or games

In addition to exhibiting one of the two patterns of symptoms, it is necessary that hyperactive/impulsive or inattentive symptoms occur in two or more settings, such as school (or work) and home. ADHD symptoms must have been present before the age of seven in order to meet these criteria for diagnosis.

Epidemiology

Attention-deficit hyperactivity disorder is one of the most common neurobehavioral disorders of childhood, and is recognized as a serious threat to public health (Centers for Disease Control and Prevention, 2007; National Institutes of Mental Health, 2007). Although prevalence rates vary depending on the sampling design and restrictiveness of the definition of ADHD used, conservative estimates suggest that between 3% and 5% of children meet the diagnostic criteria for ADHD (American Academy of Child and Adolescent Psychiatry, 1997). Prevalence rates have been reported as high as 16% in some studies (Green et al., 1999). Approximately 4.1% of adults, aged 18–44 years, are diagnosed with ADHD in a given year (Kessler, Chiu, Demler, & Walters, 2005). Boys are more likely than girls to have

ADHD; however, the estimated ratio of boys to girls with ADHD ranges from 3:1 to 9:1 (Pelham & Waschbusch, 2006). ADHD is believed to have a noticeable impact on social, economic, educational, and health care delivery systems. According to commercial data, in the year 2001, 9.7 million physician office visits were due to ADHD (Scott-Levin Associates, 2001). Using a prevalence rate of 5%, Pelham and colleagues estimated that the annual societal cost of this illness in childhood and adolescence is $42.5 billion, with a range between $36 billion and 52.4 billion (Pelham, Foster, & Robb, 2007).

Comorbidity

Children with ADHD may often meet the diagnostic criteria for other behavioral disorders. Most commonly, ADHD occurs comorbidly with oppositional defiant disorder (50–75%) and conduct disorder (20–40%; Lahey et al., 1999). Mood and anxiety disorders often overlap highly with ADHD, with rates ranging from 15% to 25% across studies (Angold, Costello, & Erkanli, 1999; Barkley, 2006). Approximately 20–30% of children who meet the criteria for a specific learning disability also meet the criteria for ADHD (Barkely et al., 2005).

Developmental Trends

Attention-deficit hyperactivity disorder is best conceptualized as a chronic, lifespan disorder. ADHD usually becomes evident in preschool or early elementary years. The median age of onset of ADHD is seven years (Kessler et al., 2005). Although estimates vary across studies, approximately 70% of childhood cases and 65% of adolescent cases persist into adulthood (Barkley, 2006). The expression of symptoms may change over time as a function of developmental and contextual factors. As they age, children may experience a relative diminution of hyperactivity and impulsivity. Attention deficits (i.e., impaired concentration, forgetfulness, disorganization) may persist as children grow older and are confronted with more challenging tasks. At various stages of development, individuals may be confronted with tasks that tax attention and concentration deficits. However, symptoms can also improve over time as children and their families develop skills.

Patient Fact Sheets and Handouts

The American Academy of Pediatrics (AAP) and the National Initiative for Children's Healthcare Quality (NICHQ; 2002) have compiled a list of tools for parents. These tools address a wide range of issues from understanding ADHD, to communicating with the school about ADHD, to developing behavioral plans to improve attention and concentration and reduce distractibility. These tools are available at http://www.nichq.org/NICHQ/Topics/ChronicConditions/ADHD/Tools/ and can be accessed free of charge by registration with NICHQ. Some helpful handouts include:

- ADHD Management Plan
- Does My Child Have ADHD?
- Educational Rights for Children with ADHD
- Evaluating Your Child for ADHD
- Homework Tips for Parents
- Working with Your Child's School

Handouts for Providers

In addition to parent handouts, the AAP and the NICHQ have also compiled a list of tools for providers. Tools for documenting encounters, billing, and treatment plans can be accessed from http://www.nichq.org/NICHQ/Topics/ChronicConditions/ADHD/Tools/. Some remarkable tools include:

- ADHD Coding Fact Sheet for Primary Care Clinicians
- ADHD Encounter Form for Clinicians
- ADHD Management Plan
- ADHD Medication Management Information
- Cover Letter to Teachers
- Document for Reimbursement
- How to Establish a School-Home Daily Report Card
- Primary Care Initial Evaluation Form
- Tips for ADHD-Related Sleep Problems

Handouts for Educators

In addition to those listed above, Impromed Medical Education provides handouts for parents and clinicians. A unique contribution of Impromed is handouts for educators, who are an integral part of comprehensive and empirically based ADHD treatment. These resources can be accessed from http://www.impromed.org/CME/adhd/enduring.asp.

- Recommended Reading for Teachers
- Recommended Websites for Teachers
- 7 Myths About AD/HD Debunked!; ADHD Background: Impact on Schools; The Role of Teachers in the Treatment and Management of ADHD – Classroom Accommodations
- When Should I Be Concerned and Refer a Student to a Clinician for an Evaluation?
- What Will a Clinician Do to Evaluate a Child for ADHD?
- What Do I Need to Know About Medications?

Clinical Assessment Tools

The AAP and the NICHQ (2002) have established guidelines for the assessment of ADHD in primary care. Briefly, these principles state that: (1) children must meet *DSM-IV* criteria to receive a formal ADHD diagnosis; (2) information about core symptoms, symptom occurrence across settings, age of onset, duration, and impairment must be gathered directly from caregivers; (3) this evidence must also be obtained directly from the classroom teacher; and (4) comorbidities must be assessed. Despite these guidelines, a large survey of primary care providers demonstrated that only 60% of physicians reported using formal diagnostic criteria for establishing a diagnosis of ADHD (Hopkins, Herrerias, Stein, & Homer, 2001).

Based on the findings regarding diagnostic practices in primary care, providers are encouraged to use formal diagnostic criteria (i.e., *DSM-IV*) when establishing a diagnosis, and to pay particular attention to the occurrence of symptoms in more than one setting and the presence of comorbid conditions. Providers are also encouraged to alert families and school personnel that there are currently no biological markers or computerized tests that allow for diagnostic specificity (AAP & NICHQ, 2002). Providers should use appropriate diagnostic tests during the evaluation process, namely direct observation, interviews with parents, children and teachers, and standardized behavior rating scales of specific ADHD symptoms (Brown et al., 2001a).

Standardized Behavior Rating Scales

The use of standardized behavior rating scales is essential for accurate diagnosis of ADHD. An accurate, well-established diagnosis is the first step to developing an effective, individualized plan of medical and behavioral treatment. Scales that measure specific ADHD symptoms are more useful in diagnosis than global indices. Although broadband rating scales have limited utility in diagnosing ADHD, they can provide useful information regarding comorbidities. The SNAP-IV and Conners' scales (1997) have performed well in discriminating children with ADHD from normal controls (Brown et al., 2001a). *DSM-IV*-based rating scales, such as those presented here, are a time-efficient and cost-effective means for gathering data in primary care.

Figure 1 shows the advantages and disadvantages of four popular rating scales. The following measures assess symptoms in accordance with *DSM-IV* diagnostic criteria, and are suitable for use in primary care (Woodard, 2006).

- ADHD Rating Scale IV (DuPaul, Power, Anastopoulous, & Reid, 1998)
- Brown Attention Deficit Disorder Scale for Children and Adolescents (Brown, 2001b)
- Conners Rating Scale – Revised (CRS-R; Conners, 1997)
- Swanson, Nolan, and Pelham Questionnaire – R (SNAP-IV; Swanson et al., 2001)

Medscape® www.medscape.com				
Scale	**Description**	**Advantages**	**Disadvantages**	**Availability**
Connors Rating Scale Revised CRS-R (3-17 years) *Multihealth Systems, Inc. Connors, 1997	A popular scale with a long history of evaluation of ADHD. Assesses a wide variety of common behavior problems (e.g., sleep, eating, and peer group problems). The revised scale updates age and gender normative data and factor structure. Available in both short and long, parent, teacher, self-report versions. Unlike other scales that are DSM-IV based, the	• DSM-IV based • Large normative base • Multiple observer forms • Abbreviated forms aid in treatment monitoring • French version	• Few items regarding comorbidities • Somewhat redundant • Full length version lengthy	www.mhs.com complete kit $265
Brown Attention Deficit Disorder Scale (BADDS) for Children and Adolescents (3-12 years, parent and teacher; 8-12 years, self-report) *Psychological Corp., Brown, 2001	BADDS measures executive functioning associated with ADHD. Also, measures developmental impairments. Separate rating scales for 3-7 years, 8-12 years, 12-18 years. The scale should be administered in an interview format, especially the parent and youth-self report. Newer DSM-IV based rating scale. Both parent and teacher form.	• Measures inattentive ADHD • Only scale that accounts for inattentive behavior as a function of age • Strong psychometrics	• Minimal data about use in clinical settings	www.addwarehouse.com complete kit $199.00
Vanderbilt ADHD Rating Scale (6-12 years, parent and teacher forms) *AAP and NICHQ, 2002	Similar to CRS-R and SNAP-IV. Assesses for comorbidities and school functioning.	• Measures co-morbidities (ODD, anxiety, depression) • Spanish and German versions • Available via Web site • Psychometrically strong scales	• Newer scales that lack sufficient data to establish their validity • Normative date from only one region in U.S. • No self-report scales	www.aap.org members $200.00 non-members $250.00
Swanson, Nolan, and Pelham IV (SNAP) (5-11 years, parent and teacher rating scale)	One of the first scales based on DSM-IV criteria. Frequently used in ADHD research.	• Scoring available on Web site • Same scale use for both parent and teacher • Measures co-morbidity	• Lack of published psychometrics and normative data • Brief assessment of co-morbidities	www.adhd.net free
Source: Pediatr Nurs © 2006 Jannetti Publications, Inc.				

Fig. 1 ADHD behavior rating scales
Accessed from http://www.medscape.com/viewarticle/ 543727_3

- Vanderbilt ADHD Rating Scale (Parent and Teacher Forms; AAP & NICHQ, 2002); available at http://www.vanderbiltchildrens.com/uploads/documents/ccdr_adhd_scale.pdf

The *Primary Care Toolkit* compiled by the AAP and the NICHQ provides resources and guidelines for the assessment of ADHD in primary care. Information regarding the toolkit is available at www.nichq.org/NICHQ/Topics/ Chronic-Conditions/ADHD/Tools/. The toolkit also provides clinicians with copies of the Vanderbilt ADHD Rating Scale, instructions for scoring, and forms for following up with teachers and parents.

Clinical Considerations

When assessing ADHD, it is important to establish that symptoms represent a pattern of behaviors that have occurred across time and contexts (e.g., home and school) for a period of at least 6 months. A thorough assessment should rely on information from parents and teachers about ADHD symptoms. Information provided by children is less useful (Pelham & Waschbusch, 2006). It is important to note that children are generally more inattentive and hyperactive than adults. Also, there is normal variability among children: some are normally more hyperactive, inattentive, and impulsive than others. In all cases, it is important to consider whether or not a child is exhibiting behavior appropriate to his or her age. It is normal for children to appear inattentive when things they are not naturally interested in are occurring. Finally, many children enjoy activity, and sometimes adults regiment their day so that there are long periods of sitting or other structured activities. This structure can make some children appear 'hyperactive' or 'impulsive' when 'bored' and 'restless' would be more accurate terms. Hyperactivity or impulsive behavior should always be judged by developmental norms.

Practice Guidelines

According to Division 53 of the American Psychological Association (2007), Behavior Parent Training, Behavioral Classroom Interventions, and stimulant medications, such as Concerta®, Metadate®, Ritalin®, and Adderall®, are well-established treatments for children with ADHD. Interventions including social skills training with generalized components and summer treatment programs are considered probably efficacious for the treatment of ADHD in children.

Division 53 (2007) reports:

Stimulant Medication
Stimulant medications such as methylphenidate (Ritalin, Concerta) and Adderall are very effective at reducing ADHD symptoms in the short-term. Stimulant medications have been found to improve children's classroom behavior, academic task completion, behavior during parent-child interactions, and performance on computer tasks assessing attention and impulsivity. Two-thirds of children with ADHD benefit from stimulant medication, while the rest either show no response or an adverse response. Common side effects include loss of appetite and insomnia. Greater improvements are generally found when medication is combined with behavior therapy.

Behavioral Parent Training
Parent training involves teaching parents behavior modification techniques that are based on social learning principles. Parents are encouraged to provide clear rules and structure in the child's environment and consistent positive and negative consequences for corresponding child behavior. Specifically, parents target and monitor problematic behaviors, reward prosocial behavior through praise, positive attention, and rewards, and decrease unwanted behavior by ignoring minor or irritating behavior (e.g., complaining, fidgeting) and using time out or removal of privileges for more serious negative behavior (e.g., fighting). BPT has been shown to be effective in improving problematic child behavior and negative parent-child interactions.

Behavioral Classroom Interventions
Classroom interventions for ADHD involve consultation with a teacher regarding the use of behavior modification strategies in the school setting. Teachers are encouraged to establish classroom rules and structure, to praise and attend to positive child behavior, ignore minor or irritating behavior, use time out for more serious behavior, and implement point or token systems. Additionally, effective classroom interventions include the implementation of a daily report card, on which specific child behaviors are targeted, and children are rewarded for meeting behavioral and academic goals. Children with ADHD are sometimes eligible for special education services or accommodations to assist them with academic or social difficulties.

Social Skills Training with Generalization Components
Given the problems in peer relationships that many children with ADHD experience, social skills training is commonly used as one component of treatment. However, little research supports the efficacy of social skills training in the treatment of ADHD. More recently, variations on social skills training that involve parents in encouraging the use of social skills outside of the clinic setting have shown more promising effects.

Summer Treatment Programs
Summer treatment programs for children with ADHD combine evidence-based ADHD treatment components, including behavioral parent training, a token or point system, positive reinforcement (i.e., praise), effective commands, time out, a daily report card, social skills training, and problem-solving skills training. These treatments are applied across recreational and academic settings in order to improve children's peer relationships, interactions with adults, academic performance, and self-efficacy. Preliminary studies suggest that summer treatment programs are effective in treating children with ADHD across many of these domains of impairment.

Publications

American Academy of Pediatrics

> Clinical Practice Guideline: Treatment of the School-Aged Child with Attention-Deficit/Hyperactivity Disorder

> Available at:
> http://aappolicy.aappublications.org/cgi/content/full/pediatrics%3b108/4/1033

American Academy of Child and Adolescent Psychiatry

> Practice Parameters for the Assessment and Treatment of Children, Adolescents, and Adults with Attention-Deficit/Hyperactivity Disorder

> Available at:
> http://www.aacap.org/page.ww?section=Practice+Parameters&name=
> Practice+Parameters

American Academy of Child and Adolescent Psychiatry

> Practice Parameter for the Use of Stimulant Medications in the Treatment of Children, Adolescents, and Adults

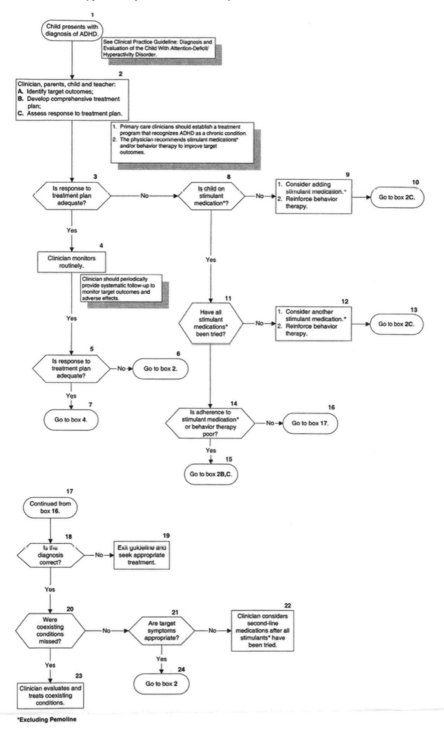

Fig. 2 Algorithm for the treatment of school-aged children with ADHD
Source: http://aappolicy.aappublications.org/cgi/content/full/pediatrics%3b108/4/1033

Available at:
http://www.aacap.org/galleries/PracticeParameters/StimMed.pdf

The AAP has provided an algorithm for the treatment of school-aged children with ADHD that synthesizes these evidence-based approaches. The algorithm is presented in Fig. 2.

Treatment Manuals and Resources for Providers

- American Academy of Pediatrics and National Initiative for Children's Health-care Quality (2002). Caring for children with ADHD: a resource toolkit for clinicians. Elk Grove, IL. Accessed on November 14, 2007from http://www.nichq.org/NICHQ/Topics/ChronicConditions/ADHD/Tools/ADHD.htm
- Barkley, R. A. (1997). *Defiant children: A clinician's manual for assessment and parent training.* (2nd ed.). New York: Guilford.
- Barkley, R. A. (1997). *Managing the defiant child: A guide to parent training* [Motion picture]. New York: Guilford.
- Barkley, R., Edwards, G., & Robin, A. (1999). *Defiant teens: A clinician's manual for assessment and family intervention.* New York: Guilford.
- DuPaul, G. J. (Writer), Stoner, G. (Writer), & Lerner, S. (Producer). (1998). *Assessing ADHD in the schools* [Motion picture]. New York: Guilford.
- DuPaul, G. J. (Writer), Stoner, G. (Writer), & Lerner, S. (Producer). (1998). *Classroom interventions for ADHD* [Motion picture]. New York: Guilford.
- Forehand, R., & McMahon, R. (2003). *Helping the noncompliant child: Family-based treatment for oppositional behavior.* (2nd ed.). New York: Guilford.

Stepped Care Treatments

Books and Workbooks

Barkley, R. A. (2000). Taking Charge of ADHD: The Complete, Authoritative Guide for Parents (Revised Edition). Guilford Press, New York: 2000

Videos and Audio Tips

The following video and audio resources are useful for providing parents with information regarding the identification of ADHD, medications, and behavioral interventions.

Living and Thriving with ADHD: A Guide for Families Video http://www.aap. org/bst/showdetl.cfm? &DID=15&Product_ID=3880&CatID=132
A Minute for Kids Audio Files http://www.aap.org/healthtopics/adhd.cfm

Attention Deficit Hyperactivity Disorder: Myths and Facts
http://www.healthology.com/hybrid-player/hybrid-asx.asp? f=children&
c=mentalhealth_adhdmyths&b=mentalhelp&sv=3&spg=RELH&han=NO&
vidAd=undefined

Attention Deficit Hyperactivity Disorder: What Every Parent Should Know
http://www.healthology.com/hybrid-player/hybrid-asx.asp?
f=adhd_comprehend&c=mentalhealth_2adhdcauses&b=mentalhelp&sv=3
&spg=&han=NO&vidAd=undefined

ADHD in School: How to Stay in the Loop http://www.healthology.com/hybrid-
player/hybrid-asx.asp? f=adhd_comprehend&c=schooladhd&b=mentalhelp
&sv=3&spg=XML&han=NO&vidAd=undefined

Helping Kids With ADHD Succeed in School http://www.healthology.com/
hybrid-player/hybrid-asx.asp? f=adhd_comprehend&c=helpadhd
&b=mentalhelp&sv=3&spg=RELH&han=NO&vidAd=undefined

Attention Deficit Hyperactivity Disorder: Tips for Parents and Teachers
http://www.healthology.com/hybrid-player/hybrid-asx.asp?
f=children&c=mentalhealth_2adhdbevtherapy&b=mentalhelp&sv=3
&spg=RELH&han=NO&vidAd=undefined

Websites

The websites included here provide comprehensive information regarding ADHD,
including diagnostic and treatment information and resources for clinicians, teachers
and parents dealing with persons with ADHD. A more comprehensive list of web-
based resources is available at http://www.nichq.org/NR/rdonlyres/CE8FA1FD-
D792-42C5-B9D8-6824C9031011/4998/25ADHDResourcesonInternet.pdf

American Academy of Child and Adolescent Psychiatry – ADHD: A Guide for
Families http://www.aacap.org/cs/adhd_a_guide_for_families/resources_for_
families_adhd_a_guide_for_families

American Academy of Pediatrics – Children's Health Topics: ADHD
http://www.aap.org/healthtopics/adhd.cfm

Children and Adults with Attention Deficit/Hyperactivity Disorder
www.chadd.org

KidsHealth.org – ADHD

Parents: www.kidshealth.org/parent/medical/learning/adhd.html
Teens: www.kidshealth.org/teen/school_jobs/school/adhd.html
Kids: www.kidshealth.org/kid/feel_better/things/ritalin.html;
www.kidshealth.org/kid/health_problems/learning_problem/adhdkid.html

National Resource Center on ADHD http://www.help4adhd.org/
National Initiative for Children's Healthcare Quality – ADHD
http://www.nichq.org/NICHQ/Topics/ChronicConditions/ADHD/

National Institute of Mental Health http://www.nimh.nih.gov/health/topics/
attention-deficit-hyperactivity-disorder-adhd/index.shtml
Therapy Advisor – ADHD http://www.therapyadvisor.com/taDisorder.aspx?
disID=27&sm=cc27

References

American Academy of Pediatrics and National Initiative for Children's Healthcare Quality (2002). *Caring for children with ADHD: A resource toolkit for clinicians.* Elk Grove, IL. Accessed on from: http://www.nichq.org/NICHQ/Topics/ChronicConditions/ADHD/Tools/ADHD.htm on November 14, 2007.

American Psychiatric Association. *Diagnostic and Statistical Manual of Mental Disorders.*4th ed. Washington, DC: American Psychiatric Association; 1994.

American Academy of Child and Adolescent Psychiatry (1997). Practice parameters for the assessment and treatment of children, adolescents, adults with attention-deficit/hyperactivity disorder. *Journal of the American Academy of Child and Adolescent Psychiatry, 36,* 85–121.

American Academy of Pediatrics (2001). Clinical practice guideline: Diagnosis and evaluation of the child with attention-deficit/hyperactivity disorder. *Pediatrics, 105,* 1158–1170.

Angold, A., Costello, E. J., & Erkanli, A. (1999). Comorbidity. *Journal of Child Psychology and Psychiatry, 40,* 57–87.

Brown, R. T., Freeman, W. S., Perrin, J. M., Stein, M. T., Amler, R. W. et al. (2001a). Prevalence and assessment of attention-deficit/hyperactivity disorder in primary care settings. *Pediatrics, 107*(3), e43 – e54.

Brown T. E. (2001b). *Brown ADD Scales for Children and Adolescents.* San Antonio, TX: Psychological Corp.

Centers for Disease Control and Prevention (2007). ADHD: A public health perspective conference. Accessed from http://www.cdc.gov/ncbddd/adhd/dadphra.htm#social on November 5, 2007.

Conners, C. K. *Conners' rating scales—revised: Instruments for use with children and adolescents.* New York, NY: Multi-Health Systems, Inc; 1997

Division 53 of the American Psychological Association: Society of Clinical Child and Adolescent Psychology and the Network on Youth Mental Health (2007). Attention Deficit/Hyperactivity Disorder—Evidence-Based Treatment Options. Accessed from: www.wjh.harvard.edu/nock/Div53/EST/index_files/Page650.htm

DuPaul, G. J., Power, T. J., Anastopoulos, A. D., & Reid, R. (1998). *ADHD rating scale-IV: Checklists, norms, and clinical interpretation.* New York: Guilford.

Green, M., Wong, M., Atkins, D., et al. (1999). Diagnosis of Attention-Deficit/Hyperactivity Disorder: Technical Review 3, Agency for Health Care Policy and Research publication 99-0050, US Department of Health and Human Services, Agency for Health Care Policy and Research, Rockville, Md.

Hopkins, M., Herrerias, C. T., Stein, M., & Homer, C. (2001). ADHD: Variations in diagnostic practices in primary care physicians: A national survey. *Abstracts of Academic Health Services Research Health Policy Meeting, 18,* 20.

National Institutes of Mental Health (2007). The numbers count: mental disorders in America. Accessed November 5, 2007, from: http://www.nimh.nih.gov/health/publications/the-numbers-count-mental-disorders-in-america.shtml

Kessler, R. C., Berglund, P. A., Demler, O., Jin, R., & Walters, E. (2005). Lifetime prevalence and age-of-onset distributions of DSM-IV disorders in the National Comorbidity Survey Replication (NCS-R). *Archives of General Psychiatry, 62*(6), 593–602.

Kessler, R., Chiu, W., Demler, O., & Walters, E. (2005). Prevalence, severity, and comorbidity of twelve-month DSM-IV disorders in the National Comorbidity Survey Replication (NCS-R). *Archives of General Psychiatry, 62*(6), 617–627.

Lahey, B. B., Miller, T. L., Gordon, R. A., & Riley A. W. (1999). Developmental epidemiology of disruptive behavior disorders. In H. C. Quay & A. C. Hogan (Eds.). *Handbook of disruptive behavior disorders*. New York: Kluwer.

Pelham, W. E., Foster, E. M., & Robb, J. A. (2007). The economic impact of attention-deficit/hyperactivity disorder in children and adolescents. *Journal of Pediatric Psychology, 32*(6), 711–727.

Pelham, W. E., & Waschbusch, D. A. (2006). Attention-deficit hyperactivity disorder (ADHD). In J. E. Fisher & W. O'Donohue (Eds.). *Practitioner's guidelines for evidence based psychotherapy*. New York: Kluwer.

Scott-Levin Associates (2001). *Physician drug and diagnosis audit*. Newton, MA: Scott-Levin Associates.

Swanson, J. M., Kraemer, H. C., Hinshaw, S. P., et al. (2001). Clinical relevance of the primary findings of the MTA: Success rates based on severity of ADHD and ODD symptoms at the end of treatment. *Journal of the American Academy of Child and Adolescent Psychiatry, 40*, 168–179.

Woodard, R. (2006). The diagnosis and medical treatment of ADHD in children and adolescents in primary care: a practical guide. *Pediatric Nursing, 32*(4), 363–370.

Behavioral Health Consultation for Coronary Heart Disease

Richard P. Schobitz, Laura L. Bauer, and Erik P. Schobitz

Coronary heart disease, also called coronary artery disease, is the most common cause of heart attacks. There are a number of causes for coronary heart disease, and many of them are related to psychological factors and lifestyle habits. In this chapter, we will discuss the role of a behavioral health consultant in working to mediate the risk for coronary heart disease or to help treat those who have already developed this condition. We will begin with an overview of coronary heart disease. This will include a description of the disease, risk factors, methods of screening used by physicians, and terminology that a behavioral health consultant will likely hear when working with patients of coronary heart disease. This overview will not be comprehensive; instead it is meant to help behavioral health consultants to better understand coronary heart disease and improve their ability to effectively communicate in the primary care setting. The chapter will then focus on specific behavioral treatments that the behavioral health consultants may wish to employ in the primary care setting. Many checklists for screening, worksheets to use by patients or the primary care staff, and descriptions of treatment are available in this chapter. This chapter is intended to be practical in nature, and the reader is encouraged to reproduce and use the included worksheets for their practice.

What is Coronary Heart Disease?

Blood vessels that bring blood to the heart are called coronary arteries. Throughout one's life, a process called atherosclerosis, or hardening of these arteries, occurs. Atherosclerosis refers to the deposition of plaques in the arteries, most notably the coronary arteries. The plaques are comprised of cholesterol, fatty deposits, and other elements. Atherosclerosis has been demonstrated in children as young as 2 years old, where the plaque first appears as a fatty streak. The process continues throughout life, progressively narrowing the arteries, reducing the blood

R.P. Schobitz (✉)
Deputy Director, Behavior Medicine Division, Office of the Chief Medical Officer, TRICARE Management Activity
e-mail: Schobitz@hotmail.com

L.C. James, W.T. O'Donohue (eds.), *The Primary Care Toolkit*,
DOI 10.1007/978-0-387-78971-2_17, © Springer Science+Business Media, LLC 2009

flow to the heart. Less blood to the heart leads to less oxygen and nutrients reaching the heart muscle. This reduction in blood flow may cause mild to severe chest pain.

Over time, the artery can become completely blocked by plaque, cutting off the blood flow and delivery of oxygen. Most commonly, a heart attack is caused by the sudden occlusion (complete blockage) of the space within the vessel wall, called lumen, with platelets. This occurs when the atherosclerotic plaque develops a tear or fissure due to turbulent blood flow. After a portion of the plaque tears off, the newly exposed area attracts blood platelets and fibrin products in an attempt to heal itself. As the platelets accumulate, the vessel lumen is progressively compromised. When the artery becomes completely occluded, the heart is deprived of blood and oxygen. The muscle experiences ischemia, and may lead to infarction, or localized tissue death. This damage, when suffered by the heart, is termed myocardial infarction or a heart attack. If perfusion is not restored within 3–6 hours, cell damage is evidenced by the leaking of cardiac enzymes troponin, myoglobin, and creatinine kinase. These enzymes can be detected in the patient's blood, and are direct evidence of a myocardial infarction.

There are a number of risk factors for coronary heart disease, some of which can be controlled while others cannot. Risk factors out of the control of the patient include older age (older than 45 years for men and older than 65 years for women) and family history of coronary heart disease. There are, however, other risk factors that the patient can control through lifestyle change. These factors include high blood cholesterol, high blood pressure, cigarette smoking, complications related to diabetes, lack of physical activity, and being overweight or obese, which can be mitigated through lifestyle change. These changes may be difficult for the patient to achieve, and thus the assistance of a behavioral health consultant as part of the treatment team may improve the patient's chances of success with lifestyle change.

Working with the primary care provider and the patient to create and implement plans for change focused on the second controllable set of risk factors is where the behavioral health consultant can have a dramatic impact on care. The roles of the behavioral health consultant may vary depending on the provider and the clinic. One possibility is to serve as an educator to the primary care physician. While behavioral modification programming is a key component in the training for most behavioral health practitioners, it is likely that medical providers working in primary care have a limited background in the foundations of behavior modification. Another role is to become directly involved as part of the treatment team. In this role, the behavioral health consultant in collaboration with the patient works toward change that will mediate risk factors for coronary heart disease. This chapter is intended to assist behavioral health consultants in either role.

Screening for Coronary Heart Disease

In this section, we will turn our focus to the screening of risk factors for coronary heart disease in primary care. We will begin with a brief description of medical assessments that primary care providers may employ in their practice. The intent of this overview is to assist behavioral health consultants in understanding the process and outcomes of these assessments. Next, we will turn to effective behavioral health screening for coronary heart disease. The intent of this section is to provide behavioral health consultants with a tool to use in the primary care clinic that will identify potential areas where behavioral change may be effective. This will lead to treatment planning, which will be discussed later in this chapter.

Assessment Tools

A number of tools exist for primary care providers to employ in the evaluation of risk factors for coronary heart disease. The Diamond Forrester method was first published in 1979. This score considers age, sex, and quality of heart disease symptoms. The tool had some limitations, in that it was only useful in a symptomatic patient; therefore, it was not necessarily generalizeable to an asymptomatic patient (Diamond & Forrester, 1979). Another tool that primary care physicians utilize is Framingham risk assessment. This tool provides the primary care physician with a risk analysis of a coronary event in the next 10 years. Patients are stratified into low risk (<10%), intermediate risk (10–20%), and high risk (>20%) (Mora et al., 2005).

Ancillary Tests

Many labs and tests are available for providers to use in determining the risks of coronary disease. Current modalities include electrocardiogram (EKG), exercise treadmill testing (ETT), cardiac stress imaging, and electron-beam computerized tomography (EBCT). The EKG is useful in determining current ischemia as well as rhythm disturbances; however, the use of EKG in screening asymptomatic patients is not supported by the literature (Jumila & Runkle, 2006). Treadmill tests can identify severe coronary artery obstruction in up to 2.7% of screened samples; however, the majority of positive results will be false positives when the patient is a low-risk patient (Fowler-Brown, Pigone, & Pletcher, 2004). In asymptomatic patients, cardiac stress imaging is reserved for patients with an abnormal exercise treadmill test. The American Hart Association (AHA) recommends that asymptomatic patients felt to be at low risk for coronary heart disease after exercise treadmill test should not have further provocative testing performed (Jumilla and Runkle, 2006). For patients with moderate to high risk and an abnormal exercise treadmill test there may be a benefit to exercise myocardial perfusion studies (Mahenthiran, Bangalore, & Yao, 2005). Many of these tests are expensive or have high false positive rates, which may lead inappropriately to more invasive tests. The United States Preventive Services Task Force (2004) recommends against routine screening with ancillary tests for asymptomatic adults at low risk for severe coronary heart disease. For asymptomatic adults at high risk of coronary heart disease, the task force neither recommends for or against the routine use of EKG, ETT, or EBCT for either the determination of severe stenosis or the prediction of cardiac events (Jumila & Runkle, 2006). Given the current data and recommendations, risk identification and abatement appears to be a good strategy for the prevention of coronary heart disease in the otherwise asymptomatic patient.

Behavioral Health Assessment for Coronary Heart Disease

Initially, when working with patients on decreasing the risk factors for coronary heart disease, we complete a brief, focused intake. The goal of this intake is to take pertinent information to make sure that any psychiatric conditions that could impact treatment planning are identified, and to determine which risk factors the treatment plan should focus on. To determine this focus, it is important to identify both areas where change is needed and made possible through the interest and motivation of the patient. We take a team approach to treatment planning. Our patients are much more likely to work toward change when they have been intimately involved in the development of their change plans rather than dictating a plan to them. To accomplish this in the 30 minutes, we allow for an initial quick session of collecting as much of information as possible. A checklist of risk factors may help streamline the initial interview. This checklist is not only a tool for the interview but also the first step in the intervention. The checklist identifies risk factors that may be the focus of lifestyle change. Often these risk factors have been measured already by the primary care physician. Reviewing the risk factors often provides a teaching moment for the behavioral health consultant, especially around cholesterol levels.

Risk Factors for Heart Disease Checklist

Have you ever had a heart attack? YES NO

For men, are you older than 45? For women, are you older than 55? YES NO

Do you have a family history of heart disease? YES NO

Do you smoke? YES NO

How often do you exercise per week?_____

What do you do for exercise?

_____

Has your physician told you are overweight? YES NO

What is your total cholesterol level?

GOOD (less than 200) BORDERLINE (between 200 and 239) HIGH RISK (240 or more)

LDL cholesterol level?

GOOD (less than 130) BORDERLINE (between 130 and 159) HIGH RISK (160 or more)

HDL cholesterol level?

GOOD (60 or more) BORDERLINE (between 40 and 60) HIGH RISK (less than 40)

On a scale of 1–10 (10 being the most stressful), how stressful is your job?_____

On a scale of 1–10 (10 being the most stressful), how stressful is the rest of your life? _____

Do you consider yourself an angry person? YES NO

Do others consider you an angry person? YES NO

Consultation for Coronary Heart Disease

We will now turn to the role of the behavioral health consultant in working with coronary heart disease. One method of consultation is to provide behavioral modification training and materials to primary care staff. This is likely to be the broadest method of assistance and consultation and can be helpful in assisting staffs in understanding the basics of behavioral change. A second and more direct method of providing consultation would be to work directly with the primary care physician in order to prepare him or her to assist the patient with behavioral change. The references available at the end of this chapter may be helpful as you educate the physician on developing a behavioral plan. It will be important to educate the provider on the importance of follow-up and the need to check in with the patient on any planned 'homework' on each follow-up. The final method is for the behavioral health consultant to directly work with the patient as part of the health care team. In this role, the behavioral health consultant is active in assisting the patient to identify lifestyle habits that may be in need of change, focusing on areas the patient is interested and willing to work toward change, and developing a plan for change. A key task for the behavioral health consultant is to communicate the plan to the primary care physician.

Effective consultation and treatment of risk factors for coronary heart disease may involve interventions focused on reducing stress, reducing anger, increasing fitness, reducing weight, and smoking cessation. Brief interventions for each of these factors will be discussed now and tools for practice in a primary care setting will be provided. Obesity and smoking cessation are discussed elsewhere in this book, and will only be briefly discussed here. The reader is encouraged to refer to those chapters for greater details on interventions focused on mediating these risk factors for coronary heart disease.

Stress and anger have both been identified as factors that may increase the risk for coronary heart disease (Kawachi, Sparrow, Spiro, Vokonas, & Weiss, 1996). Brief cognitive behavioral techniques may be useful in the primary care setting in order to assist patients in controlling their levels of stress and anger. The first step in helping patients to reduce stress in their lives is to help them identify sources of stress in their lives. For many patients, the question "What are the sources of stress in your life?" will suffice. For others, it may be helpful to ask the patients to keep a simple diary of the events of their days and tracking the level of stress or anger each event has attached to it. The following is an example of such a diary that can be used as a handout in primary care.

Stress Diary

Day of the week:_____

Please list the three most important tasks that you have completed today. After each, please rate the level of stress associated with that task on a 1–10 scale. For this scale, 1 is the least stressful task you can imagine (e.g., taking a nap) and 10 is the most stressful (e.g., making life-altering decisions for you and your family).

Task 1:

_____
_____
_____
_____
_____

Levels of stress (1–10):_____

Task 2:

_____
_____
_____
_____

Levels of stress (1–10):_____

Task 3:

_____

_____

_____

_____

_____

Levels of stress (1–10):_____

Please make sure to bring this form in your follow-up appointment!

We use this type of log in two different ways in our primary care clinic. Responses to the log may help to target brief, solutions-focused interventions. For example, if a patient has identified a stressful or anger provoking activity in their life, it may be beneficial to challenge the patient to decide whether participation in that activity is worth the negative impact on their mood. If the task or activity is important, another possibility is to work with the patient to develop strategies for coping with the stress related to the activity. By helping the patient to identify that they are under stress as a result of certain tasks may allow for the development of ideas to reduce the stress around those activities. The 'ah ha' moment may appear in this brief session that will allow the patient to restructure their tasks in order to reduce stress. Many times, this is a major step in assisting patients to reduce stress and anger.

A second technique that may be useful in the primary care setting is to take the brief cognitive behavioral approach of investigating the cognitions or thoughts related to each activity that may have led the activity to be seen as stressful. For example, a patient mentions fighting traffic in order to make it to work on time as a stressful activity. The type of solution-focused intervention listed above may lead the behavioral health consultant to work with the patient to brainstorm on alternatives that would reduce the need to drive in traffic. Such ideas may include alternative routes or methods of transportation, leaving earlier, etc. A brief cognitive behavioral approach may be as simple as asking the patient to report what thoughts were going through their mind while in traffic, asking them to consider the rationality of such thoughts, and encouraging them to counter their thoughts with calmer thoughts.

The worksheet may help in asking patients to identify stressful or 'hot' thoughts and replace them with calmer or 'cool' thoughts. Getting the patient to practice the identification of stress- or anger-producing thoughts and replacing these thoughts with calmer thoughts is a key to developing this technique as an automatic process, which in turn reduces the distress the patient perceives. Encouraging daily practice is a key in this intervention. There are many other cognitive therapy techniques that may be useful in therapy, but in our primary care clinic we tend to prefer the simplest and least time-consuming of interventions to match the pace of the primary care setting.

Another intervention that we often use in our clinic to help patients control their level of stress is the teaching of relaxation exercises. There are a number of methods

Hot Thoughts / Cool Thoughts

Please complete this worksheet listing your stressful or HOT thoughts on the left side during the day. After identifying the HOT thought, please list one or more calming or COOL thoughts that may reduce the level of stress you are experiencing.

HOT Thoughts	COOL Thoughts

of relaxation that are described in the literature. When introducing relaxation as a stress management technique, our focus is on helping the patient to find the technique that will work for them. Often a patient will be able to recall different methods that help them relax, such as yoga, exercise, or even simply time alone. If the patient provides the strategy that will work for them then the follow-up questions we ask are: "Are you doing this relaxing activity?" "If not, what is getting in the way?" "How do you schedule relaxing time into your day?" "What can keep you away from relaxing, and how do we work around potential issues?" For patients with a preferred relaxation methods we take a behavioral approach and develop a plan for scheduling relaxation for the patient in a way that will work. Setting realistic goals is the key as early success tends to lead our patients to continue with any behavioral change program.

While some patients do have relaxation strategies that have worked for them in the past, others may be looking to the behavioral health consultant for relaxation training. There are a number of types of relaxation exercises that clinicians use in practice. The two that we rely on are diaphragmatic breathing and progressive muscle relaxation. Instruction worksheets are provided hereunder to use with your patients. In teaching relaxation to patients, the first step is to discuss the appropriate setting. Ideally the patient should practice in a comfortable room, dressed in loose clothing, and with limited distraction. The location and time for relaxation practice is built into the plan, and problem-solving around possible interruptions or distractions is included. During the introductory session of relaxation exercise, the patient may acknowledge that it is likely to be more challenging to relax in the clinic with the clinician present than it will be at home. The key is to develop a plan with the patient, identifying potential barriers to implementation and working around these barriers. We have included instructions on diaphragmatic breathing and progressive muscle relaxation that may be reproduced for patient use in your clinic.

Deep Breathing

A regular practice of relaxation exercises has been shown to decrease one's symptoms of stress. The following technique, diaphragmatic or deep breathing, is a simple yet effective way of increasing your level of relaxation.

Instructions

1. First create a calm environment by adjusting lighting, avoiding noise, wearing loose clothing, etc. Lie comfortably on your back. Many people prefer to do this exercise in bed, but any flat surface that is comfortable would do. Place one hand on your chest and the other on your abdomen, right beneath your rib cage.
2. Inhale slowly and deeply through your nose. Your goal is to breathe as deeply into your lungs as you can. You should feel your stomach push against your lower hand. The hand on your chest should move as little as possible.
3. Once you have inhaled, pause briefly. Next, exhale slowly through your nose and/or mouth.
4. At first, do ten full breaths making sure to keep a slow pace. Try not to rush. As you become more comfortable, increase the total amount of time to at least five minutes. Over time, breathing in this fashion will become easier and more automatic.

Progressive Muscle Relaxation

The first step in progressive muscle relaxation is to create a relaxing environment. Set time aside for your relaxation 'appointment,' reduce distractions, set room temperature and lighting to comfortable levels, and wear loose clothing. Lie down or sit in a comfortable position and close your eyes. As you begin progressive muscle relaxation, it is important to develop a passive attitude. It is difficult to relax if you are having anxiety provoking thoughts such as "I have to relax right now," or "I only have a few minutes and I need to focus on relaxing as fast as I can."

If these thoughts do come, simply acknowledge them as normal and okay, and let them go.

Now it is time to begin the progressive relaxation session. To do this you should simply tense and relax different muscle groups:

1. Toes: Curl your toes as tightly as you can for five seconds and then relax.
2. Feet: Bend your ankles toward your body as far as you can for five seconds and then relax.
3. Thighs: Tighten your thigh muscles by pressing your legs together as tightly as you can for five seconds and then relax.
4. Hips and buttocks: Tighten your hip and buttock muscles for five seconds and then relax.
5. Shoulders: Shrug your shoulders up to your ears for five seconds and then relax.
6. Upper arms: Bend your elbows. Tense your biceps for five seconds and then relax.
7. Hands: Extend your arms in front of you. Clench your fists tightly for five seconds then relax.
8. Back: Arch your back five seconds and then relax.
9. Stomach: Tighten your stomach muscles for five seconds and then relax.
10. Face: Wrinkle your forehead and close your eyes as tightly as you can and then relax.

Diet, Exercise, and Smoking

Tools for diet, exercise, and smoking have been covered extensively in other chapters of this book. Here, we will provide the readers with a brief overview of risk factors and treatments for coronary heart disease. One risk factor for coronary heart disease is elevated cholesterol, specifically elevated low-density lipoprotein (LDL) and decreased high-density lipoprotein (HDL). Lowering the level of LDL cholesterol will reduce the build-up of plaque in arteries. In order to do so, the patient will need to monitor his or her intake of foods high in cholesterol and saturated fat. Adding certain foods to the diet, especially those rich in soluble fiber, is another effective method for reducing LDL cholesterol. We work with patients to make specific goals for dietary change, and always ask the patient to keep a log or food diary when attempting to change. In session, we develop a plan and then ask the patient about potential barriers. We ask the patient to track any challenges that they face when attempting to make a change for discussion next session. This allows for problem-solving around the program. For many patients we also place a consult to a nutritionist who can provide important guidance and can create a plan specific to that individual.

In addition, we work with patients to increase exercise as exercise and diet both help to control weight which can place extra stress on the heart. We encourage the patient to talk with their primary care physician and the patient to develop and implement plans for change. The exercise we suggest are always specific to the patient. Suggesting a patient participate in a form of exercise that they will dislike reduces the chance that the patient will continue that exercise program for an extended time. Instead, we find it important to develop a realistic plan for change that is more likely to work for the patient and that includes a discussion of potential barriers and solutions to these barriers. We will briefly discuss our behavioral interventions to improve diet and exercise here and more information on these topics is located in the obesity chapter of this book.

Diet and exercise changes need to be closely coordinated with the primary care provider who may also consult with other specialties such as nutrition care. Many patients at risk for coronary artery disease will likely begin a supervised program at the treating hospital or health clinic. The behavioral health consultant can be a valuable part of the treatment team as the patient prepares to move their treatment to their home. Developing goals, identifying barriers, and making concrete plans for implementation are keys to the long-term success of the exercise program.

Aerobic exercises such as walking and biking help heart and other muscles. We develop an exercise plan with our patients that includes the types of aerobic exercise that they are most likely to continue. We work with the patient to choose the type of exercise, the frequency of exercise, and the duration in order to set the patient on the best path toward success. A key question we ask is "What is realistic for you?". We also always ask, "What could get in the way of you completing these exercises?" Planning for real-life barriers is a must in behavioral intervention programming, and it is an integral part of our treatment planning.

Many patients have limited experience with exercise programming; thus, it is very important to discuss the proper intensity of the exercise. An easy technique to determine if a patient is starting out with too high an intensity is the talk test. We encourage the patient to talk to themselves or others as they exercise. If the patient can converse while exercising, they are likely exercising at about the proper intensity. If the patient is too out of breath to talk in a comfortable manner, they are likely exercising at too high an intensity. Remember, the goal is long-term change. If a patient works out one time at so high an intensity that they are miserable, the chances of continuing the program are likely reduced. Of course, there are also physical risks inherent to overexertion as well. Other signs of overexertion include lightheadedness, dizziness, nausea, chest pain or pressure, pain in the arms, shoulder, jaw, or back, racing heart beat, difficulty catching breath, or extreme fatigue. It is important to remind the patient to watch for any of these signs and stop exercising if they occur.

In addition to developing an exercise program, dietary changes may also be needed in order to mediate the risk for coronary heart disease. Proper diet is discussed elsewhere in this book. Here, we will focus on three areas where the behavioral health consultant may wish to focus with respect to coronary heart disease: reducing fat, reducing sodium, and reading food labels.

Reducing the intake of fat, especially saturated fat, may help to lower the cholesterol levels. A lower fat diet may also help the patient to reduce weight, thus lower risk for heart disease. Some points we make with our patients include switching to low fat versions of the foods they like to eat, such as low fat dressings, mayonnaise, etc. We also suggest avoiding fried foods, eating low fat or fat-free dairy products, and choosing fish, white meat poultry or lean read meat. When cooking, we suggest the patient steam or broil their foods.

Two much sodium (salt) can also raise blood pressure in some people. We suggest the patient talk with their primary care provider about the need to reduce sodium intake, and a general goal for our patients is to limit sodium to 2400 milligrams maximum per day. In order to reduce the intake of salt, we suggest avoiding high salt meals and snacks, choosing fresh or unprocessed frozen foods, and using alternative spices such as lemon, garlic, pepper, etc. We also suggest that the patient to put the salt shaker away.

Choosing a low-fat, low-sodium diet is unlikely to be successful if the patient does not know how to read food labels. We keep a few food labels from actual products in our clinic in order to work with the patient to help them understand how to read the labels and make the best choices when shopping.

Finally, smoking is also a risk factor for coronary artery disease. By implementing the smoking cessation interventions described in the smoking cessation chapter of this book a patient reduces this risk.

The behavioral health consultant is an important part of the primary care treatment team. There are a number of areas that the consultant can make an impact in assisting patients in making health behavior changes. By partnering with the primary care provider and the patient, the behavioral health consultant can successfully implement the tools outlined in this chapter and elsewhere in this book to assist in making lifestyle changes that will reduce the risk for coronary heart disease.

Additional Resources

The American Heart Association; available at http://www.americanheart.org

- A great place to start. Resources on signs and symptoms of heart problems, healthy lifestyles, specific information for health care providers, information tailored for children, links to resources in your area, and a lot more.

Cardiology 101: Your one stop resource for the basics on heart disease and cardiology; available at http://heartdisease.about.com/cs/starthere/l/bl101.htm

- About.com's heart disease web page provides a nice glossary of terms that should be very helpful for anyone new to working with coronary heart disease. Other sections include the basics of heart disease, preventing heart disease, living with heart disease, and much more.

My Heart Central.Com; available at http://www.healthcentral.com/heart-disease

- Site includes information about lifestyle change, explanations of different medical treatments for heart disease, diagrams of the heart that may be useful in educating patients, links to other resources, and a lot more. Patients can also watch videos on heart disease at this site.

National Heart Lung and Blood Institute; available at http://www.nhlbi.nih.gov

- From the National Institutes of Health, a highlight of this website includes a section dedicated to health professionals. In this section, the behavioral health consultant can browse clinical practice guidelines, health information and publications, continuing education, and much more.

Heart Disease Guide, WebMD; available at http://www.webmd.com/heart-disease/guide/heart-disease-coronary-artery-disease

- This site may already be familiar to patients. Its question-and-answer format may be less overwhelming for some patients, and much of the information is bulleted, and pictures and diagrams are included.

References

Diamond, G., & Forrester J. (1979). Analysis of probability as an aid in the clinical diagnosis of Coronary Artery Disease. *NEJM*, 3000.

Fowler-Brown A., Pigone M., & Pletcher M. (2004). Exercise tolerance testing to screen for coronary heart disease; a systematic review for the technical support for the US Preventive Services Task Force. *Annals of Internal Medicine, 140*(4).

Kawachi, I., Sparrow, D., Spiro, A., Vokonas, P., & Weiss, S. (1996). The Normative Aging Study.*Circulation, 94.*

Jumila, J., & Runkle, G. (2006). Coronary Artery Disease Screening, Treatment, and Follow up. *Primary Care: Clinics in Office Practice, 33*(4).

Mahenthiran J., Bangalore S., & Yao S. (2005). Comparison of prognostic value of stress echocardiography in patients with suspected coronary artery disease.*American Journal of Cardiology, 96*(5).

Mora, S., Redberg, R. Sharrett, R., & Blumenthal, R. (2005). Enhanced risk assessment in asymptomatic individuals with exercise testing and framingham risk scores. *Circulation, 112,*

United States Preventive Services Task Force (2004). Screening for Coronary Heart Disease: Recommendation Statement. *Annals of Internal Medicine, 140*(7).

Smoking

Dianne Lavin

What is Nicotine Dependence?

Nicotine dependence is characterized by tolerance to nicotine and withdrawal symptoms when tobacco use is discontinued (American Psychiatric Association, 2000). Nicotine can be found in smokeless tobacco products, cigars, and cigarettes. Cigarette smoking is the focus of this chapter as it represents the most addictive and popular form of nicotine use. Smoking delivers nicotine to the brain within seconds; hence, dependence develops from rapid and frequent reinforcement. Over time, a smoker develops tolerance, finding it necessary to increase both the dose and frequency of nicotine use. Withdrawal symptoms include craving, dysphoria, irritability, anxiety, restlessness, impaired concentration, insomnia, craving for sweets, and weight gain (American Psychiatric Association, 2000).

Basic Facts About Cigarette Smoking

Cigarette smoking is the most preventable cause of morbidity and death in the United States. One in every five Americans dies annually as a result of cigarette smoking, representing approximately 438,000 deaths across the nation (CDC, 2002). Nearly 45.3 million adults smoke in the United States, and reportedly, these individuals will spend $88.8 billion dollars on tobacco products; $82 billion dollars will be spent on cigarettes alone, (CDC, 2007). As a known carcinogen, tobacco smoke increases the risk of dying from lung cancer by 23 times in men and by 13 times in women (US Department of Health and Human Services, 2004).

D. Lavin (✉)
Schofield Barracks Family Practice Clinic, Schofield Barracks, HI, USA
e-mail:ddlavin001@hawaii.rr.com

L.C. James, W.T. O'Donohue (eds.), *The Primary Care Toolkit*,
DOI 10.1007/978-0-387-78971-2_18, © Springer Science+Business Media, LLC 2009

Malignancies related to smoking arise in the lung, bladder, kidney, mouth, esophagus, pancreas, stomach, cervix, and blood (US Department of Health and Human Services, 2004). Moreover, tobacco use leads to stroke, coronary artery disease, and chronic obstructive lung disease.

Currently, 23% of high-school aged Americans smoke (CDC, 2006). Each day, 4000 teenagers initiate smoking, and 1140 young people become habitual smokers, most taking their first puff prior to the age of 14 (Substance Abuse and Mental Health Services Administration, 2005). Currently, 10% of high school males use smokeless tobacco products (CDC, 2005). Teens who use smokeless tobacco are more likely to develop a cigarette habit (US Department of Health and Human Services, 1994).

There is no risk-free level of exposure to secondhand smoke. Second-hand smoke increases the risk of heart disease by 25–30% and lung cancer by 20–30% (US Department of Health and Human Services, 2006). Secondhand smoke contains toxic substances; a number of these chemicals are known carcinogens (US Department of Health and Human Sciences, 2000). Women who smoke during pregnancy are twice as likely to develop complications, thus increasing the risk of delivering prematurely by 30% (CDC, 2007). Females who smoke are also more likely to deliver low-birth-weight infants, resulting in greater infant morbidity and death (CDC, 2007). Female smokers increase their risk of infertility by 30% (CDC, 2007). Sixty percent of children are exposed to second-hand smoke which predisposes them to develop respiratory infections, ear problems, and asthma (US Department of Health and Human Services, 2006). Infants who are exposed to secondhand smoke are at greater risk of dying from sudden infant death syndrome (US Department of Health and Human Services, 2006).

Screening for Smoking in the Primary Care Setting

It has been shown that clinicians often fail to address smoking cessation with their patients. Reportedly, only 15% of patients who smoke are offered assistance in order to quit their habit (Fiore et al., 2000) and only 3% receive follow-up care to address this problem (CDC, 2000). At the same time, 70% percent of current adult smokers have expressed a desire to quit this habit (CDC, 2002). In 2006, 44.2% (19.2 million) of adult smokers renounced their habit for at least one day, and 45.7 million adults were reported to be former smokers (CDC, 2006).

Cigarette smoking is the single most preventable cause of premature death and morbidity. Therefore it is critical that every primary care patient be screened for tobacco use, and candidates thus identified are counseled on tobacco cessation on a regular basis regardless of whether the patient has expressed a desire to quit. Evidence suggests a dose–response relationship exists between the number of times smoking cessation is addressed with a patient and the patient's abstinence from tobacco. Brief tobacco counseling for 3 minutes or less has also been shown to enhance abstinence rates (VA/DoD, 2004), and treatments which offer both behavioral counseling and pharmacologic treatment result in quit rates of 20–25% (Surgeon General's Report-Reducing Tobacco Use: Managing of Nicotine Addiction, 2000).

Moreover, collaborative tobacco cessation counseling involving multiple members of the primary health care team has been shown to increase abstinence rates (VA/DoD, 2004). The primary health care team includes often multiple providers, the physician or primary care provider (PCP), the behavioral health provider (BHP), nurses, pharmacists, and medical assistants. Potentially, the patient can receive a brief tobacco cessation message from each clinician. However, these efforts must be coordinated; hence the BHP is available for designing and implementing a system-wide, evidence-based smoking cessation program, staff training, consultation, referral, and provision of individual and group interventions in a primary health care setting.

The 5A's approach is the most well known and widely disseminated approach to identify and counsel patients on quitting a tobacco habit. The 5A's approach consists of *asking, advising, assessing, assisting, and arranging* treatment for tobacco use and dependence (Fiore et al., 2000).

- **Ask** – systematically identify tobacco users at every visit.
- **Advise** – strongly urge all tobacco users to quit.
- **Assess** – determine willingness to quit.
- **Assist** – aid the patient in quitting tobacco habit.
- **Arrange** follow-up contact with the patient.

Adapted from Fiore, M.C., Bailey, W.C., & Cohen S.J., et al., *Treating Tobacco Use and Dependence*. Quick Reference Guide for Clinicians, Rockville, MD: U.S. Department of Health and Human Services. Public Health Service. October 2000.

Asking each patient if they smoke or use tobacco at every visit

Asking involves identifying patients who use tobacco products by inquiring about their tobacco use. The patient is asked, "Do you smoke and do you want to quit?" Documentation can be included as an expansion of the patient's vital signs. Additionally, former smokers should be asked if they continue to be tobacco-free, offering them assistance as needed and recognizing their effort in maintaining abstinence. Previous attempts to quit should be recorded as well. Obtaining a smoking history will assist in determining the degree of tobacco addiction as well as obstacles to quitting the habit.

Vital signs:

BP: _____/_____ HR:_____ R:_____ T:_____

WT:_____ HT:_____ BMI:_____

Tobacco Use: Current _____

Past_____Never_____

Past
Quits:_____

Adapted from Fiore, M.C., Bailey, & W.C., Cohen, S.J., et al.,
Treating Tobacco Use and Dependence . Quick Reference
Guide for Clinicians. Rockville, MD: U.S. Department of
Health and Human Services. Public Health Service. October 2000.

Advise each smoker to quit this habit

The patient is then advised to quit smoking in a *clear*, *strong*, and *personalized* approach. The message may be brief but should be personalized to the client in order to make the message more relevant to the tobacco user. The patient is advised to quit smoking and counseled on the risks and costs of continuing to smoke.

- *Clear:* "I think it is important for you to quit now, and I can assist you."
- *Strong:* "Quitting is the most important thing you can do to protect your health."
- *Personalized:* Relate tobacco use to one's current and future health, impact on family and children, social and economic costs, and motivation and willingness to quit.

Adapted from Fiore, M.C., Bailey, W.C., & Cohen, S.J., et al., *Treating Tobacco Use and Dependence.* Quick Reference Guide for Clinicians. Rockville, MD: U.S. Department of Health and Human Services. Public Health Service. October 2000.

Assess each smoker to determine if they are willing to quit

During the assessment phase, the patient is asked: "How willing are you to quit now (i.e., the next 30 days)?" If the patient expresses a desire to quit, the patient is advised to set a quit date within the next month. If the patient indicates that he or she intends to quit in the near future, assistance to quit is initiated. For those patients who are unwilling to quit sometime during the next 6 months, a motivational intervention is used to encourage change. Lastly, for those patients who have quit, treatment consists of support and relapse prevention.

5-Stage Trans-theoretical Model of Behavior Change

- *Precontemplation:* The patient has no plan to quit their tobacco habit.
- *Contemplation:* The patient is thinking about quitting their tobacco habit within the next 6 months.
- *Preparation:* The patient is attempting change toward quitting their tobacco habit within the next 30 days.
- *Action:* The patient is working on quitting their tobacco habit.
- *Maintenance:* The patient is maintaining abstinence from tobacco use.

Prochaska, J. & DiClemente, C. (1983). Stages and process of self-change of smoking: toward an integrative model of change. Journal of Consulting and Clinical Psychology, 51(3), 390-95.

Enhancing patient's motivation to quit smoking

According to the 5-stage trans-theoretical model of behavior change (Prochaska & DiClemente, 1983), the process of change involves successfully navigating through a series of stages in order to implement permanent behavioral change. The model is often used to describe health-seeking behavioral change and is considered useful because interventions can be matched to the stage of change (Acton, Prochaska, Kaplan, Small, & Hall, 2001; Prochaska, DiClemente, & Norcross, 1992; Prochazka, 2000). The *Stages of Change* (Cancer Prevention Research Center, 1991) measure is a self-report tool designed to assess a patient's stage of change. The *Readiness-to-Change Ruler* provides another useful tool depicting the stages of change as well as the roles of both the patient and the provider.

Patients in the *precontemplation* stage are generally unwilling to quit their tobacco habit and do not see their habit as a problem. Appropriate interventions include education on the benefits of quitting and the health risks of continuing their smoking habit. Those patients *contemplating* change tend to be ambivalent about continuing their habit and their list of pros and cons for quitting or continuing to smoke are generally balanced. The 5R's Motivational Intervention (Fiore et al., 2000) is used to enhance the patient's ambivalence about his or her tobacco habit and to motivate the patient toward tobacco cessation.

The 5R's Motivational Intervention

- *Relevance:* Provider presents a personalized message on why quitting is relevant to the patient's health status, family, past quitting experience, and barriers to quitting.

- *Risks:* Patient asked to identify acute and long-term health risks and consequences of tobacco use related to self and others.
- *Rewards:* Patient asked to identify the benefits of discontinuing tobacco use, i.e., improvement in health, saving money, good feeling about self.
- *Roadblocks:* Patient asked to identify barriers to quitting, i.e., withdrawal symptoms, weight gain, and lack of support.
- *Repetition:* Repeat, repeat, and repeat at each and every visit.

Adapted from Fiore, M.C., Bailey, W.C., & Cohen, S.J., et al., *Treating Tobacco Use and Dependence.* Quick Reference Guide for Clinicians. Rockville, MD: U.S. Department of Health and Human Services. Public Health Service. October 2000.

The *Fagerstrom Test for Nicotine Dependence* (Heatherton, Kozlowski, Frecker, & Fagerstrom, 1991) is perhaps the most popular tool available to determine the level of one's tobacco dependence due to its brevity (six questions), easy scoring, and adequate psychometric properties. If the patient indicates that he or she is currently a tobacco user, the *Fagerstrom Test for Nicotine Dependence* can be incorporated into the assessment process, both as a measure of addiction and as a tool to foster ambivalence.

Fagerstrom Test for Nicotine Dependence

1. How soon after waking up do you smoke your first cigarette?
2. Do you find it difficult to refrain from smoking in places where it is forbidden?
3. Which cigarette would you hate most to give up?
4. How many cigarettes do you smoke per day?
5. Do you smoke more frequently during the first hours after waking up than during the rest of the day?
6. Do you smoke even if you are so ill that you stay in bed most of the day?

Adapted from Heatherton, T.F., Kozlowski, L.T., Frecker, R.C., & Fagerstrom, K.O., The Fagerstrom Test for Nicotine Dependence : a revision of the Fagerstrom Tolerance Questionnaire. British Journal of Addiction, 1991;86(9): 1119-1127.

Similar tools include the The Hooked on Nicotine Checklist (DiFranza, J. et al., 2002), a psychometrically sound, 10-item scale designed to measure tobacco dependence and lost autonomy over tobacco. The *Cigarette Dependence Scale* is a 12-item scale that provides a measure of tobacco dependence as well as loss of control, withdrawal, and compulsion to smoke (Etter, LeHouezec, & Perneger, 2003). The *Decisional Balance* (Cancer Prevention Research Center, 1991) measure provides an assessment of the balance between the pros and cons of continuing to smoke and the pros and cons of quitting. The *Self-Efficacy/Temptation scale* (Cancer Prevention Research Center, 1991) is a self-help tool that provides a measure of the patient's perceived ability to stop smoking and resist the temptation to relapse moreover, the scale can be used to identify more adaptive coping tools, enhancing the patient's ability to resist the urge to somke and boost self-efficacy. .

Assist the patient in quitting tobacco habit

For those patients preparing to quit setting a quit date and providing supportive counseling and strategies for quitting is appropriate. The quit date, ideally scheduled in two weeks, provides a target date and an interval of time during which the patient can prepare for cessation. One session of brief counseling (less than 3 minutes) has been shown to increase abstinence rates, which go up dramatically as the length and frequency of counseling increases (VA/DoD, 2004).

A *minimal counseling* intervention is generally focused on the practical aspects of cessation to include coping with urges, withdrawal symptoms, and medications. In general, minimal counseling involves one session of 3-minute duration (VA/DoD, 2004). A personal quit plan can be initiated and examples can be found on the internet. In general, a quit plan should include the quitting date, personal reasons for quitting, sources of social support and encouragement, routine changes, and coping strategies to avoid triggers and ride-out urges. The patient is asked to review and identify past attempts to quit noting successful strategies and factors that led to relapse. Self-help materials are an appropriate intervention at any stage of change. Self-help materials are not only time-efficient for clinicians but most importantly, reinforce tobacco-cessation counseling (VA/DoD, 2004). Moreover, the combination of self-help materials and advisement by a health provider appears to be more effective in motivating patients to quit smoking than does advisement from a health care provider alone (Janz et al., 1987). Numerous sources for self-help materials and tobacco cessation treatment modules can be found on the internet, available in the public domain. Additionally, depending on the needs of the patient population and the resources available, the patient can be referred to tobacco cessation programs in the community.

Intensive counseling has been shown to be more effective than brief interventions. Recommendations suggest that intensive counseling takes a total contact time greater than 30 minutes provided in four or more sessions, each lasting more than 10 minutes (Fiore et al., 2000). Intensive counseling is effective because of repeated contact and can be conducted via individual sessions, in groups, or proactive telephone programs (quit lines). Overall treatments should be adapted for special needs populations to include patients who are pregnant, adolescents, and those with comorbid diagnoses (VA/DoD, 2004), and should incorporate strategies aimed at preventing relapse. Moreover, the materials must be language-appropriate and culturally sensitive.

Pharmacotherapy has become a mainstay in tobacco cessation treatment, and it is recommended that all smokers who are attempting to quit who are actively working on cessation and for those maintaining cesstion be offered appropriate pharmacotherapy (Fiore et al., 2000). Exceptions to this recommendation include those individuals who are pregnantor breastfeeding, adolescents, those with medical comorbidities, or who smoke less than 10 cigarettes a day. First-line pharmacotherapy includes nicotine replacement therapy (NRT) and Wellbutrin (bupropion). NRT comes in a variety of formulations as shown in the following box.

First-line Pharmacotherapy for Smoking Cessation

> Wellbutrin, Zyban (bupropion)
> Nicotine gum
> Nicotine inhaler
> Nicotine nasal spray
> Nicotine patch

Second-line Pharmacotherapy for Smoking Cessation

> Clonidine
> Nortriptyline

Adapted from Fiore, M. C., Bailey, W. C., & Cohen, S. J., et al., *Treating Tobacco Use and Dependence*. Quick Reference Guide for Clinicians. Rockville, MD: US Department of Health and Human Services. Public Health Service, October 2000.

Arranging follow-up contact with patient to prevent relapse

The US Department of Health and Human Services (Fiore et al., 2000) recommends that the patient be contacted one week and then one month following the quit date either in person or by telephone contact. Particularly relevant to the patient is education and support in regard to withdrawal symptoms. Successful cessation should be appreciated; relapse should be approached as a learning experience and challenges and problems should be identified. If appropriate, the patient can be referred to more intensive treatment.

Effective Consultation and Liaison for this Problem

In the 'intermittent care strategy,' the patient receives services from the BHP and the PCP in turn (O'Donohue, Cummings, Cucciare, Runyan, & Cummings, 2006). Thus, the BHP counsels the patient in regard to cognitive and behavioral strategies to quit smoking and maintain abstinence, and the PCP is available to provide pharmacotherapy to assist with cessation. Through consultation with the PCP and members of the primary health care team, the patient's progress can be monitored and treatment modified as appropriate. As a case manager, the BHP ensures that all appropriate smoking cessation resources are readily available to the patient additionally, the BHP serves as a liaison to community health resources. Dialogue with the patient can occur by phone contact or during brief visits; the patient's fears and concerns as well as successes are reviewed, and the patient is offered support and assistance as needed to enhance and maintain cessation.

Links and Tools for Behavioral Health Providers

- Fact Sheets – Smoking: http://www.cdc.gov/nccdphp/publications/factsheets/Prevention/smoking.htm
- Fact Sheets – Tobacco/Smoking Cessation: http://www.cancer.gov
- Fagerstrom Test for Nicotine Dependence: http://ww2.heartandstroke.ca/DownloadDocs/PDF/Fagerstrom_Test.pdf
- No Butts About It...Tobacco Stinks!: http://www.ama-assn.org/ama/upload/mm/15/tobacco_module.pdf
- Rapid Estimate of Adult Literacy in Medicine, Revised (REALM-R): http://www.adultmeducation.com/index.html
- Readiness-to-Change Ruler: http://www.tobaccoteacher.com/readytoquit poster.pdf
- Smoking – Decisional Balance Measure (Cancer Prevention Research Center, 1991): http://www.uri.edu/research/cprc/Measures/Smoking07.htm
- Smoking – Self-Efficacy/Temptation Measure (Cancer Prevention Research Center, 1991): http://www.uri.edu/research/cprc/Measures/Smoking07.htm
- Smoking – Stages of Change Measure (Cancer Prevention Research Center, 1991): http://www.uri.edu/research/cprc/Measures/Smoking07.htm
- Standardized Measures for Youth Tobacco Users (National Cancer Institute Measures Guide for Youth Tobacco Research): http://dccps.nci.nih.gov/tcrb/guide_measures.html
- The Cigarette Dependence Scale: http://dccps.nci.nih.gov/tcrb/cds_5.html
- The Hooked on Nicotine Checklist: http://fmchapps.umassmed.edu/honc/TOC.htm

Self-Help Resources for Smokers Who Wish to Quit

- http://www.americanheart.org/presenter.jhtml? identifier=3048036: Cost of smoking calculator
- http://www.ashp.org/s_ashp/bin.asp?CID=2038&DID=6458&DOC=FILE.PDF: Smoking Cessation Educational Kit

- http://www.ashp.org: Decisional balance worksheet
- http://www.cdc.gov/tobacco/quit_smoking/index.htm: Support in quitting, a quit plan, educational materials, and referrals to local resources
- http://www.ffsonline.org: Freedom From Smoking®; online smoking cessation clinic
- http://www.helpguide.org/mental/quit_smoking_cessation.htm: Non-profit online site to assist with smoking cessation
- http://www.lungusa.org: Online tobacco cessation treatment module; Click on 'Quit' and then 'FFS online program'
- http://www.quitline.com: Washington State Department of Health, worksheet for a tobacco quit plan, 1-800-Quit-Now to speak with a quit coach
- http://www.smokefree.gov: Brochures for download, telephone contact, and support worldwide
- http://www.smokefree.gov/pubs/clearing_the_air.pdf: Clearing the Air: Quit Smoking Today booklet
- http://www.surgeongeneral.gov/tobacco/: Patient brochures for download
- http://www2.mdanderson.org/depts/aspire: Interactive activities and support materials to help teens reach their smoking cessation goal developed
- http://www.uri.edu/research/cprc/measures.htm#Smoking: Smoking assessment measures

Referral and Stepped Care for Special Populations of Smokers

Certain populations such as those with mood, anxiety, and substance abuse disorders may present particular challenges to the primary care team, requiring referrals to specialty care or implementing more intensive treatment along the continuum of stepped care. Nicotine dependence, for example, is more common among those with mood, anxiety, and other mental disorders (APA, 2000; Grant, Hasin, Chou, Stinson, & Dawson, 2004), and major depression is associated with the progression of occasional smoking to daily smoking (Breslau et al., 1998). Escalating symptoms of depression during cessation may trigger relapse (Burgess et al., 2002). Alcohol use and smoking are often linked (Dierker, Avenevoli, Stolar, & Merikangas, 2002); therefore, treating substance use and depression prior to addressing tobacco use may be more appropriate. The BHP can address barriers to treatment progress and determine if more intensive therapies are appropriate, making referrals to external providers and agencies as needed.

The design and implementation of maternal smoking cessation interventions could be enhanced with (1) integration and communication between women's health care providers and services and (2) addressing the relationship between lower maternal education and smoking, depression, alcohol use, modifying the behavior of other smokers in the household, and making nicotine replacement more available during pregnancy and early parenthood (Kahn, Certain, & Whitaker, 2002). Weight concerns have been recognized as a major obstacle in tobacco cessation, particularly among women (Cooper, Dundon, Hoffman, & Stoever, 2005; Clark, et al., 2004). Weight-concerned female smokers appear to have a distorted view of smoking as a means of weight management (White, McKee, and O'Malley, 2007). Cognitive behavioral treatment to address dysfunctional beliefs regarding eating, body shape, and weight has been shown to be more effective than treatment focusing on dieting and weight loss (Levine, Marcus, & Perkins, 2003; Perkins, Conklin, & Levine, 2008; Perkins, et al., 2001). Additionally, dieting during cessation has been shown to be counterproductive; rather, weight loss should not take place until the patient has maintained tobacco abstinence for at least 6 months or, preferably, 1 year (Perkins, Conklin, & Levine, M., 2008). Referrals for nutritional counseling can provide strategies for healthy calories, snacking, and fluid and fiber intake. Additionally, exercise combined with NRT may delay weight gain and increase functional exercise capacity during cessation (Prapavessis, et al., 2007).

References

Acton, G. S., Prochaska, J., Kaplan, A., Small, T., & Hall, S. (2001). Depression and stages of change for smoking in psychiatric outpatients. *Addictive Behaviors, 26*, 621–631.

American Psychiatric Association (2000). *Diagnostic and Statistical Manual of Mental Disorders*, (4th ed., Text Revision). Washington, DC: American Psychiatric Association.

Boardman, T., Catley, D., Mayo, M., & Ahluwalia, J. (2006). Self-efficacy and motivation to quit during participation in a smoking cessation program. *International Journal of Behavioral Medicine, 12*(4), 266–272.

Breslau, N., Peterson, E., Schultz, L, Chilcoat, H., & Andreski, P. (1998). Major depression and stages of smoking. *Archives of General Psychiatry, 55*, 161–166.

Burgess, E. S., Brown, R. A., Kahler, C. W., Niaura, R., Abrams, D. B., Goldstein, M. G., et al. (2002). Patterns of change in depressive symptoms during smoking cessation: who's at risk for relapse? *Journal of Consulting & Clinical Psychology, 70*(2), 56–61.

Centers for Disease Control and Prevention (2002a). Annual Smoking-Attributable Mortality, Years of Potential Life Lost, and Productivity Losses-United States, 1997-2001. *Morbidity and Mortality Weekly Report, 51*(14), 300–303.

Centers for Disease Control and Prevention (2007). *Economic Facts about US Tobacco Use and Tobacco Production Fact Sheet*, http://www.cdc.gov/tobacco/data_statistics/Factsheets/economic_facts.htm

Centers for Disease Control and Prevention (2007). *Preventing Smoking and Exposure to Second-hand Smoke Before, During, and After Pregnancy*. National Center for Chronic Disease Prevention and Health Promotion.

Centers for Disease Control and Prevention (2002b). Cigarette Smoking Among Adults—United States, 2000. *Morbidity and Mortality Weekly Report, 51*(29), 642–645.

Centers for Disease Control and Prevention (2006). Cigarette Smoking Among Adults—United States, 2006. *Morbidity and Mortality Weekly Report, 56*(44), 157–1161.

Centers for Disease Control and Prevention (2006). Cigarette Use Among High School Students-United States, 1991– 2005. *Morbidity and Mortality Weekly Report, 55*(26), 724–726.

Centers for Disease Control and Prevention (2005). Tobacco Use, Access, and Exposure to Tobacco in Media Among Middle and High School Students—United States, 2004. *Morbidity and Mortality Weekly Report, 4*(12): 297–301.

Clark, M., Decker, P., Offord, K., Patten, C., Vickers, K., Croghan, I., et al. (2004). Weight concerns among male smokers. *Addictive Behaviors, 29*, 1637–1641.

Cooper, T., Dundon, M., Hoffman, B., & Stoever, C. (2005). General and smoking cessation related weight concerns in veterans. *Addictive Behaviors, 31*, 722–725.

Dent, L. A., Harris, K. J., & Noonan, C. W. (2007). Tobacco interventions delivered by pharmacists: a summary and systematic review. *Pharmacotherapy, 27*(7):1040–51.

Dierker, L., Avenevoli, S., Stolar, M., & Merikangas, K. R. (2002). Smoking and depression: An examination of mechanisms of comorbidity. *American Journal of Psychiatry, 159*, 947–953.

DiFranza, J. R., Savageau, J. A., Fletcher, K., Ockene, J. K., Rigotti, N. A., McNeill, A. D., et al. (2002). Measuring the loss of autonomy over nicotine use in adolescents. *Archives of Pediatric and Adolescent Medicine, 156*, 397–403.

Etter, J. F., LeHouezec, J., & Perneger, T. V. (2003). A self-administered questionnaire to measure addiction to cigarettes: the cigarette dependence scale. *Neuropsychopharmacology, 28*(2), 359–370.

Fiore, M. C., Bailey, W. C. , Cohen, S. J., et al. (2000). *Treating tobacco use and dependence. Quick reference guide for clinicians.* Rockville, MD: US Department of Health and Human Services. Public Health Service. October 2000. Available at: http://www.surgeongeneral.gov/tobacco/clinpack.html.

Grant, B., Hasin, D., Chou, S., Stinson, F., & Dawson, D. (2004). Nicotine dependence and psychiatric disorders in the united states. *Archives of General Psychiatry, 61*, 1107–1115.

Heatherton, T. F., Kozlowski, L. T., Frecker, R. C., & Fagerstrom, K. O. (1991). The fagerstrom test for nicotine dependence : a revision of the fagerstrom tolerance questionnaire. *British Journal of Addictions, 86*(9), 1119– 1127.

Janz, N., Becker, M., Kirscht, J., Eraker, S., Billi, J., & Woolliscroft, J. (1987). Evaluation of a minimal-contact smoking cessation intervention in an outpatient setting. *American Journal of Public Health, 77*, 805–809.

Kahn, R., Certain, L., & Whitaker, R. (2002). A reexamination of smoking before, during, and after pregnancy. *American Journal of Public Health, 92*(11), 1801– 1808.

LeFoll, B. & George, T. (2007). Treatment of tobacco dependence: integrating recent progress into practice. *Canadian Medical Association Journal, 177*(11), 1373– 1380.

Levine, M., Marcus, M., & Perkins, K. (2003). Women, weight, and smoking: a cognitive behavioral approach to women's concerns about weight gain following smoking cessation. *Cognitive and Behavioral Practice, 10*, 105–111.

O'Donohue, W., Cummings, N., Cucciare, M., Runyan, C., & Cummings, J. (2006). *Integrated Behavioral Health Care: a guide to effective intervention.* Amherst, New York: Humanity Books.

Perkins, K., Conklin, C., & Levine, M. (2008). *Cognitive-behavioral therapy for smoking cessation: a practical guidebook to the most effective treatments.* New York: Taylor & Francis Group, LLC.

Perkins, K., Marcus, M., Levine, M., D'Amico, D., Miller, A. Broge, M., et al. (2001). Cognitive-behavioral therapy to reduce weight concerns improves smoking cessation outcome in weight-concerned women. *Journal of Consulting and Clinical Psychology, 69*(4), 604–613

Prapavessis, H., Cameron, L., Baldi, J. C., Robinson, S., Borrie, K., Harper, T., et al. (2007). The effects of exercise and nicotine replacement therapy on smoking rates in women. *Addictive Behaviors, 32*(7), 1416–1432.

Prochaska, J. (1981) Self-efficacy and smoking cessation maintenance: A preliminary report. *Cognitive Therapy and Research, 5*(2), 175–187

Prochaska, J., & DiClemente, C. (1983). Stages and process of self-change of smoking: toward an integrative model of change. *Journal of Consulting and Clinical Psychology, 51*(3), 390–95.

Prochaska, J., DiClemente, C., & Norcross, J. (1992). In search of how people change: applications to addictive behaviors. *American Psychologist, 47*(9), 1101–1114.

Prochazka, A. (2000). New developments in smoking cessation. *Chest, 117*, 169–175.

Shadel, W. G., & Cervone, D. (2006). Evaluating social-cognitive mechanisms that regulate self-efficacy in response to provocative smoking cues: an experimental investigation. *Psychology of Addictive Behaviors, 20*(1), 91–96.

Shiffman, S., West R. J., & Gilbert, D. G.(2004). Recommendation for the assessment of tobacco craving and withdrawal in smoking cessation trials. *Nicotine & Tobacco Research, 6*(4), 599–614.

Sheahan, S., & Free, T. (2005). Counseling parents to quit smoking. *Pediatric Nursing, 31*(2), 98–109.

Substance Abuse and Mental Health Services Administration. (2005). *Results From the 2005 National Survey on Drug Use and Health.*, NSDUH Series H-27, DHHS Publication No. SMA 05–4061, Rockville, MD: Office of Applied Studies.

Tonstad, S., Tonnesen, P., Hajek, P., Williams, K., Billing, C., & Reeves, K. (2006). Effect of maintenance therapy with varenicline on smoking cessation. *Journal of the American Medical Association, 296*(1), 64–71.

US Department of Health and Human Services (2005). 11th report on carcinogens. *National Toxicology Program,* http://ntp.niehs.nih.gov/ntp/roc/eleventh/profiles/s176toba.pdf.

US Department of Health and Human Services (1994). *Preventing Tobacco Use Among Young People: A Report of the Surgeon General.* Atlanta, GA: US Department of Health and Human Services, Public Health Service, Centers for Disease Control and Prevention, National Center for Chronic Disease Prevention and Health Promotion, Office on Smoking and Health.

US Department of Health and Human Services (2000). *Reducing Tobacco Use: A Report of the Surgeon General.* Atlanta, Georgia: US Department of Health and Human Services, Centers for Disease Control and Prevention, National Center for Chronic Disease Prevention and Health Promotion, Office on Smoking and Health.

US Department of Health and Human Services (2004). *The Health Consequences of Smoking: A Report of the Surgeon General.* Atlanta, Georgia: US Department of Health and Human Services, Centers for Disease Control and Prevention, National Center for Chronic Disease Prevention and Health Promotion, Office on Smoking and Health, 2004.

US Department of Health and Human Services (2006). *The Health Consequences of Involuntary Exposure to Tobacco Smoke: A Report of the Surgeon General.* Atlanta, Georgia: US Department of Health and Human Services, Centers for Disease Control and Prevention, Coordinating Center for Health Promotion, National Center for Chronic Disease Prevention and Health Promotion, Office on Smoking and Health.

Velicer, W. F, Prochaska, J. O., Fava, J. L., Norman, G. J., & Redding, C. A. (1998) Smoking cessation and stress management: Applications of the transtheoretical Model of behavior change. *Homeostasis, 38,* 216–233. (Cancer Prevention Research Center, Detailed Overview of the Transtheoretical Model, http://www.uri.edu/research/cprc/TTM/detailedoverview.htm).

Veterans Administration, Department of Defense (2004). *VA/DoD clinical practice guideline for the management of tobacco use.* Washington (DC): Department of Veteran Affairs.

White, M., McKee, S., & O'Malley, S. (2007). Smoke and mirrors: magnified beliefs that cigarette smoking suppresses weight. *Addictive Behaviors, 32*(10): 2200–2210

Pediatric Obesity

Brie A. Moore and Amanda Drews

Clinical Definition

Body mass index (BMI; weight in kilograms divided by the square of the height in meters) is the most common measure of weight status, and is considered a reliable indicator of body fatness for most children and teens (Center for Disease Control and Prevention, 2007). Overweight children are commonly defined as those aged between 2 and 20 years with a BMI value greater than the 95th percentile for their age and sex (Center for Disease Control and Prevention, 2007). Children with a BMI value falling between the 85th and 95th percentiles for their age and sex are characterized as 'at-risk for overweight' (Center for Disease Control and Prevention, 2007).

Epidemiology

A few decades ago, childhood obesity was a rare condition. In the 1960s, one in every 24 children aged 6–11 years was overweight (National Center for Health Statistics, 2002). With the exception of few early researchers (e.g., Bacon & Lowrey, 1967), the treatment of pediatric obesity has also historically received little professional attention. Currently, because of the availability and widespread use of energy-dense foods and increasingly sedentary lifestyles, the prevalence of childhood obesity in the United States continues to rise at an alarming rate (Horgen & Brownell, 2002). Over the last 30 years, the percentage of overweight children has more than tripled (National Center for Health Statistics, 2002). In the United States, an estimated 19% children aged 6–11 years are classified as overweight (Ogden et al., 2006). Childhood obesity affects both sexesand in children of all ages, with Mexican-American, African-American, and Native American children particularly at risk (Dietz, 2004).

B.A. Moore (✉)
CareIntegra, Inc., University of Nevada, Reno, NV, USA
e-mail: brieamoore@yahoo.com

L.C. James, W.T. O'Donohue (eds.), *The Primary Care Toolkit*,
DOI 10.1007/978-0-387-78971-2_19, © Springer Science+Business Media, LLC 2009

Comorbidity

Physical Comorbidities and Developmental Trends

Childhood obesity is associated with significant health problems, and is an important early risk factor for both child and adult morbidity and early mortality. Children who are inactive and overweight are more likely to have high blood pressure,
abnormal insulin and cholesterol concentrations, and more abnormal lipid profiles.
In some populations, children with obesity now account for as much as 50% of type
2 diabetes mellitus, a metabolic disorder related to obesity and sedentary lifestyles
and historically rare in children (Fagot-Campagna et al., 2000). These changes
increase the risk of early disability and death from heart disease, kidney disease,
and other organ damage (Young-Hyman et al., 2001). Other important complications include asthma and sleep apnea, skeletal and joint problems, liver disease, and
gastrointestinal complications. A recent population-based cohort study with 276,835
children found that higher childhood BMI values are associated with an elevated risk
of coronary heart disease in adulthood, with this risk increasing as children grow
older (Baker, Olsen, & Sorensen, 2007).

Psychological Comorbidities

The psychological stress of social stigmatization imposed on overweight children
may be as damaging as medical morbidities. Comorbidities may include poor self-
esteem, body image disturbances, depression, social isolation, difficulty with peer
relationships, and poor academic achievement (Ebbeling, 2002). Childhood obesity
poses an unprecedented burden in terms of children's physical and psychological
health and future healthcare costs.

Patient Fact Sheets and Handouts

- The Surgeon General's Call to Action to Prevent and Decrease Overweight
  and Obesity: Overweight in Children and Adolescents; available at http://www.
  surgeongeneral.gov/topics/obesity/calltoaction/factsheet06.pdf

  ○ Feeding Your Toddler
  ○ Encouraging a Healthy Weight for Your Child
  ○ Eating and Exercising: What Works for You?

- NICHQ Healthy Care for Healthy Kids Toolkit – Family Information Tools;
  available at http://www.nichq.org/NICHQ/Topics/PreventiveCare/Obesity/Tools/
  familyinformation.htm

  ○ Parenting Tips

- Jump Up & Go!
  - Nutrition Tips
  - Family Friendly Recipes
  - Activity Tips
  - Go Walking Tips
  - Resources

○ Patient Education Tools

- Serving Portion by Age and Gender
- Drink Comparison Handout
- Food Portions Exercise

Tools for Providers

- NICHQ Healthy Care for Healthy Kids Office Tools; available at http://www.nichq.org/NICHQ/Topics/PreventiveCare/Obesity/Tools/managementandtreatmentoffice.htm

  ○ Encounter Documentation Tool
  ○ Patient Registry
  ○ Coding and Fact Sheet for Primary Care Pediatricians
  ○ Pediatric Coding Companion
  ○ Levels of Billing: Coding and Reimbursement for Children with Abnormal Weight Gain in Primary Care

- NICHQ Healthy Care for Healthy Kids Assessment and Diagnosis Tools; available athttp://www.nichq.org/NICHQ/Topics/PreventiveCare/Obesity/Tools/HCHKAssesmentanddiagnosis.htm

  ○ Body Mass Index Charts for Boys and Girls of Age 2–20 years
  ○ Algorithm for Approach for Prevention & Management of Overweight Children 2 to12 Years Old Blood Pressure Levels for the 90th and 95th Percentiles of Blood Pressure for Boys and Girls of Age 1 17 Years

Clinical Assessment Tools

The development of effective prevention and intervention strategies for childhood obesity will require a robust appreciation for biological, genetic, psychological, sociocultural, and environmental factors that are important to the etiology of this chronic condition (American Academy of Pediatrics, 2003). A necessary intervening step between understanding the etiology of childhood obesity and the treatment of it, however, is a thorough and multifaceted assessment. The following domains should be included in a comprehensive primary care assessment.

Body Mass Index

The measurement of BMI, a ratio of height to weight, represents the first critical step to the assessment and treatment of childhood obesity. The American Academy of Pediatrics, in their 2003 policy statement, endorsed "[r]outine assessments. . .of excessive weight relative to linear growth. . ." throughout childhood (p. 426). This position, reaffirmed by the Academy in 2006, and subsequently used to inform the expert recommendations of the NICHQ Childhood Obesity Action Network in 2007, that BMI should be calculated *and plotted on pediatric growth charts* at well-child visits and tracked for significant change over time for all children aged 2–18 years. Pediatric growth charts are readily available online at http://www.cdc.gov/nchs/about/major/nhanes/growthcharts/charts.htm. Together with calculating children's BMIs, plotting the indices allows pediatric practitioners to determine whether pediatric patients fall within the 'normal weight,' 'at-risk for overweight,' or 'overweight' category. The term 'overweight' is applied when the BMI of a child exceeds the 95th percentile for their age and sex. The 'at-risk for overweight' descriptor is applied for a child falling between the 85th and 95th percentiles for their age and sex (Center for Disease Control and Prevention; CDC, 2007). Perrin, Finkle, and Bejamin (2006) recommend plotting BMI on color-coded charts. They offer that the technique flags a child's risk for both the pediatrician and the parent in a clear stoplight coding assigned to normal weight (green), at risk (yellow), and overweight (red) as in the familiar asthma action plan.

Familiarity with the above guidelines, however, does not guarantee that pediatric staff will consistently calculate and plot pediatric BMI. Recently, Larsen, Mandleco, Williams, and Tiedeman (2006) reported that nurse practitioners working in family practice or general pediatric settings, despite being aware of childhood obesity prevention guidelines, were not consistently using the BMI-for-age index to screen for child obesity. Thus, pediatric care settings are charged with the task of ensuring that staff is not only aware of obesity practice guidelines but also that they are routinely and appropriately implemented. This is particularly important given the recent and increasing evidence that parents and clinicians do not consistently and accurately identify their overweight children (or patients) as being overweight (e.g., Carnell, Edwards, Croker, Boniface, & Wardle, 2005; He & Evans, 2007; Spurrier, Magarey, & Wong, 2006).

Family History

A thorough family history is also important to a comprehensive assessment of pediatric obesity. In particular, it is recommended that pediatric practitioners assess the presence of obesity in the child's first degree relatives as well as any history of cardiovascular disease, type 2 diabetes, and/or cancer in first- or second-degree relatives (Deitz & Robinson, 2005).

Focused Review of Systems

As part of routine physical examination and review of systems, pediatricians are encouraged to assess for potential complications of overweight in a deliberate and targeted manner. In Table 1, the signs and symptoms of conditions associated with obesity are summarized. Attention to these potential conditions is warranted as part of the review of systems for at-risk and overweight youngsters.

Diet

The fourth crucial component of a comprehensive obesity assessment is a detailed dietary history. Deitz and Robinson (2005) encourage pediatric practitioners to inquire about caretakers who feed their pediatric patients as well as about foods in the patients' diets that are high in calories and low in nutritional value that can be reduced, eliminated, or replaced. Additionally, they recommend that practitioners assess children's eating patterns, including the timing, content, and location of meals and snacks. Likewise, information regarding the family climate surrounding meals and eating should be gathered. This is particularly important in light of emerging evidence that parental behaviors, specifically over-controlling and rejecting behavior, may contribute to overweight in children. Paternal behaviors perceived by children as rejecting, the use of controlling discipline styles, verbal prompting to eat at mealtime, attentiveness to non-eating behavior, and close

Table 1 Symptoms and signs of conditions associated with obesity

Symptoms	Signs
Anxiety, school avoidance, social isolation (depression)	**Poor linear growth** (hypothyroidism, Cushing's syndrome, Prader-Willi syndrome)
Polyuria, polydipsia, weight loss (type 2 diabetes mellitus)	**Dysmorphic features** (genetic disorders, including Prader-Willi syndrome)
Headaches (pseudotumor cerebri)	**Acanthosis nigricans** (NIDDM, insulin resistance)
Night breathing difficulties (sleep apnea, hypoventilation syndrome, asthma)	**Hirsutism and excessive acne** (polycystic ovary syndrome)
Daytime sleepiness (sleep apnea, hypoventilation syndrome, depression)	**Violaceous striae** (Cushing's syndrome)
Abdominal pain (gastroesophageal reflux, gall bladder disease, constipation)	**Papilledema, cranial nerve VI paralysis** (pseudotumor cerebri)
Hip or knee pain (slipped capital femoral epiphysis)	**Tonsillar hypertrophy** (sleep apnea)
Oligomenorrhea or amenorrhea (polycystic ovary syndrome)	**Abdominal tenderness** (gall bladder disease, GERD, non-alcoholic fatty liver disease (NAFLD))
	Hepatomegaly (NAFLD)
	Undescended testicle (Prader-Willi syndrome)
	Limited hip range of motion (slipped capital femoral epiphysis)
	Lower leg bowing (Blount's disease)

Source: NICHQ Childhood Obesity Action Network Expert Recommendations

parental monitoring may decrease children's ability to self-regulate energy intake and, therefore, their ability to maintain or lose weight (e.g., Arredondo et al., 2006; Klesges, Stein, Eck, Isbell, & Klesges, 1991; Stein, Epstein, Raynor, Kilanowski, & Paluch, 2005).

Obtaining detailed information regarding contextual variables (i.e., caretakers, type of food, and timing and location of meals and snacks) relevant to a child's eating can directly reflect the type of preventive health information provided to parents and caretakers. Ellyn Satter, an internationally known expert on feeding and eating, developed the 'division of responsibility in feeding' paradigm (Satter, 2007) that addresses parents' and children's roles in managing the variables involved in the feeding process. She asserts that parents are responsible for the *what, when,* and *where* of eating while children are responsible for *how much* and *whether*.

More specifically, Satter identifies parents' feeding jobs as:

- choosing and preparing the food
- providing regular, scheduled meals and snacks
- making eating times pleasant
- showing children what they have to learn about food and mealtime behavior
- not letting children graze for food or beverages between meal and snack times
- letting children grow up to get a physique that is right for them

Children, on the other hand, do the job of eating. This includes:

- eating the amount of food they need
- learning to eat the foods their parents eat
- growing predictably
- learning to behave well at the table

To the extent that pediatric practitioners are able to obtain detailed information about children's diets and contextual variables surrounding meal and snack times, their ability to provide helpful, preventive information that could increase the probability that children are able to self-regulate their energy intake and, thereby, maintain a healthy weight is greatly enhanced.

Activity Level

The Surgeon General's Call to Action to Prevent and Decrease Overweight and Obesity recommends that children accumulate at least 60 minutes of moderate physical activity most days of the week and reduce the amount of time spent on sedentary activities like watching television or playing video games to less than 2 hours per day (USDHHS, 2007). In accordance with these guidelines, pediatric practitioners are encouraged to inquire about children's activity level as part of their comprehensive obesity assessment. Deitz and Robinson (2005) recommend that specific attention be paid to the following:

- barriers to walking or riding a bike to school
- total time spent at play

- frequency, duration, and intensity of activity during school recess and physical education
- participation in active after-school and weekend activities
- total screen time (television, videotapes and DVDs, and video games) per day

Laboratory Testing

Guidelines for the laboratory portion of a comprehensive pediatric obesity assessment have been put forth by numerous experts; these vary slightly with regard to the criteria pediatricians might use as indicators for the specific tests. A fasting profile of lipoprotein, insulin, and glucose levels, for example, has been recommended by some experts for all overweight children (e.g., Barlow & Deitz, 1998). More recently, the NICHQ Childhood Obesity Action Network's expert committee recommended the following laboratory testing guidelines:

- For BMI 85–94 percentile *without* risk factors

  o Fasting lipid profile

- For BMI 85–94 percentile at age 10 years and older *with* risk factors

  o Fasting lipid profile
  o ALT and AST
  o Fasting glucose

- For BMI ≥ 95 percentile at age 10 years and older

  o Fasting lipid profile
  o ALT and AST
  o Fasting glucose
  o Other tests as indicated by health risks

Risk factors present in children of age 10 years and older with a BMI between 85 and 94 percentiles include a history of type 2 diabetes in a first- or second-degree relative, non-White race, and/or conditions associated with insulin resistance, such as acanthosis nigricans, hypertension, dyslipidemias, or polycystic ovary syndrome.

Psychosocial Adjustment

For at-risk and overweight children, it may be prudent to include an assessment of current psychosocial and emotional functioning as part of routine care. Although the literature is somewhat mixed, there have been numerous reports of higher rates of psychopathology among overweight children, particularly those that are seeking treatment for overweight as compared to normal weight children. Overweight youngsters have been described as having lower self-esteem and greater difficulties with depression, anxiety, impulse control, and perceived cognitive and athletic inability (Braet & van Strien, 1997; Britz, Siegfried, Ziegler, & Lamertz, 2000; Epstein, Klein, & Wisniewski, 1994; Erermis et al., 2004; Friedman & Brownell, 1995; McElroy et al., 2004) as compared to their normal weight peers. Although more research in this area is sorely needed, addressing comorbid psychiatric and behavioral issues may prove effective in diminishing resistance, enhancing short- and long-term treatment efficacy, and improving the quality of life for overweight pediatric patients.

Parental Readiness to Change

Parental readiness to change has also been suggested as a potentially important aspect of pediatricians' assessment and prevention of pediatric overweight. Perrin et al. (2006) recommended the inclusion of a question (like the following) in the intake survey to be completed by parents in the pediatric waiting room:

How do you feel about making some changes to help your child eat healthy or be active?

– I am *not* interested in making changes at this time.
– I am *not* ready to make changes yet, but want to talk more.
– I am ready to make some changes now and would like help.
– I am already helping my child eat healthy or be more active, and I don't feel there is much more to do.

Some authors suggested, for example, that if, after assessing readiness to change, a pediatrician determines that a family is not ready for and/or not interested in making changes to their diet and physical activity routines, she or he can 'plant the seed' about the importance of the topic and return to it at a different time when the family is more ready. In contrast, if a family reports that they are interested in making changes, they should promptly be engaged in a conversation about how to get started with requisite lifestyle changes. Motivational interviewing is recommended for ambivalent families to improve the success of action planning (NICHQ, 2007). Patient-centered counseling is discussed as a key strategy in the Expert Committee Recommendations – Step 1, as highlighted below.

Practice Guidelines

The Expert Committee Recommendations on the Assessment, Prevention, and Treatment of Child and Adolescent Overweight and Obesity (2007) and the Child-hood Obesity Action Network's associated Implementation Guide identify three key steps to address pediatric obesity: (1) Obesity Prevention at Well-Care Visits (Assessment and Prevention); (2) Prevention Plus Visits (Treatment); and (3) Going Beyond Your Practice (Prevention and Treatment). As clinical guidelines for assessment have already been addressed, Step 1 will be briefly discussed, emphasizing on prevention strategies. Next, recommendations and implementation guidelines for Steps 2 and 3 will be presented. Tools for providers for implementing these recommendations are available at http://www.nichq.org/NICHQ/Topics/ Preventive Care/Obesity/Tools/managementandtreatmentcarepartnershipreport

Step 1 – Obesity Prevention at Well-Care Visits (Assessment and Prevention):

- Assess all children of age 2–18 years for obesity at all well-care visits.

  ○ Leaders should provide education to staff and colleagues to help implement obesity prevention.

- After a thorough assessment (as described earlier), provide consistent, evidence-based messages for all children regardless of their weight.

  ○ Use the Maine Collaborative 5-2-1-0 message:

    ▪ 5 servings of fruits and vegetables each day
    ▪ 2 hours or less of 'screen time' each day (i.e., TV, computers, games)
    ▪ 1 hour or more of physical activity (moderate to vigorous activity)
    ▪ 0 servings of sweetened beverages (e.g., juice, sodas)

      • Encourage an authoritative parenting style in support of increased physical activity and reduced TV viewing.
      • Discourage restrictive parenting style regarding child's eating.
      • Encourage parents to be good role models and address lifestyle as a family issue rather than the child's own problem.

  ○ Other recommendations include:

    ▪ Remove television from children's bedrooms.
    ▪ Eat breakfast every day.
    ▪ Limit eating out, especially fast food.
    ▪ Have regular family meals.
    ▪ Limit portion sizes.

- Use 'empathize, provide, elicit' to improve the effectiveness of your counseling.

  ○ Patient-centered counseling approaches, such as motivational interviewing (Rollnick & Miller, 1995), can help families recognize and resolve ambivalence. Resistance is minimized with this approach, as counseling techniques prompt families to independently generate personally relevant strategies for healthy lifestyle change.

    ▪ Sample dialogue:

      • Your child's height and weight may put him at increased risk of developing diabetes or heart disease at a very early age. What do you make of this? Would you be interested in talking more about ways to reduce your child's risk?

- Some different ways to reduce your child's risk are.... Do any of these seem like something your family could work on, or do you have other ideas?
- Where does that leave you? What you might need to be successful?

Step 2 – Prevention Plus Treatment:

- Develop an office-based approach for follow up of overweight and obese children.

  ○ Expert Committee Recommendations promote a staged approach for children of age 2–19 years whose BMI values fall within the 85th and 94th percentiles with risk factors and for children whose BMI is equal to or greater than the 95th percentile.

    ■ Stage 1 = Prevention Plus

      - Family visits with a physician trained in pediatric weight management and behavioral counseling (individual or group).
      - Implement prevention strategies described earlier, such as the 5-2-1-0 plan.
      - Establish a weight loss target (see Table 2).

Table 2 Weight loss targets

	BMI 85-94%ile No Risks	BMI 85–94%ile With Risks	BMI 95–98%ile	BMI ≥ 99%ile
Age 2–5 years	Maintain weight velocity	Decrease weight velocity or weight maintenance	Weight maintenance	Gradual weight loss of up to 1 pound a month if BMI is very high (>21 or 22 kg/m^2)
Age 6–11 years	Maintain weight velocity	Decrease weight velocity or weight maintenance	Weight maintenance of gradual loss (1 pounds per month)	Weight loss (average is 2 pounds per week)*
Age 12–18 years	Maintain weight velocity; after linear growth is complete, maintain weight	Decrease weight velocity or weight maintenance	Weight loss (average is 2 pounds per week)*	Weight loss (average is 2 pounds per week)*

*Excessive weight loss should be evaluated for high risk behaviors.
Source: Childhood Obesity Action Network (2007); available at http://www.nichq.org/NR/rdonlyres/7CF2C1F3-4DA3-4A00-AE15-4E35967F3571/5316/COANImplementationGuide62607FINAL.pdf

- Implement 'Stage 2: Structured Weight Management' if no improvement in weight, BMI or weight velocity in 3–6 months, and if the family is ready to make changes.

○ To implement these recommendations, the Obesity Action Network recommends the use of the following clinical management support tools, which are available at http://www.nichq.org/NICHQ/Topics/PreventiveCare/Obesity/Tools/managementandtreatmentoffice.htm

  ■ Presentation of health education materials
  ■ Administration of behavioral risk assessment and self-monitoring tools
  ■ Action planning and goal-setting tools
  ■ Clinical documentation tools
  ■ Counseling protocols
  ■ Involvement of other health professionals such as dietitians, psychologists, and health educators

    - Secondary goals include improving self-esteem and self-efficacy (confidence)

- Use motivational interviewing to improve the success of action planning.

  ○ Patient-centered counseling techniques (as discussed earlier) are an effective approach to address childhood obesity prevention and treatment. Motivational interviewing is particularly effective for ambivalent families, and can also be used for action planning.

    ■ For example, instead of telling patients what changes to make, elicit 'change talk' from them, taking their ideas, strengths, and barriers into account.

Step 3 – Going Beyond Your Practice (Prevention and Treatment):

- Advocate improved access to healthy lifestyles in your community and schools:

  ○ Physicians, allied healthcare professionals, and professional organizations are recommended to advocate Federal government to increase physical activity intervention programs in schools.
  ○ Physicians, allied healthcare professionals, and professional organizations are recommended to support efforts to preserve and enhance parks as areas for physical activity, including walking and bicycle paths, and promoting families' use of these and other community resources.

    ■ The Obesity Action Network provides advocacy tools and resources and information regarding multifaceted community interventions at http://www.nichq.org/NICHQ/Topics/PreventiveCare/Obesity/Tools/Communityresourcestools.htm

- Identify and promote community services that encourage healthy lifestyles.

o Physicians, allied healthcare professionals, and professional organizations are recommended to promote physical activity at schools and in child care settings (including after-school programs), by asking children and parents about activity in these settings during routine office visits.

■ The Obesity Action Network recommends Public Health Departments and Parks and Recreation as good places to start looking for community programs and resources.

- Identify or develop more intensive weight management interventions for families who do not respond to Prevention Plus.

o The Expert Committee's recommendations include the following staged approach for children of age 2–19 years whose BMI is between the 85th and 94th percentiles with risk factors and for children whose BMI is 95th percentile or above:

■ Stage 2 – Structured Weight Management

• Family visits with a physician or health professional specifically trained in weight management. Monthly visits can be individual or group.

■ Stage 3 – Comprehensive, Multidisciplinary Intervention

• Multidisciplinary team with experience in childhood obesity. Frequency is often weekly for 8–12-weeks with follow-up.

■ Stage 4 – Tertiary Care Intervention

• Medications (e.g., sibutramine, orlistat), very-low-calorie diets (VLCDs), weight control surgery (e.g., gastric bypass or banding). Recommended for select patients only when provided by experienced programs with established clinical or research protocols. Gastric banding is in clinical trials and is not currently approved by FDA.

Treatment Manuals

Handbooks

- Fairburn, C. G. & Brownell, K. D. (2002). *Eating disorders and obesity, second edition: A comprehensive handbook*. New York, New York: Guilford.
- O'Donohue, W. T., Moore, B. A., & Scott, B. J. (2007). *Handbook of pediatric and adolescent obesity treatment*. New York, NY: Routledge.
- Wadden, T. & Stunkard, A. J. (2004). *Handbook of obesity treatment*. New York, NY: Guildford.

Clinical Guides

- Cooper, Z., Fairburn, C. G., & Hawker, D. M. (2004). *Cognitive-behavioral treatment of obesity: A clinician's guide*. New York, NY: Guilford.
- Hassink, S. G. (2006). *A clinical guide to pediatric weight management and obesity*. Lippincott: Williams & Wilkins.
- Sothern, M. S., Gordon, S. T., & von Almen, T. K. (2006). *Handbook of pediatric obesity: Clinical management*. Boca Raton: CRC Press.

Stepped Care Treatments

Books

For Parents

- American Academy of Pediatrics & Hassink, S. G. (2006). *A Parent's guide to childhood obesity: A roadmap to health*. American Academy of Pediatrics.
- Trim Kids: The proven 12-week plan that has helped thousands of children achieve a healthier weight

Workbooks

- Craighead, L. (2006). *The appetite awareness workbook: How to listen to your body and overcome bingeing, overeating, & obsession with food*. Oakland, CA: New Harbinger.
- Johnson, S. & Mellin, L. (2002). *Just for Kids! (Obesity Prevention Workbook)*. CA: Balboa.
- Latner, J. & Wilson, T. *Self-Help approaches for obesity and eating disorders: Research and practice*. New York, NY: Guildford.
- Mellin, L. (2000). Shapedown. CA: Balboa.

  ○ Parent, children, pre-teen, and teen workbooks available

Online Assessment Resources

- BMI calculator: http://apps.nccd.cdc.gov/dnpabmi/Calculator.aspx
- Growth charts allow for longitudinal tracking of BMI; available at http://www.cdc.gov/nchs/about/major/nhanes/growthcharts/charts.html

Education and Treatment Websites

- American Academy of Pediatrics: http://www.aap.org/obesity
- American Dietetic Association: http://www.eatright.org

- American Obesity Association: http://www.obesity.org/subs/childhood
- BAM! Body and Mind: http://www.bam.gov
- CDC: http://www.cdc.gov
- Fit & Healthy Kids: http://www.fitandhealthykids.com

Websites for School and Community-Based Action

- Alliance for a Healthier Generation: http://www.healthiergeneration.org/
- California 5 a Day: http://www.dhs.ca.gov/ps/cdic/cpns/ca5aday/default.htm
- Snackwise: http://www.nationwidechildrens.org/GD/Templates/pages/childrens/ hwn/HWNLongContent.aspx?page=6146
- CDC – Key Strategies to Prevent Obesity at School: http://www.cdc.gov/Healthy Youth/keystrategies/index.htm

Other Tools

- Expert Committee Recommendations on the Assessment, Prevention, and Treatment of Child and Overweight and Obesity, 2007: An Implementation Guide from the Childhood Obesity Action Network; available at http://www. nichq.org/NR/rdonlyres/7CF2C1F3-4DA3-4A00-AE15-4E35967F3571/5316/ COANImplementationGuide62607FINAL.pdf
- NICHQ; available at http://www.nichq.org/NICHQ/Programs/ConferencesAnd Training/ChildhoodObesityActionNetwork.html

References

American Academy of Pediatrics (2003) Policy statement: Prevention of pediatric overweight a and obesity *Pediatrics, 112*, 424–430.

American Academy of Pediatrics (2007) AAP publications retired or reaffirmed, October 2006 *Pediatrics, 119*, 405.

Arredondo E. M., Elder J. P., Ayala G. X., Campbell N., Baquero B., & Duerksen S. (2006) Is parenting style related to children's healthy eating and physical activity in Latino families? *Health Education Research: Theory & Practice, 21*, 862–871.

Baker, J., Olsen, L., & Sorensen, T. (2007). Childhood body mass index and the risk of coronary heart disease in adulthood. *New England Journal of Medicine, 357*(23), 2329–2337.

Bacon, G. E., & Lowery, G. H. (1967). A clinical trial of fenfluramine in obese childern. *Current Therapeutic Research Clinical Experimental, 9*, 626–630.

Barlow S. E., & Deitz W. H. (1998) Obesity evaluation and treatment: Expert committee recommendations. *Pediatrics, 102*,e29.

Braet C., & van Strien T. (1997) Assessment of emotional, externally induced and restrained eating behavior in nine to twelve year old obese and non-obese children. *Behaviour Research and Therapy, 35*, 863–873.

Britz B., Siegfried W., Ziegler A., & Lamertz C. (2000) Rates of psychiatric disorder in a clinical Study Group of adolescents with extreme obesity and in obese adolescents ascertained via a population based study. *International Journal of Obesity and Related Metabolic Disorders : Journal of the International Association for the Study of Obesity, 24*, 1707–1714.

Carnell S., Edwards C., Croker H., Boniface D., & Wardle J. (2005) Parental perceptions of overweight in 3–5 year olds. *International Journal of Obesity, 29*, 353–355.

Center for Disease Control and Prevention (2007) About BMI for children and teens. Available at: http://www.cdc.gov/nccdphp/dnpa/bmi/childrens_BMI/about_childrens_BMI.htm

Deitz W. H., & Robinson T. N. (2005) Overweight in children and adolescents. *The New England Journal of Medicine, 352*, 2100–2109.

Dietz, W.H. (2004). Overweight in childhood and adolescence. *New England Journal of Medicine, 350*(9), 855–857.

Ebbeling, C. B., Pawlak, D., & Ludwig, D. (2002). Childhood obesity: Public-health crisis, common sense cure. *Lancet, 10*(360), 473–483.

Epstein L. H., Klein K. R., & Wisniewski L. (1994) Child and parent factors that influence psychological problems in obese children. *International Journal of Eating Disorders, 15*, 151–157.

Erermis S., Cetin N., Tamar M., Bukusoglu N., Akdcniz F., & Goksen D. (2004) Is obesity a risk factor for psychopathology among adolescents? *Pedatrics International, 46*, 296–301.

Fagot-Campagna, A., Pettitt, D., Engelgau, M., Burrows, N., Geiss, L., Valdez, R., et al. (2000). Type 2 diabetes among North American children and adolescents: An epidemiologic review and a public health perspective. *Journal of Pediatrics, 136*(5), 664–672.

Friedman M. A., & Brownell K. D. (1995) Psychological correlates of obesity: moving to the next research generation. *Psychological Bulletin, 117*, 3–20.

He M., & Evans A. (2007) Are parents aware that their children are overweight or obese? Do they care? *Canadian Family Physician, 53*, 1493–1499.

Horgen, K.B. & Brownell, K.D. (2002). Confronting the toxic environment; Environmental, public health actions in a world crisis. In T. A. Wadden & A. J. Stunkard (Eds.). *Handbook of obesity treatment* (pp. 95–106). New York: Guilford Press.

Klesges R. C., Stein R. J., Eck L. H., Isbell T. R., & Klesges L. M. (1991) Parental influence on food selection in young children and its relationships to childhood obesity. *The American Journal of Clinical Nutrition, 71*, 1054–1061.

Larsen L., Mandleco B., Williams M., & Tiedeman M. (2006) Childhood obesity: Prevention practices of nurse practitioners. *Journal of the American Academy of Nurse Practitioners, 18*, 70–79.

McElroy, S. L., Kotwal, R., Malhotra, S., Nelson, E. B., Keck, P. E., & Nemeroff, C. B. (2004). Are mood disorders and obesity related? A review for the mental health professional. *Journal of Clinical Psychiatry, 65*, 634–651.

National Center for Health Statistics (2002). Retrieved on September 2, 2008 from http://www.cdc.gov/nchs/nhanes.htm

Ogden C. L., Carroll M. D., Curtin L. R., McDowell M. A., Tabak C. J., & Flegal K. M. (2006). Prevalence of overweight and obesity in the United States, 1999–2004. *Journal of the American Medical Association, 295*, 1549–1555.

Perrin E. M., Finkle J. P., & Bejamin J. T. (2006). Obesity prevention and the primary care pediatrician's office. *Current Opinion in Pediatrics, 19*, 354–361.

Rollnick S., & Miller, W. R. (1995). What is motivational interviewing? *Behavioural and Cognitive Psychotherapy, 23*, 325–334.

Satter, E. (2007). Ellyn Satter's division of responsibility in feeding. Available at: http://www.ellynsatter.com/

Stein, R. I., Epstein, L. H., Raynor, H. A., Kilanowski, C. K., & Paluch, R. A. (2005). The influence of parenting change on pediatric weight control. *Obesity Research, 13*, 1749–1755.

Spurrier N. J., Magarey A., & Wong C. (2006) Recognition and management of childhood overweight and obesity by clinicians. *Journal of paediatrics and child health, 42*, 411–418.

United States Department of Health and Human Services [USDHHS] (Updated on January 11, 2007) The Surgeon General's Call to Action to Prevent and Decrease Overweight and Obesity: Overweight in Children and Adolescents. Available at: http://www.surgeongeneral. gov/topics/obesity/calltoaction/fact_adolescents.htm

Young-Hyman, D., Schulundt, D. G., Herman, L., Deluca, F., & Counts, D. (2001). Evaluation of the insulin resistance syndrome in 5- to 10-year-old overweight/obese African-American childern. *Diabetes Care, 24*, 1359–1364.

Somatization in Primary Care

Michael A. Cucciare and Jason Lillis

What is Somatization?

In health care settings, the term somatization refers to the association between medically unexplained symptoms related to psychological distress and medical help-seeking behavior (Kroenke, Spitzer, & Williams, 2002). Patients presenting with somatization (or somatizers) have been characterized as having physical or medical problems that are physical manifestations of emotional conflicts (O'Donohue, Cummings, Cucciare, Cummings, & Runyan, 2006). Dr. Nicholas Cummings suggests that these emotional conflicts are often unconscious and translated into physical symptoms such as headaches, gastrointestinal problems, and pain. He further points out that the relationship between physical complaints and emotional problems can vary. For example, some somatizers may experience physical complaints or illness that is primarily the result of emotional problems, whereas others may have a physical illness that is exacerbated by their emotional conflicts (O'Donohue et al., 2006).

Before we proceed any further, it is important to define and clarify the terms used in this chapter. The term 'somatization' is often used synonymously with other phrases to describe patients presenting with physical complaints of no identifiable medical etiology. Some of those phrases include 'medically unexplained symptoms,' 'functional disorder,' and 'functional somatic symptoms' (Rosendal, Fink, Flemming, & Olesen, 2005). Given its prevalent use in the literature, we will use the term somatization and the phrase 'medically unexplained symptoms' synonymously.

The *Diagnostic and Statistical Manual of Mental Disorders – Fourth Edition* (*DSM-IV*) classifies somatization disorder as one of the five somatoform disorders that have, as a common feature, "...the presence of physical symptoms that suggest a general medical condition (hence the term somatoform) and are not fully explained by a general medical condition, by the direct effects of a substance, or by another mental disorder (e.g., panic disorder)" (p. 445). Recent estimates show that 39%

M.A. Cucciare (✉)
VA Palo Alto Health Care System, and Stanford University School of Medicine CA 94025, USA
e-mail: cucciare@hotmail.com

L.C. James, W.T. O'Donohue (eds.), *The Primary Care Toolkit*,
DOI 10.1007/978-0-387-78971-2_20, © Springer Science+Business Media, LLC 2009

patients in primary care meet the diagnostic criteria for a somatoform disorder, the most commonest being somatization disorder (5.3% prevalence) (Toft et al., 2005).

Somatization disorder is rarely recognized in primary care. Therefore, it is important that providers of both physical and mental health services are able to recognize somatization in patients presenting with physical symptoms. To meet *DSM-IV* criteria for somatization disorder, the patient must have a history of many physical complaints over a period of several years which have resulted in significant impairment in social, occupational, or other important domains of functioning (p. 449). The patient must have had four pain events (e.g., head, chest), two gastrointestinal symptoms (e.g., nausea, vomiting), one sexual problem (e.g., erectile dysfunction), and one pseudoneurological symptom (e.g., impaired coordination, double vision) that either (1) cannot be attributed to a general medical condition or substance or (2) manifest in excess than would be expected from a medical condition (determined by history, physical examination, and/or laboratory findings) (American Psychiatric Association, 1994, p. 450).

Basic Facts About Somatization

Sociodemographic Characteristics and Prevalence

Somatization disorder affects both men and women with lifetime prevalence being 0.2 to 2% in women and 0.2% in men (American Psychiatric Association, 1994), and these individuals tend to have low socioeconomic status, less educated, often unemployed, living on a pension, sick pay, or poor social security (Fink, Sorensen, Engberg, Holm, & Munk-Jorgensen, 1999). The prevalence rates of somatization are considerably higher in primary care. Toft et al. (2005) found that 5% of men and 13% of women presenting to primary care met the diagnostic criteria for somatization disorder, with as high as a 40% lifetime prevalence rate for both men and women (Feder et al., 2001; Toft et al., 2005).

As many as 22% of patients presenting to primary care meet the criteria for 'abridged' somatization disorder (at least four persistent and impairing medically unexplained symptoms in men and six in woman) (Feder et al., 2001). Patients can also present to primary care with medically unexplained symptoms but not meet the criteria for either full-blown or abridged somatization disorder. It has been reported that as many as three of four patients presenting with medically unexplained symptoms fall into the latter category (Smith & Gardiner, 2006).

Comorbidity

Along with depression and anxiety, somatization is the most common psychiatric problem seen in primary care (Kroenke, 2000; Ormel et al., 1994; Spitzer et al., 1994). The most common comorbid psychiatric conditions include major depressive, panic, and substance-related disorders and histrionic, borderline, and antisocial personality disorders (American Psychiatric Association, 1994). After adjusting for age and gender, the most common physical complaints in somatizing patients are limb pain, trouble sleeping, feeling tired/having low energy, and nausea/gas/indigestion (Feder et al., 2001). Two-thirds of psychiatric problems are observed exclusively in primary care patients reporting somatization (Keely et al., 2004; Kroenke, 2004). Unfortunately, somatization often goes undetected in primary care resulting in comorbid psychiatric conditions, which also remain undetected (Smith & Gardiner, 2006).

Health Care Utilization

Somatizers place a great strain on our health care system as they are associated with higher health care costs and consumption of increased resources when compared to patients presenting with the next two most common psychological problems (c.g., depression or anxiety) in primary care (Hahn et al., 1996; Smith, 1994). Somatizing patients account for approximately $256 billion of health care a year after adjusting for comorbid conditions (Barsky, Orav, & Bates, 2006). They use more outpatient and inpatient health care (Smith & Gardiner, 2006), primary and specialty care, and have more emergency room visits than non-somatizing patients (Barsky et al., 2006).

Health Care-Seeking Characteristics

Somatizers are often described as 'difficult' patients due to their tendency to 'doctor-shop,' consult multiple health care providers for the same problem(s), use emergency services at high rates, and often failing to keep scheduled appointments (Barsky et al., 2006). These patients commonly present to primary care with physical complaints that are not easily (if at all) ameliorated by medical care, resulting in dissatisfaction with the health care setting, the system, and the provider (Barsky et al.).

Assessment of Somatization

What Should Be Ruled Out?

When assessing somatization, one should rule out physical complaints due to a coexisting medical condition(s); and psychiatric conditions that are associated with physical complaints such as schizophrenia, anxiety disorders (e.g., panic, generalized anxiety disorder, and post-traumatic stress disorder), and mood disorders (e.g., depressive disorders) (Kroenke, Spitzer, DeGruy, & Swindle, 1998). A physician should be consulted when a medical condition is thought to be contributing to the presence of what are suspected of being medically unexplained physical symptoms.

What Is Involved in Effective Assessment?

A thorough assessment of somatization in primary care involves screening for the presence, number, and severity of somatic symptoms, the degree to which the patient is bothered by these symptoms, a thorough medical history and exam to determine whether the somatic, complaints are due to a general medical condition(s), anxiety (e.g., panic and generalized anxiety disorder), and depressive disorders (as these disorders typically present with somatic symptoms), substance use, and/or the presence and severity of psychosocial stressors.

It is important that providers distinguish between patients presenting with somatization and patients who are experiencing and communicating distress as physical complaints. Lipowski (1988) argues that the latter is a normal human reaction to stress, and should not be considered abnormal. This presentation becomes abnormal when patients attribute their physical distress (resulting from psychological distress) to a physical problem and thus seek medical diagnosis and treatment. Bridges and Goldberg (1985) suggest that providers look for the following when attempting to identify somatization in primary care:

- Medical help-seeking for physical manifestations of psychological distress with no presentation of psychological symptoms
- Attributing somatic complaints to undiagnosed physical problems (e.g., disease or cardiac problems)
- Somatic complaints that justify diagnosis of a psychological problem when examined by a mental health professional
- Treatment of psychological problem results in the reduction or absence of somatic complaints

Assessment Instruments for Screening, and Diagnosing Somatization in Primary Care

There are several brief, psychometrically sound measures that can be used to identify and diagnose somatization in primary care. A brief description of each measure is provided below.

Patient Health Questionnaire-15

The Patient Health Questionnaire (PHQ)-15, based on the self-administered version of PRIME-MD, contains 15 questions to assess somatization (Barsky, et al., 2006; Kroenke et al., 2002; see Appendix A in this chapter). Research has demonstrated strong internal reliability and convergent and discriminate validity. Kroenke et al. demonstrated that as PHQ-15 scores increase, corresponding decreases in functional status are also observed. Furthermore, increased PHQ-15 scores are shown to be related to increased symptom-related difficulties (e.g., number of sick days) and health care utilization (see Kroenke et al.). Each item in PHQ-15 takes a score from 0 ('not bothered at all') to 2 ('bothered a lot') and has cut-off scores of 5, 10, and 15, representing low, medium, and high somatic symptom severity, respectively.

12-Item Somatization Scale of the Symptom Checklist-90

The Symptom Checklist (SCL)-90 is a self-administered, psychometrically sound instrument used to assess a broad range of symptoms associated with various psychological problems (Derogatis & Cleary, 1977). It contains various subscales that assess symptoms related to such problems as somatization, obsessive-compulsive disorder, depression, and anxiety. The somatization scale contains ;items and can be used separately from the rest of the test to assess somatization in primary care (Fink et al., 1999; Toft et al., 2005). The SCL-90 can be used in both adolescents and adults and can be administered through paper and pencil, computer, audio cassette, or Internet. It is available in several languages, and may be purchased online from Pearson Assessments (http://www.pearsona sessments.com/tests/scl90r.htm).

Somatic Symptom Index

The Somatic Symptom Index (SSI) is an 11-item, self-report questionnaire that assesses the presence of common somatic symptoms (Aronson, Barrett, & Quigley, 2006). The SSI contains items that are based on *DSM-III* somatization symptoms, and was originally developed to identify abridged or sub-threshold somatization disorder (Escobar, Rubio-Stipec, Canino, & Karno, 1989). The focus on abridged somatization disorder was done for two primary reasons – more patients present with abridged somatization disorder (than the full-blown version); and identifying the abridged version often maintains the predictive value of full-blown diagnosis (Escobar et al., 1989). The SSI has strong psychometric properties including high internal consistency (Aronson et al., 2006) and strong validity as it has been shown to accurately identify 98% of individuals meeting criteria of somatization disorder in community samples (Swartz et al., 1986). The cut-off scores for the presence of abridged somatization disorder are 4 and 6 or more somatic symptoms for men and women, respectively (Escobar et al. 1989).

Evidence-based Treatment of Somatization

Several interventions have been shown to be effective in reducing somatization (e.g., reducing severity and frequency of medically unexplained symptoms), including pharmacotherapy, provider psychoeducation, patient reattribution training, and cognitive behavioral therapy (CBT). A brief discussion of each of these interventions is provided in the following section.

Pharmacotherapy

Research supports the use of antidepressants as an effective treatment for somatization. A review of 94 clinical trials that targeted a variety of symptom presentations (e.g., headache, fibromyalgia, gastrointestinal problems, pain, chronic fatigue, and general somatization) showed a reduction of medically unexplained symptoms after the use of antidepressants (see O'Malley et al., 1999). Major outcomes included reduced pain and headaches; a reduction in the total number of symptoms and symptom(s) intensity; enhanced well-being and functional status (i.e., increased ability to perform self-care-related behaviors and other physical activities). The results of the review showed that patients treated with tricyclic antidepressants, antiserotonin antidepressants, or selective reuptake inhibitors were three times more likely to experience improvements in physical symptoms when compared to patients treated with a placebo-control (O'Malley et al., 1999). However, there was no reliable difference across classes of antidepressants and no way to determine whether the effect was due to the treatment of an underlying psychiatric condition, improvement in the ability to manage pain, or alteration in neurotransmitters that were thought to have contributed to the experience of somatization (O'Malley et al., 1999).

Provider Consultation

A series of studies demonstrate the use of consultation letters to be effective in helping primary care physicians treat patients with medically unexplained symptoms (e.g. Dickinson et al., 2003; Smith et al., 2006; Smith, Monson, & Ray, 1986; Smith, Rost, & Kashner, 1995). Each of these studies identified somatizing patients in primary care and randomly assigned physicians to receive a care recommendation letter or conduct treatment as usual. Findings show that consultation letters were effective at reducing both patients' physical symptoms (e.g., frequency and severity of pain or headaches) and medical care costs but, generally, had no effect on reducing psychological symptoms such as depression.

The consultation letters consisted of general recommendations on how to identify and treat somatizers presenting to primary care.

1. The patient should be regularly scheduled for brief appointments in primary care with urgent appointments avoided if possible.
2. The physician should look closely for signs of a disease rather than simply taking the patient's report of symptoms at face.
3. Hospitalization, surgery, or diagnostic procedures should be avoided unless indicated by physical abnormalities.
4. Patient symptoms should be viewed as part of an unconscious process rather than telling the patient that the problem is 'all in your head.' (recreated from Dickinson et al., 2003).

Reattribution Training

Reattribution training (RT) aims to normalize patients' interpretations of bodily symptoms, modify their beliefs about causes of their symptoms, and treat the underlying psychological problems (e.g., depression) that can contribute to the presence of medically unexplained symptoms (Morriss & Gask, 2002). Although RT was not effective in reducing physical complaints, patients reported an increased ability to conduct daily physical activity and a reduction in comorbid psychological problems such as depression and anxiety (Morriss et al., 1999). RT appears to be most effective for patients who are willing to consider that their symptoms may be influenced by psychological/emotion factors. RT appears to also improve physicians' awareness of medically unexplained symptoms (Rosendal, Bro, Fink, Christensen, & Olesen, 2003) and reduce negative attitudes toward somatizing patients (Christensen, Rosendal, Nielsen, Kallcrup, & Olen, 2003).

Reattribution training involves:

1. Taking a relevant history of physical symptoms, psychosocial difficulties, and beliefs about the cause of patients' symptoms and conducting a focused physical examination of these symptoms.
2. Providing feedback with a tentative explanation that physical symptoms may be linked to psychosocial and lifestyle factors.
3. If the patient is open to this interpretation, provide more detailed education about the physiological or temporal link between psychosocial or lifestyle problems and the symptom (recreated from Morriss & Gask, 2002).

Cognitive Behavioral Therapy

A recent review of the literature found CBT to be effective in treating somatizing patients (Kroenke & Swindle, 2000). The authors reviewed 31 controlled trials that targeted a variety of symptom presentations (e.g., chronic fatigue, irritable bowel, pain, and general somatization) and employed a range of intervention techniques (e.g., relaxation training, behavioral activation, and cognitive therapy). Results indicated that group and individual CBT was effective in reducing physical symptoms and improving functional status. Major outcomes included reduced pain, reduced total number of symptoms, reduced intensity of physical symptoms, and improved ability to perform self-care, self-maintenance, and physical activities.

Some primary care providers may find it challenging to administer CBT to somatizing patients given the lack of (a) time available to treat psychological problems in primary care and (b) adequate training in CBT. In such cases, it may be more pragmatic to refer somatizing patients to specialty mental health care or a collocated behavioral health provider. The latter scenario is perhaps most efficient as many somatizing patients (and most patients with psychological problems, in general) fail to show up for initial appointments to specialty mental health care. For primary care providers interested in delivering aspects of CBT in primary care settings, we provide a brief description of some of the main components below (also see Woolfolk & Allen, 2006). Resources for providers interested in learning more about how to administer the specific components discussed below are provided after this section.

Clinical trials that demonstrated the effectiveness of CBT in treating somatization in primary care have shown relaxation training, behavioral activation, and cognitive restructuring to be crucial in reducing the presence and frequency of physical symptoms associated with somatization (Kroenke & Swindle, 2000).

Relaxation Training

The technique of relaxation has become so popular and widely used that some have called it the 'aspirin' of psychotherapy (Russo, Bird, & Masek, 1980). Relaxation can take many forms including yoga, meditation, diaphragmatic breathing (also known as belly breathing) to name a few. Perhaps the most common forms of relaxation in psychotherapy are progressive muscle relaxation, guided imagery, and diaphragmatic breathing. All three relaxation techniques are conceptually simple to understand and can be taught relatively quickly (see Ferguson, 2003).

Progressive muscle relaxation training involves a muscular tense-release procedure targeting various muscle groups throughout the body. A patient is directed to move through each muscle group slowly, while tensing and releasing the muscles to produce a relaxing effect. Progressive muscle relaxation can be delivered in script, CD, or audio file format (Bernstein, Borkovec, & Hazlett-Stevens, 2000). Guided imagery involves focusing one's attention on auditory stimuli. For example, a patient might listen to a therapist's voice while being directed to picture what is being said in his/her mind. The effect is often positive and can reduce a wide variety of psychological and physical symptoms. This relaxation technique requires little training, though practice is important (see Weil, 2004). Diaphragmatic Breathing is simply a deep breathing technique designed to increase the intake of oxygen for the purpose of reducing the impact of emotional distress. Diaphragmatic breathing or "belly" breathing as it is sometimes referred is a personal favorite of the authors as it can be taught to patients in as little as 1 minute and used in a wide variety of settings (including while driving) (see Appendix B for diaphragmatic breathing instructions). Ferguson (2003) outlines four recommendations for primary care providers interested in conducting relaxation training:

(a) *Identify the setting* – providers should choose a room that is quiet and has little probability of being used during the time the patient is engaging in relaxation. The room should (at minimum) consist of a comfortable chair, and ideally a fan or noise maker to drown out any outside sound. Patients should be instructed to be dressed comfortably during relaxation training.

(b) *Providing a rationale* – patients should receive a rational for relaxation to promote motivation to engage in this procedure. In presenting the rationale, providers should review clients problem behaviors (e.g., stress, anxiety, pain) and how they relate to stress and arousal, discuss how relaxation can serve as a coping strategy for managing a variety of uncomfortable emotional experiences, provide the patient with an overview of the specific procedure being taught (e.g., diaphragmatic breathing or progressive muscle relaxation), and emphasize the role of the provider as a coach and the need for practicing relaxation outside of the health care setting to obtain maximum benefits.

(c) *Pre-post assessment* - It is important for patients to complete both an initial and post assessment of stress level. Most patients report changes in the level of stress/arousal soon after the completion of a relaxation exercise. Capturing self-reported changes in relaxation is important as it may increase patients' motivation to continue the procedure at different settings. Self-rating of relaxation levels can be brief and should be done regularly (see Appendix C for an example of a rating form).

(d) *Relaxation training* – Most relaxation techniques (e.g., diaphragmatic breathing) can be taught relatively quickly. When teaching this technique, it is recommended that providers schedule a 30–50 minute session separate from the original visit to allow for enough time to properly teach the exercise and answer any questions patients might have. This separate session provides clinicians an opportunity to understand and describe any presenting complaint(s) (e.g., pain, headaches, stress, etc) the patient might have and present how levels of stress and arousal may contribute to the experience of these physical symptoms (i.e., rationale for relaxation).

This session should also provide adequate time to allow patients an opportunity to practice the taught exercise and have any questions addressed during that time. If appropriate, providers should schedule a follow-up appointment after patients have had an opportunity to practice on their own (e.g., 2–4 weeks after the initial appointment). Follow-up appointment may take the form of in-person or phone session, depending on the provider's and patient's availability.

Behavioral Activation

The second main component of CBT treatment for somatization is behavioral activation (BA). In general, BA is a strategy for increasing patients' engagement in pleasant activities (Martell, Addis, & Jacobson, 2001). BA was originally developed from a conceptualization of depressed patients that described these individuals as having an imbalance of punishing and reinforcing stimuli in their lives (i.e., more punishing than reinforcing stimuli – pleasant events). This conceptualization of the etiology of depression explains that depressed patients often experience an event that triggers an emotional response, resulting in a pattern of avoidance and isolation. Using the example of somatization, a patient may experience a headache that leads to a feeling of sadness, which in turn results in the patient canceling an activity with a friend. The intention of using BA is to promote patients engaging in activities even when physical or emotional barriers are present (Addis, Martell, & Jacobson, 2001).

There are two important keys to teaching patients how to engage in BA. The first key is for the clinician to provide a rationale for this aspect of treatment clearly explaining the relationship between activity and mood. Second, it is important that the patient track his or her behavioral activity through self-monitoring to demonstrate this relationship. This might take the form of a chart that includes all of the hours in a day and provides enough room for the patient to record (a) what he or she did during that time, (b) how they felt during that activity, and (c) the intensity of the feeling during each hour. This provides both the clinician and the patient with an opportunity to record demonstrations between what the the patient does and how it may influence how they feel, which may serve to enhance patient's motivation to continue engaging in BA. Common goals of this treatment component include getting the patient to increase their number of daily, positive activities (e.g., a 5-minute walk, making a cup of tea, calling a friend, etc.) in a manner that is appropriate for their lifestyle.

Cognitive Restructuring

Cognitive restructuring is concerned with altering patients' negative ways of thinking to improve their mood and ways of behaving. Cognitive restructuring is a core concept (and set of techniques) of CBT which has been shown to be effective in treating patients presenting with somatization (see Nezu, Nezu, & Lombardo, 2001, for a review). CBT is built on the assumption that emotional distress and behavioral problems are greatly impacted by distorted thinking patterns and pervasive negative interpretations of life events (Ellis, 2003). In their review, Nezu et al. demonstrates how negative thought patterns, behaviors, and emotions impact a patient's experience of medically unexplained physical symptoms. For example, negative ways of thinking (e.g., catastrophizing – "It is terrible I have this pain; I must really be sick") may make symptoms worse, and may also impact how patients feel (e.g., increased depression and sadness) and behave (e.g., decreased physical activity, increased medical help-seeking). Cognitive restructuring is therefore focused on (a) helping patients understand the relationship between their actions, thinking patterns, and emotions; and (b) providing patients with strategies for altering negative ways of thinking to change how they think, feel, and behave (Ellis, 2003). Some of the key elements of cognitive restructuring are as follows (see Dobson & Hamilton, 2003; Ellis, 2003, for a thorough description of these elements):

1. Discussing the interaction between dysfunctional thinking, negative feelings, and behavioral patterns.
2. Identifying core beliefs or negative thoughts (e.g., "I'll never be a good father") that play a role in the patient's mood disturbances or negative behavior patterns.
3. Testing thoughts or beliefs empirically (i.e., seeking the evidence).
4. Helping the patient learn ways to logically dispute dysfunctional thoughts (e.g., "I do not have to win at everything in order to prove I'm worthy of approval").
5. Develop rational coping statements and say them over and over (e.g., "When my heart is beating quickly, it doesn't mean I'm dying or sick").

6. Change 'musts' to 'preferences' (e.g., "I must never feel ill" versus "I would prefer that I did not have a headache").
7. Do cost–benefit analysis of actions stemming from dysfunctional thoughts (i.e., "Do I really need to visit the doctor every time I have a headache?").
8. Test thoughts behaviorally (create a reasonable behavioral task that will allow a thought or belief to be tested; decide on relevant criteria for evaluation).

Provider Resources

There are a wide variety of resources available to providers in the form of books, audios, and websites that can assist in the treatment of somatization in primary care. For example, there are popular books available that contain detailed content on CBT for treating somatization disorder. Some of the most popular are (all of which can be purchased from Amazon.com):

- Woolfolk, R. L., & Allen, L. A. (2006). *Treating somatization: a cognitive-behavioral approach.* New York: The Guilford Press.

  This book presents a CBT approach to treating somatization and related problems. It also contains case examples and reproducible appendices containing useful handouts and forms.

- O'Donohue, W. T., Fisher, J. E., & Hayes, S. C. (Eds.), *Cognitive behavioral therapy: applying empirically supported techniques in your practice.* Hoboken, NJ: John Wiley & Sons.

  This volume contains a wide variety of evidence-based practice guidelines for providers interested in delivering aspects of CBT, including cognitive restructuring, behavioral activations, relaxation, and self-monitoring.

- Addis et al. (2001). *Depression in context: strategies for guided action.* New York: Norton.

  This book provides an in-depth look at behavioral strategies for treating depression with a special focus on behavioral activation.

- Bernstein et al. (2000). *New directions in progressive relaxation training: a guidebook for helping professionals.* Westport, CT: Praeger Publishing.

  This is a user-friendly guide for providers interested in learning techniques for teaching patients relaxation strategies for managing stress and other uncomfortable emotions.

- O'Donohue, W. T., & Levensky, E. (2006). *Promoting treatment adherence: a practical handbook for health care providers.* New York: Sage.

  This book covers an important topic of treatment adherence. It discusses the cutting-edge research and theory and provides practical recommendations for providers interested in promoting treatment adherence among their patients.

Effective Self-Help TreatmentResources

There several self-books and audio materials that contain information on the preceding treatments. Three of the most popular self-help books providing evidence-based recommendations for treating chronic somatic complaints include (all of which can be purchased through Amazon.com):

- Asmundson, G. J. G., & Taylor, S. (2005). *It's not all in your head: how worrying about your health could be making you sick - and what you can do about it.* New York: Guilford Press.
- Barsky, A. J. & Deans, E. C. (2006). *Stop being your symptoms and start being yourself: the six-week mind-body program to ease your chronic symptoms.* New York: Collins.

There are also three popular self-help books available for teaching patients cognitive restructuring and relaxation. These books/audio materials include:

- Burns, D. D. (1999a). *Feeling good: the new mood therapy* (2nd Ed). New York: Plume.
- Burns, D. D. (1999b). *The feeling god handbook.* New York: Plume.
- Lewinsohn, P. M., Munoz, R. F., Youngren, M. A., & Zeiss, A. M. (1992). *Control your depression.* New York: Fireside/Simon & Schuster.
- Weil, A. (2004). *Self-healing with guided imagery: how to use the power of your mind to heal your body* (Audio CD). Sounds True Publishing.

Useful Websites that provide information on the risk factors, symptoms, and treatment of somatization and self-help materials for treating depression, obtaining social support, and managing stress include:

- US National Library of Medicine and the National Institutes of Health – Information on Somatization: http://www.nlm.nih.gov/medlineplus/ency/article/000955.htm
- New York University Medical Center – Information on Somatization: http://www.med.nyu.edu/patientcare/library/article.html?ChunkIID=96749
- University of Pennsylvania – Authentic Happiness: http://www.authentic happiness.sas.upenn.edu/

- HealthPlace.com – Online Support Groups: http://www.healthyplace.com/site/support_groups_hp.asp
- MindTools – Stress Management Self-Help: http://www.mindtools.com/smpage.html

Appendix A[1]

Patient Health Questionnaire 15 – Item Somatic Symptom Severity Scale			
During the past 4 weeks, how much have you been bothered by any of the following problems	Not bothered at all	Bothered a little	Bothered a lot
a. Stomach pain	☐	☐	☐
b. Back pain	☐	☐	☐
c. Pain in arms, legs, or joints, knees, hips, etc.	☐	☐	☐
d. Menstrual cramps or other problems with periods (for women)	☐	☐	☐
e. Headaches	☐	☐	☐
f. Chest pain	☐	☐	☐
g. Dizziness	☐	☐	☐
h. Fainting spells	☐	☐	☐
i. Feeling your heart pound or race	☐	☐	☐
j. Shortness of breath	☐	☐	☐
k. Pain or problems during sexual intercourse	☐	☐	☐
l. Constipation, loose bowels, or diarrhea	☐	☐	☐
m. Nausea, gas, or indigestion	☐	☐	☐
n. Feeling tired or having low energy	☐	☐	☐
o. Trouble sleeping	☐	☐	☐

Appendix B[2]

Instructions for Diaphragmatic Breathing

1. Sit comfortably in a chair with your feet flat on the ground.
2. Put one hand on your stomach.
3. Slowly inhale through your nose.
4. As you inhale, feel your stomach expand with your hand. If your chest expands, try to focus your next breath so that your stomach expands instead.

---

[1] Adapted from Kroenke et al., 2002, p. 266.

[2] Instructions for diaphragmatic breathing can be provided verbally to patients and/or recorded on CD so that patients can practice outside of the session.

5. Take slow, deep breaths and continue to feel your stomach expand until it becomes natural.
6. Once you have perfected breathing with your stomach, focus your breathing so that it follows the following three steps:

   a. a. Inhale for a count of two seconds.
   b. b. Hold your breath for two seconds.
   c. c. Exhale for a count of two seconds.

7. Repeat for 1–5 minutes.

Appendix C: Self-Report Rating Scale – Relaxation

Instructions: Please use the following scale to rate your current level of relaxation – circle 1 to indicate that you feel extremely relaxed (e.g., like a wet noodle); circle 5 to indicate that you feel extremely stressed (e.g., stiff as a board).

1	2	3	4	5
"Wet noodle"				" Stiff as a board"

References

Addis, M., Martell, C., & Jacobson, N. S. (2001). *Depression in Context: Strategies for Guided Action.* New York: Norton.

American Psychiatric Association. (1994). *Diagnostic and Statistical Manual of Mental Disorders– Fourth Edition.* Washington, DC: American Psychiatric Association.

Aronson, K. R., Barrett, L. F., & Quigley, K. (2006). Emotional reactivity and the overreport of somatic: sensitivity or negative reporting style? *Journal of Psychosomatic Research, 60,* 521–530.

Asmundson, G. J. G., & Taylor, S. (2005). *It's not all in your head: how worrying about your health could be making you sick - and what you can do about it.* New York: Guilford Press.

Barsky, A. J., & Deans, E. C. (2006). *Stop being your symptoms and start being yourself: the six-week mind-body program to ease your chronic symptoms.* New York: Collins.

Barsky, A. J., Orav, E. J., & Bates, D. W. (2006). Distinctive patters of medical care utilization in patients who somatize. *Medical Care, 44*(9), 803–811.

Bernstein, D. A., Borkovec, T., & Hazlett-Stevens, H. (2000). *New directions in progressive relaxation training: a guidebook for helping professionals.* Westport, CT: Praeger Publishing.

Bridges, K. W., & Goldberg, D. P. (1985). Somatic presentation of DSM-III psychiatric disorders in primary care. *Journal of Psychosomatic Research, 29,* 563–569.

Burns, D. D. (1999a). *Feeling good: the new mood therapy*(2nd. Ed). New York: Plume.

Burns, D. D. (1999b). *The feeling god handbook.* New York: Plume.

Christensen, K. S., Rosendal, M., Nielsen, J. M., Kallerup, H., & Olen, F. (2003). Outreach visits. Choice of strategy for interviewing general practitioners. *Ugeskr Laeger, 165,* 1456–1460.

Derogatis, L. R., & Cleary, P. A. (1977). Confirmation of the dimensional structure of the SCL – 90: A study in construct validation. *Journal of Clinical Psychology, 33,* 981–989.

Dickinson, W. P., Dickinson, L. M., deGruy, F. V., Main, D. S., Candib, L. M., & Rost, K. (2003). A randomized clinical trial of a care recommendation letter intervention for somatization in primary care. *Annals of Family Medicine, 1,* 228–235.

Dobson, K. S., & Hamilton, K. E. (2003). Cognitive restructuring: behavioral tests of negative cognitions. In W. T. O'Donohue, J. E. Fisher, & S. C. Hayes (Eds.), *Cognitive behavioral therapy: Applying empirically supported techniques in your practice* (pp. 84–88). Hoboken, NJ: John Wiley & Sons.

Ellis, A. (2003). Cognitive restructuring of the disputing of irrational beliefs. In W. T. O'Donohue, J. E. Fisher, & S. C. Hayes (Eds.), *Cognitive behavioral therapy: Applying empirically supported techniques in your practice* (pp. 79–83). Habokin, NJ: John Wiley & Sons.

Escobar, J. I., Rubio-Stipec, M., Canino, G., & Karno, M. (1989_. Somatic Symptom Index (SSI): a new and abridged somatization construct. Prevalence and epidemiological correlates in two large community samples. *The Journal of Nervous and Mental Disorders, 177*(3), 140–146.

Feder, A., Olfson, M., Gameroff, Fuentes, M., Shea, S., & Lantigua, R. A., et al. (2001). Medically unexplained symptoms in an urban general medical practice. *Psychosomatic, 42*(3), 261–268.

Ferguson, K. E. (2003). Relaxation. In W. T. O'Donohue, J. E. Fisher, & S. C. Hayes (Eds.), *Cognitive behavioral therapy: applying empirically supported techniques in your practice* (pp. 330–340). Hoboken, NJ: John Wiley & Sons.

Fink, P., Sorensen, L., Engberg, M., Holm, M., & Munk-Jorgensen, P. (1999). Somatization in primary care: prevalence health care utilization and general practitioner recognition.

Hahn, S. R., Kroenke, K. Spitzer, Williams, J. B. W., Brody, D., Linzer, M., et al. (1996). The difficult patient in primary care: prevalence, psychopathology, and impairment. *Journal of General Internal Medicine, 11*, 1–8.

Kroenke, K. (2000). Somatization in primary care: it's time for parity. *General Hospital Psychiatry, 22*, 141–143.

Kroenke, K. (2004). The interface between physical and psychological symptoms. Primary care companion. *Journal of Clinical Psychiatry, 5*(suppl 7), 11–18.

Kroenke, K., Spitzer, R. L., DeGruy, F. V., & Swindle, R. (1998). A symptom checklist to screen for somatoform disorders in primary care. *Psychosomatics, 39*, 263–272.

Kroenke, K., Spitzer, R. L., & Williams, J. B. W. (2002). The PHQ-15: validity of a new measure for evaluating the severity of somatic symptoms. *Psychosomatic Medicine, 64*, 258–266.

Kroenke, K. & Swindle, R. (2000). Cognitive-behavioral therapy for somatization and symptom syndromes: A critical review of controlled clinical trials. *Psychotherapy and Psychosomatics, 69*, 205–215.

Lewinsohn, P. M., Munoz, R. F., Youngren, M. A., & Zeiss, A. M. (1992). *Control your depression.* New York: Fireside/Simon & Schuster.

Lipowski, Z. J. (1988). Somatization: the concept and its clinical application. *American Journal of Psychiatry, 145*, 1358–1368.

Martell, C. R., Addis, M. E., & Jacobson, N. S. (2001). *Depression in context, statistics for guided action.* New York: W.W. Norton.

Morriss, R. K., & Gask, L. (2002). Treatment of patients with somatized mental disorder: Effects of reattribution training on outcomes under direct control of the family doctor. *Psychosomatics, 43*, 394–399.

Morriss, R. K., Gask, L., Ronalds, C., Downes-Grainger, E., Thompson, H., & Goldberg, D. (1999). Clinical and patient satisfaction outcomes of a new treatment for somatized mental disorder taught to general practitioners. *British Journal of General Practice, 49*, 263–267.

Nezu, A. M., Nezu, C. M., & Lombardo, E. R. (2001). Cognitive behavioral therapy for medically unexplained symptoms: a critical review of the treatment literature. *Behavior Therapy, 32*, 537–583.

O'Donohue, W. T., Cummings, N. A., Cucciare, M. A., Cummings, J., & Runyan, C. (2006). *Integrated behavioral health care: a guide to effective intervention.* New York: Prometheus Books.

O'Donohue, W. T., & Levensky, E. (2006). *Promoting treatment adherence: A practical handbook for health care providers.* New York: Sage.

O'Malley, P. G., Jackson, J.l., Santoro, J., Tomkins, G., Balden, E., & Kroenke, K. (1999). Antidepressant therapy for unexplained symptoms and symptom syndromes. *The Journal of Family Practice, 48*, 980–990.

Ormel, J., Von Korff, M., Ustun, T. B., Pini, S., Korten, A., & Oldehinkel, T. (1994). Common mental disorders and disability across cultures: results from the WHO Collaborative Study on Psychological Problems in General Health Care. *Journal of the American Medical Association, 272*, 1741–1748.

Rosendal, M., Bro, F., Fink, P., Christensen, K. S., & Olesen, F. (2003). Diagnosis of somatization: Effect of an educational intervention in a cluster randomized controlled trial. *British Journal of General Practice, 53*, 917–922.

Rosendal, M., Fink, P., Flemming, B., & Olesen, F. (2005). Somatization, heartsink patients, or functional somatic symptoms? *Scandinavian Journal of Primary Health Care, 23*, 3–10.

Russo, D. C., Bird, B. L., & Masek, B. J. (1980). Assessment issues in behavioral medicine, *Behavioral Assessment, 2*, 1–18.

Smith, G. R. (1994). The course of Somatization and its effects on utilization of health care resources. *Psychosomatics, 35*, 263–267.

Smith, R. C., & Gardiner, J. C. (2006). Administrative database screening to identify somatizing patients. *Medical Care, 44*(9), 799–802.

Smith, R. C., Gardiner, J. C., Lyles, J. S., Sirbu, C., Dwamena, F. C., Hodges, A., et al. (2006). Exploration of DSM-IV criteria in primary care patients with medically unexplained symptoms. *Psychosomatic Medicine, 67*, 123–129.

Smith, G. Jr., Monson, R. A., & Ray, D. C. (1986). Psychiatric consultation in somatization disorder: A randomized controlled study. *New England Journal of Medicine, 314*, 1407–1413.

Smith, G. R., Rost, K., & Kashner, T. M. (1995). A trial of the effect of a standardized psychiatric consultation on health outcomes and costs in somatizing patients. *Arcives of General Psychiatry, 52*, 238–243.

Spitzer, R. L., Williams, J. B. W., Kroenke, K., Linzer, M., deGruy, F. V., Hahn, S. R., et al. (1994). Utility of a new procedure for diagnosing mental disorders in primary care: the PRIME-MD 1000 study. *Journal of the American Medical Association, 272*, 1749–1756.

Swartz, M., Hughes, D., George, L., Blazer, D., Landerman, R., & Bucholz, K. (1986). Developing a screening index for community studies of somatization disorder. *Journal of Psychiatric Research, 20*, 335–343.

Toft, T., Fink, P., Oernboel, E., Christensen, K., Frostholm, L., & Olesen (2005). Mental disorders in primary care: prevalence and co-morbidity among disorders. Results from the Functional Illness in Primary Care (FIP) study. *Psychological Medicine, 35*, 1175–1184.

Weil, A. (2004). *Self-healing with guided imagery: how to use the power of your mind to heal your body*(Audio CD). Sounds True Publishing.

Woolfolk, R. L., & Allen, L. A. (2006). *Treating somatization: A cognitive-behavioral approach*. New York: The Guilford Press.

Index

Note: The letter *t* and *f* in the index refers to *tables* and *figures* respectively
For example 86*t* refers to *table* in page 86 and 215*f* refers to *figure* in page 215

Printed in the United States of America